Cutaneous Manifestations of Child Abuse and Their Differential Diagnosis

Robert A.C. Bilo • Arnold P. Oranje
Tor Shwayder • Christopher J. Hobbs

Cutaneous Manifestations of Child Abuse and Their Differential Diagnosis

Blunt Force Trauma

Springer

Authors
Robert A.C. Bilo, M.D.
Department of Forensic Medicine
Netherlands Forensic Institute
The Hague, Netherlands

Arnold P. Oranje, M.D., Ph.D.
Department of Paediatric Dermatology
Erasmus MC - Sophia
Rotterdam, Netherlands

Tor Shwayder, M.D.
Director of Pediatric Dermatology
Department of Dermatology
Henry Ford Hospital
Detroit, Michigan
USA

Christopher J. Hobbs, M.D.
St. James's University Hospital
Leeds, United Kingdom

Contributing Authors of Chapter 9
Frans Bel, RMF
Medical Photographer
Erasmus MC - Sophia
Rotterdam, The Netherlands

Andre van den Bos
Medical Forensic Photographer
Netherlands Forensic Institute
Department of Forensic Medicine
The Hague
The Netherlands

Hubert G.T. Nijs
Netherlands Forensic Institute
Department of Forensic Medicine
Section Forensic Pediatrics
The Hague
The Netherlands

Illustrations by
Pieter Van Driessche
Netherlands Forensic Institute
Department of Forensic Medicine
The Hague
The Netherlands

ISBN 978-3-662-52062-8 ISBN 978-3-642-29287-3 (eBook)
DOI 10.1007/978-3-642-29287-3
Springer Heidelberg New York Dordrecht London

Printed on acid-free paper

Springer is part of Springer Science+Business Media (www.springer.com)

Foreword

About 80,900,000 Results in 0.11 s

If you google the term "child abuse," you will get over 80 million hits in less than 1 s. If you search in "PubMed," you will find more than 30,000 hits in the medical literature. Child abuse has many appearances and is often difficult to recognize by professionals like physicians and police despite the availability of an enormous amount of professional literature.

We are all in shock when we hear about child abuse. We are willing to accept the existence of child abuse in our professional lives, but in our private lives we still assume that it is rare and does not exist in our neighborhoods. From recent statistics, however, it is known that each year 1 in 20–30 children in the Netherlands will be victim of some form of child abuse. Looking at these numbers and considering the short- and long-term effects on children, families, and society, it is important that child abuse is recognized as soon as possible. Despite or maybe because of the huge amount of publications, many physicians do not have enough knowledge, experience, and the right tools for recognizing child abuse in an early stage.

With the introduction of forensic pediatrics at the Netherlands Forensic Institute (NFI) in 2008, we decided not only to focus on forensic cases and case reports but also on education and training of professionals in the field of forensic medicine, healthcare, civil and criminal justice, for example, pediatricians, family physicians, forensic doctors, other medical disciplines, police, and prosecutors.

Physical violence against children can lead to many different physical findings, for example, unexplained fractures. In 2010, Bilo, Robben, and van Rijn published a book in which the forensic aspects of fractures in children are discussed in an accessible way.[1] It describes the differential diagnosis of fractures. It has become a reference book worldwide for child protection professionals.

"Cutaneous manifestations of child abuse" by Bilo, Oranje, Shwayder, and Hobbs is an important addition to the former book, because it discusses injuries caused by the most prevalent form of physical violence against children: blunt-force trauma like hitting, kicking, biting, twisting, and pinching.

---

[1] Bilo RAC, Robben SGF, van Rijn RR (2010) Forensic aspects of paediatric fractures – differentiating accidental trauma from child abuse, 1st edn. Springer, Berlin/Heidelberg

It contains a comprehensive description of the differential diagnosis of suspicious cutaneous findings.

I am convinced this book will become a worldwide reference book for professionals working with children. In the end, children and families will benefit.

The Hague, Netherland Dr. Ellen van Berkel

Preface

My Skin Is Only the Top Layer of the Problem...

In July 1995, Irene A. Crosby wrote an article for the Archives of Dermatology, titled "My skin is only the top layer of the problem." She described the problems she encountered as a patient with atopic dermatitis: *"As a dermatologist, you see many patients with atopic dermatitis. There are a lot of us. We come to you in the arms of anxious parents who feel personally responsible for our agony and look to you for absolution of their erroneously perceived guilt. Regardless of how your atopic patients arrive, we all expect a cure in short order. Sometimes we heal, but often we do not. At this point, you and your patients like me are often thrown into an uneasy symbiosis where each unfairly blames the other for the chronicity of the disease."* As a patient with atopic dermatitis, she wants to be treated in a respectful and proper way.

The same accounts for victims of child abuse. Just replace "dermatologist" by "doctor" and "atopic dermatitis" by "a suspicion of child abuse" and you read a fascinating introduction that could have been written by a victim of child abuse: *"As a doctor, you see many patients with a suspicion of child abuse. There are a lot of us."* At the same time, the quote shows some of the quandaries of physicians who are confronted with a suspicion of child abuse, because a physician practically always examines a child when one parent is or both parents are present: *"We come to you in the arms of anxious parents who feel personally responsible for our agony and look to you for absolution of their erroneously perceived guilt..."* The parent who accompanies the child is not necessarily the parent who abused the child and does not always know what happened, but will feel guilty even when unjustly accused of child abuse. When "dermatologist" is replaced by pediatrician and/or pediatric dermatologist, a fascinating introduction arises that clarifies the role of these disciplines in the diagnosis as well as in the differential diagnosis of skin findings whenever a suspicion of child abuse arises.

The skin is the most accessible organ of the body and is therefore easy to observe for anybody. The skin is also the primary target organ to become damaged in physical abuse of children. Furthermore, skin findings may be encountered in all types of child abuse. Therefore, these findings often play a central role in the recognition of child abuse. These abnormalities can be observed by well-trained physicians and by untrained bystanders. Nevertheless, the interpretation of skin lesions is primarily the task of physicians in general and (pediatric) dermatologists in particular and is not always simple. In recent years, many reports have been published on pediatric (dermatological) disorders and accidental injuries that were unjustly regarded as physical signs of child abuse. Knowledge of the differential diagnosis of unexplained or apparent skin findings is essential for an accurate diagnosis, sometimes even vital because errors in either direction (false positive and false negative) can be disastrous.

Doctors do have a specific role in the medical diagnosis of cases of physical violence and neglect, sexual abuse, and artificial disorders like pediatric condition falsification (formerly known as Munchausen's syndrome by proxy), factitious disorders (formerly known as Munchausen's syndrome), and self-mutilation. When a suspicion of child abuse arises because of physical findings, it is important to avoid jumping to conclusions. No physical sign or symptom is in itself an absolute proof of child abuse. The combination of physical findings, a thorough medical history, and the determination of the child's developmental level allows a well-trained physician to conclude whether a story told by the parents is consistent with the findings in the child. In other words, a suspicion of child abuse arising from physical abnormalities must be approached in the same way as any other medical problem:

- Formulating and testing a differential diagnosis (including a detailed history)
- Undertaking additional (e.g., laboratory) investigations
- Establishing a definite diagnosis

Therefore, it is essential that the physical examination is done by well-trained physicians, and in case of skin findings in cooperation with an experienced (pediatric) dermatologist.

Robert A.C. Bilo
Arnold P. Oranje
on behalf of
Tor Shwayder and
Chris Hobbs

Acknowledgements

Many colleagues and friends helped us to write this book. We will not be able to mention them all. Some of them we would like to thank in person for their contributions to this book.

Firstly, Pieter Van Driessche, M.D., forensic (neuro) pathologist. He used one of his many talents to create the hand-drawn illustrations in this book.

Secondly, André van den Bosch, Frans Bel, and Huub Nijs for their chapter on forensic photography.

Furthermore (in alphabetical order and among others), Ellen van Berkel, Daan Botter, Geertje Hoogenboom, Wouter Karst, Bela Kubat, Arjo Loeve, Ann Maes, Hans van der Meijden, Rick van Rijn, Vidija Soerdjbalie, B. Tank, Eddy de Valck, Dirk Van Varenbergh, Peter Varkevisser, Rob Visser, and Mayonne van Wijk.

Last but not least, we would like to express our appreciation for everybody who (unknowingly) contributed to this book by providing photographs to the World Wide Web and placing these photographs in the setting of the public domain. Most figures were derived from the archives of the Netherlands Forensic Institute, the Erasmus MC - Sophia and the Henry Ford Hospital.

Contents

General Aspects of Physical Abuse and Neglect

1

1.1 Defining Child Abuse, Physical Abuse, and Neglect

There is no universal definition of child abuse or of any of its subtypes (Table 1.1). Definitions vary according to their function, for example, whether used for political, cultural, sociological, scientific, or legislative purposes. They may also vary from concise and to the point to comprehensive and more descriptive. The American Humane Association (2000) defines child abuse concisely as "harm resulting from inappropriate or abnormal childrearing practices". The definition of the World Health Organization (2006a) is more descriptive and also includes the various types of child abuse into their definition: "child abuse or maltreatment constitutes all forms of physical and/or emotional ill-treatment, sexual abuse, neglect or negligent treatment or commercial or other exploitation, resulting in actual or potential harm to the child's health, survival, development or dignity in the context of a relationship of responsibility, trust or power."

Physical abuse of a child is defined as the deliberate physically violent behavior toward a child, committed by parents, care providers, and other known (such as brothers, sisters, acquaintances, and teachers) and unknown individuals. Child abuse is very rarely caused by the last group of unknown individuals. This behavior leads to actual or potential physical harm that is the result of the interaction, or lack of an interaction, which should reasonably be within the control of a parent or person in a position of responsibility, power, or trust (WHO 2006a). The severity of the behavior may range from frequent physically aggressive behavior, such as beating, punching, kicking, biting, and burning with or without visible injuries and/or scars, that is not life-threatening to a single incident with severe life-threatening and even lethal consequences.

Hobbs (1999) defined physical abuse from the perspective of the child: "a physically abused child is any child who receives (received) physical injury (or injuries) as a result of acts (or omissions) on the part of his parents or guardians. This includes the actual or probable physical injury to a child or the failure to prevent physical injury (or suffering) to a child, including deliberate poisoning, suffocation and pediatric condition falsification."

Neglect is the failure to provide for the needs of the child in every aspect of a child's life: health, education, emotional development, nutrition, shelter and safe living conditions, within the context of resources generally considered available to the family or caretakers, and causes or has a

Table 1.1 Types of child abuse in clinical practice

- Physical abuse
- Neglect, including physical neglect and other types of negligent behavior
- Sexual abuse
- Psychological/emotional abuse
- Pediatric condition falsification/fictitious disorder by proxy/medical child abuse (US terminology)/fabricated or induced illness (UK terminology) (formerly known as Munchausen syndrome by proxy)

R.A.C. Bilo et al., *Cutaneous Manifestations of Child Abuse and Their Differential Diagnosis*,
DOI 10.1007/978-3-642-29287-3_1, © Springer-Verlag Berlin Heidelberg 2013

high probability of causing harm to the child's health or physical, mental, spiritual, moral, or social development. This includes the failure to properly supervise and protect children from harm to the best of one's ability (WHO 2006b).

As a result of the aggressive or negligent behavior, the child may suffer injuries. However, the absence of physical injuries at physical examination does not exclude the existence of physical abuse or neglect since not all physically violent or negligent behavior will result in apparent physical injuries. Moreover, not all physical injuries are noticed at the moment they are present or, when they are present, they may not be recognized by the person examining the child.

1.2 Epidemiology of Physical Abuse

1.2.1 Physical Abuse

Official reports about the epidemiology of physical abuse will underestimate the scale of the problem. It is now and will be in the future impossible to establish the exact incidence and prevalence of child abuse in general and physical abuse in particular. This is due to several issues, like definitional problems, including the defining of child abuse related to the function of the definition (Sect. 1.1), study design, and studied populations, and in particular to the fact that child abuse is underreported due to its occult occurrence (Keenan and Leventhal 2009).

Definitional problems are mainly created by the fact that no universal definition exists and that the definition of child abuse in general and of physical abuse more specifically may vary from concise and to the point to comprehensive and more descriptive. There may also be a difference in the scope of the definition: the narrower the definition, the lower the incidence and prevalence will be. If physical abuse is defined as an act of a carer leading to physical injuries (e.g., slapping, beating, or kicking, leading to bruises and abrasions), the incidence and prevalence will be lower than in a situation in which the act in itself is defined as physical abuse and in which the defining of physical abuse does not depend on the finding of injuries but on the chance that physical or other, for example, emotional injury may occur.

This also means that it will be impossible to give a reliable estimate of the underreporting. Estimates vary from one to two unrecognized cases for each reported case (American Humane Association 2000) up to possibly as many as four unrecognized cases for each known case (Oosterlee et al. 2009).

According to the 2007 UNICEF report on child well-being in Europe and Northern America, the United States and the United Kingdom ranked lowest with respect to the well-being of their children (UNICEF 2007). The Netherlands ranked the highest according to the same report. Despite the difference in ranking, there seem to be similarities in the incidence and prevalence of child abuse in the Netherlands on the one side and the United States and the United Kingdom on the other side.

In 1998, Straus published the data of a survey in which they asked parents in the United States how they disciplined their children (Straus et al. 1998). From this survey, an estimated rate of physical abuse of 49 per 1,000 children (1:20) was obtained when the following kinds of behavior were included in the definition of child abuse: hitting the child with an object other than on the buttocks and/or kicking and/or beating the child and/or threatening the child with a knife or gun. In 2000, about three million cases of suspected child abuse were reported in the United States (American Humane Association 2000). About 1 in 4 reports was confirmed (12.2 per 1,000 children). A more recently published study in the United States (2008) again illustrates the influence of differences in definitions on incidence and prevalence data: about 1 in 50 children fell victim of a nonfatal form of child abuse (assault, neglect, and/or abuse) (CDC 2008).

In the United States, about 1 in every 4 or 5 abused children is a victim of physical assault (National Committee to Prevent Child Abuse 1998), and about 10% of all children under the age of 5 who visit an emergency department with injuries do have non-accidental injuries resulting from assault or neglect (Holter and Friedman 1968).

Child abuse (physical violence, neglect, and sexual abuse) was reported as a possible cause in 2–25% of the children who required medical care for burns (Hight et al. 1979; Deitch and Staats 1982; Jones and Pickett 1987; Purdue et al. 1988; Andronicus et al. 1998). After bruises and burns, fractures are the most prevalent injuries in child abuse (McMahon et al. 1995; Cramer 1996). Often (maybe even as many as 1 in 5 victims) fractures are the first sign of child physical abuse (Sinal and Stewart 1998). More than 30% of children evaluated in the emergency department because of suspected abuse appear to have fresh and/or healing fractures (Hyden and Gallagher 1992). In children less than 1 year old, 50–75% of all fractures are reported to be sustained by physical abuse or neglect (King et al. 1988; Leventhal et al. 1993).

In the United Kingdom, as in many other countries such as the USA and the Netherlands, it is still common practice to use physical methods to control children, including hitting, slapping, and kicking (Smith et al. 1995; Cawson et al. 2000). Smith (1995) found that 15% of all children had been severely punished defined as the use implements and occurring over a protracted period of time, (potentially) causing physical or psychological damage. They also found that 9 out of 10 children had been hit at some time in their life and that the frequency with which they were hit decreased with age (hit more than once per week: 38% at 4, 27% at 7, and 3% at 11 years of age). In the United Kingdom, 7–9% of all children had been physically assaulted (hereby physical assault was certainly considered if clinically visible injuries were encountered) (Cawson et al. 2000). These percentages are comparable to the data of Straus (1998) on physical abuse in the United States.

In the Netherlands (almost 16 million inhabitants with a birth figure of 180,000 births per year), it is expected that each year somewhere between 100,000 and 160,000 minors will fall victim to child abuse (van IJzendoorn et al. 2007; Lamers-Winkelman et al. 2007).

Van IJzerendoorn (2007) used data, collected in 2005, to estimate the prevalence of child abuse in the Netherlands. These data were collected by more than 1,100 carefully selected professionals working in various health care, child care, and educational institutions in society across all major regions of the Netherlands. The informants were carefully instructed in the use of a uniform definition of child abuse and of a uniform registration system for child abuse. Also the registrations of all Dutch Child Protection Services in 2005 were included. Van IJzerendoorn estimated that the prevalence in the Netherlands may be 30 cases of child abuse per 1,000 children. About 1 in 5 abused children was victim of physical abuse. The results of the second prevalence study by the same research group showed comparable data (Alink et al. 2011).

Lamers-Winkelman (2007) used a questionnaire to interview 1,845 adolescents from 14 randomly selected secondary schools. Of the interviewed adolescents, 1 in 3 indicated that they had experienced an event in their lives which may be regarded as a form of child abuse (serious psychological aggression by parents, domestic violence (including physical abuse), perceived physical conflicts between parents, sexual abuse, and/or severe neglect). Nearly 20% appears to have experienced one form or another of child abuse during the past 12 months before the interview. One out of fifteen adolescents reported to have been a victim of a combination of different forms of child abuse during the past 12 months before the interview.

Another Dutch study focused on the effects of infant crying on parental actions ($n = 3{,}259$, aged 1–6 months) showed that 5.6% of the parents reported that they had smothered, slapped, or shaken their baby at least once because of their crying (Reijneveld et al. 2004).

Child abuse occurs in all social classes in the United Kingdom, although identified cases predominate in poor and disadvantaged families. Postcode-derived deprivation scores confirmed that subdural hematoma or effusion following non-accidental injury occurred in all socioeconomic quintiles of the population but was more common in the least affluent populations compared with the most affluent (Hobbs et al. 2005). Van IJzerendoorn (2007) found that the risk for child abuse increases almost sevenfold in families with very low-educated parents. When both parents were unemployed, the risk increases at least fivefold. In families with parents from ethnic minorities, the risk for child abuse is about 3.5 times larger, but when their lower educational level is taken into account, the risk becomes much smaller. In families with single parents and in larger families (three or more children), the risk of child abuse and neglect doubles (van IJzendoorn et al. 2007).

Children most at risk of serious or fatal injuries due to child abuse and neglect are young, preverbal children (including infants). Children with any kind of disability have child abuse rates 3–4 times that of non-disabled children (Sullivan and Knutson 2000). The relationship between disabilities and abuse is complex. One should always consider that a disability is not only a risk factor for abuse but may also be the outcome of abuse, for example, in abusive head trauma.

1.2.2 Injury-Related Fatalities

The most prevalent causes of death and physical disabilities in children under the age of 15 are injuries by accidental and by non-accidental causes. According to the WHO, annually about 27,900 children will die of their injuries in Europe, which is equivalent to 36% of all deaths (WHO 2006b). Of these, 24,700 (89%) are due to accidental injuries and 3,200 (11%) are non-accidental (violence-related and self-inflicted) (Table 1.2). For every child who dies, there are several thousand victims of injury or violence who live with varying degrees of disability or psychological scarring. The WHO cites a Dutch study, which concludes that for every death from home- and leisure-related injuries, there are about 160 hospital admissions and 2,000 emergency department visits. If these figures are generalized for all injury-related deaths in Europe, this would translate into 4.5 million hospital admissions and 56 million emergency department visits (WHO 2006b).

The WHO defines as strongly associated risk factors for childhood injuries: poverty, single parenthood, low maternal education, low maternal age at birth, poor housing, large family size, and parental alcohol and substance abuse (WHO 2006b). These factors contribute to unsafe environments and risky behavior. The gender of the child also plays a role; boys are more at risk than girls. After the age of 1 year, all injury rates are higher for boys than for girls. Under 5 years of age, the rates for boys are 30% higher than for girls; however, this increases to 200% higher between 5 and 14 years of age (WHO 2006b). One should bear in mind that in injury-related fatalities, the differentiation between death due to "true" accidental causes, preventable death due to a momentary lapse in supervision, and preventable death due to "true" neglect will demand a comprehensive investigation of the circumstances.

Table 1.2 Deaths in relative percentage of total numbers from injury categorized by cause in the WHO European Region

Cause	%
Road traffic	23
Drowning	17
Poisoning	7
Self-inflicted	6
Violence	5
Fires	5
Falls	4
Other injury causes (incl. choking, smothering, venomous animals, electrocution, firearm incidents, war)	33

Children <15 years, 2002 (WHO 2006b)

In 2002, the World Health Organization concluded the following on fatal child abuse worldwide (WHO 2002):

> In 2000 there were an estimated 57,000 deaths attributed to homicide among children under the age of 15 years. Global estimates of child homicide suggest that infants and very young children are at greatest risk, with rates for the 0 to 4-year-old age group more than double those of 5 to 14-year-olds. The risk of fatal abuse for children varies according to the income level of a country and region of the world. For children under 5 years of age living in high-income countries, the rate of homicide is 2.2 per 100,000 for boys and 1.8 per 100,000 for girls. In low- to middle-income countries, the rates are 2–3 times higher (6.1 per 100,000 for boys and 5.1 per 100,000 for girls). The highest homicide rates for children under 5 years of age are found in the WHO African Region (17.9 per 100,000 for

boys and 12.7 per 100,000 for girls). The lowest rates are seen in high-income countries in the WHO European, Eastern Mediterranean and Western Pacific Regions. Many child deaths, however, are not routinely investigated and postmortem examinations are not carried out, which makes it difficult to establish the precise number of fatalities from child abuse in any given country. (Cited from the report)

1.2.3 The Relevance of Unreliable Data

Although precise definition of child abuse is difficult and measures of incidence and prevalence inevitably are imprecise, child abuse is clearly a major societal and health problem (Sect. 1.3.2). It also is one of the leading causes of child mortality.

In his report following the violent death of Victoria Climbié on February 25, 2000, Lord Laming writes on the incidence and prevalence of child abuse: "I have no difficulty in accepting the proposition that this problem (deliberate harm to children) is greater than that of what are generally recognized as common health problems in children, such as diabetes mellitus or asthma" (Laming 2003).

1.3 Clinical Features

1.3.1 Signs and Symptoms of Child Abuse and Neglect

The wide range of clinical presentations, symptoms, signs, and radiological features of physical abuse and neglect includes (Hobbs et al. 1999):

- Injuries arising from abusive and negligent behavior
- Signs of neglect, for example, infestation, lack of hygiene or care, failure to thrive, gross and untreated obesity, vitamin deficiencies from poor or inappropriate diet, injuries from lack of supervision, delayed development and poor educational attainment, cold injury, untreated medical conditions, and lack of educational opportunity
- Behavioral problems
- Emotional signs
- Other signs and symptoms, for example, skin lesions caused by self-mutilation or unexplained symptoms of illness in an otherwise healthy child which defies diagnosis

Because of this wide range of signs and symptoms, the evaluation of suspected child abuse demands multidisciplinary cooperation, involving welfare agencies, health professionals, and civil/criminal justice systems. Within the health care for children, it demands the cooperation between different pediatric disciplines, like forensic pediatrics, community pediatrics, pediatric dermatology, and pediatric radiology. Examples of the importance of cooperation in case of physical findings and their differential diagnosis are shown in Figs. 1.1, 1.2, 1.3, 1.4, 1.5, 1.6, 1.7, and 1.8 and in the following chapters.

1.3.2 Long-Term Consequences of Child Abuse

The health consequences of all forms of child abuse are long-standing and serious (Table 1.3) (WHO 2002). Apart from death or handicap following injuries such as brain injury or abdominal trauma, most effects are seen in the child's emotional and intellectual development. Also, it has a negative effect on the social functioning and general well-being of the child in his or her life for

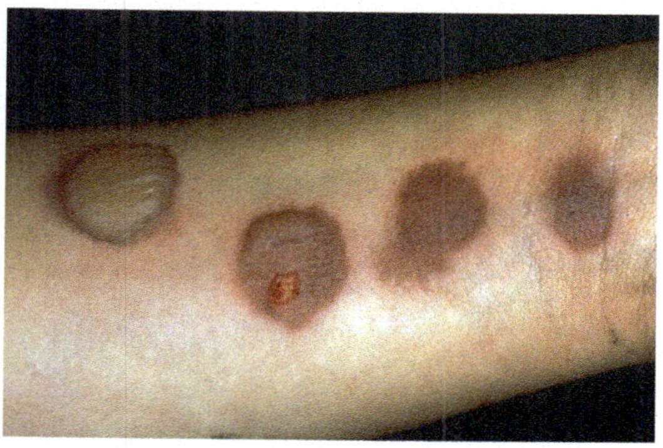

Fig. 1.1 Cigarette burns due to self-mutilation (= Fig. 2.38)

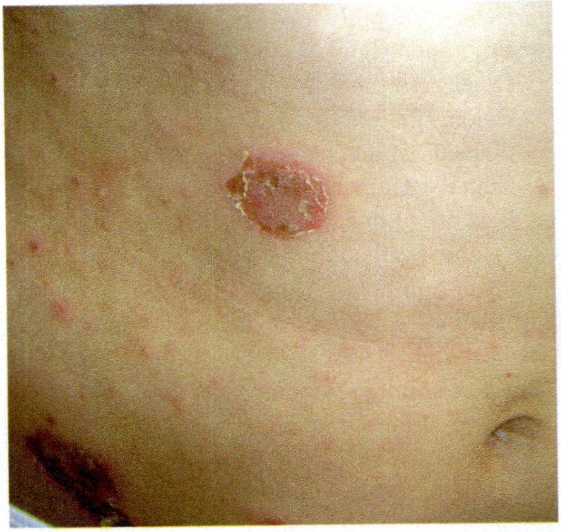

Fig. 1.2 Impetigo in the differential diagnosis of cigarette burns

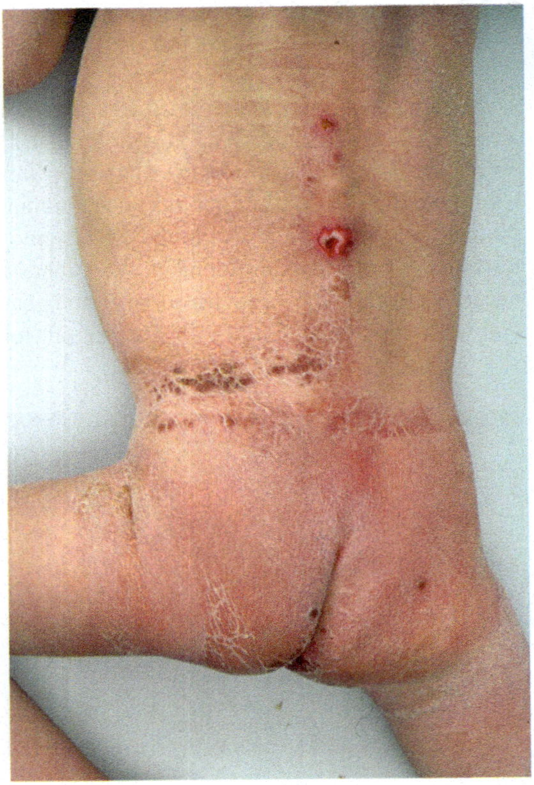

Fig. 1.3 Severe diaper dermatitis due to neglect

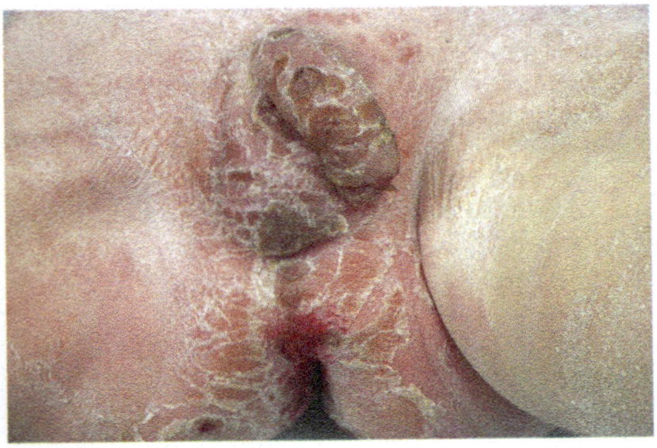

Fig. 1.4 Same child as in Fig. 1.3

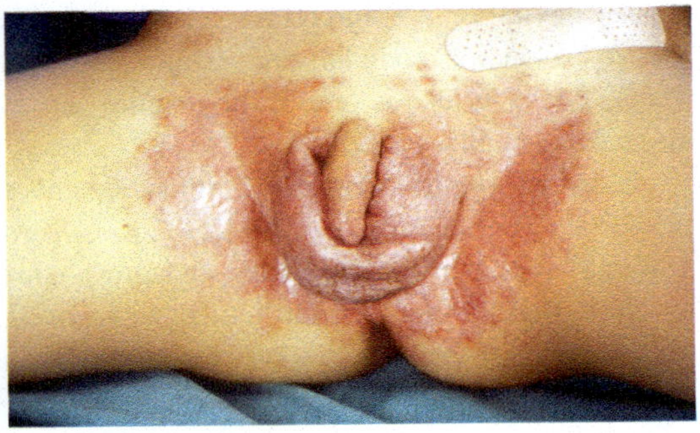

Fig. 1.5 Linear IgA disease in the differential diagnosis of diaper dermatitis

decades to come. The relationship between health-risk behavior and disease in adulthood and the extent of exposure to childhood emotional, physical, or sexual abuse and domestic dysfunction was described in the ACE study (Felitti et al. 1998). The study found a strong-graded relationship between the extent of exposure to abuse or domestic dysfunctioning during childhood and multiple risk factors for several of the leading causes of death in adults. These included alcoholism, drug abuse, depression, and suicide. Other adverse outcomes included smoking, high numbers of sexual intercourse partners, poor self-related health, sexually transmitted disease, physical inactivity, and severe obesity. There also appeared to be a connection with ischemic heart disease, cancer, chronic lung disease, skeletal fractures, and liver disease.

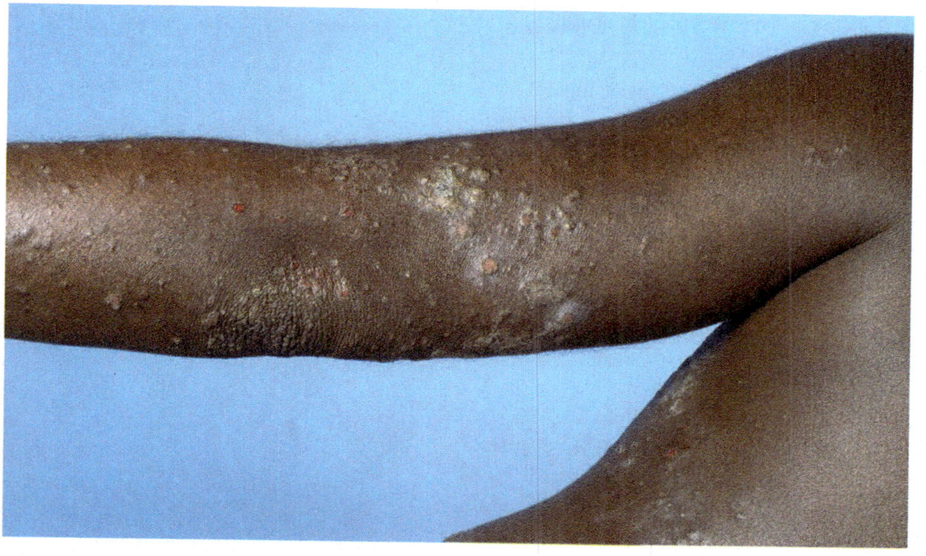

Fig. 1.6 Eczema in neglect

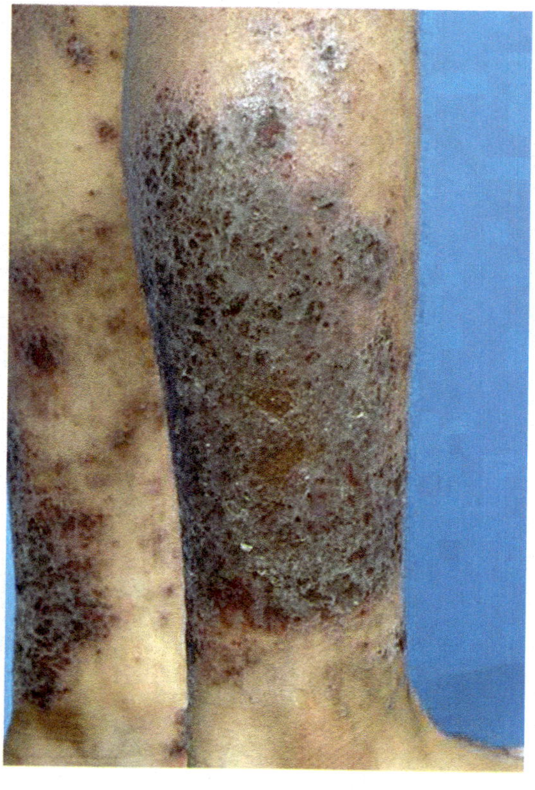

Fig. 1.7 Eczema in neglect

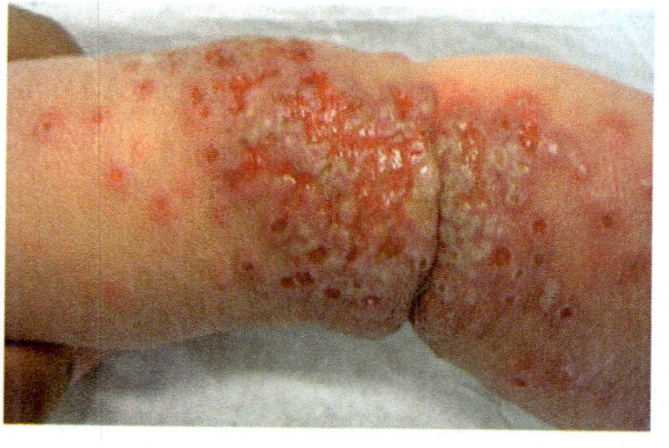

Fig. 1.8 Eczema herpeticum as differential diagnosis of neglect

1.4 Child Abuse and the Rights of Children

From a contemporary point of view, one may state that child abuse has been present throughout history in all societies and cultures. From a historical point of view, however, one should realize that the behavior that nowadays is defined as child abuse was not recognized as such in earlier

Table 1.3 Health consequences of child abuse

Consequences	
Physical	• Abdominal/thoracic injuries • Brain injuries/injuries to the central nervous system • Bruises and welts • Burns and scalds • Disability • Fractures • Lacerations and abrasions • Ocular damage
Sexual and reproductive	• Reproductive health problems (e.g., infertility) • Sexual dysfunction • Sexually transmitted diseases, including HIV/AIDS • Unwanted pregnancy
Psychological and behavioral	• Alcohol and drug abuse • Cognitive impairment • Delinquent, violent, and other risk-taking behaviors • Depression and anxiety • Developmental delays • Eating and sleep disorders • Feelings of shame and guilt • Hyperactivity • Poor relationships • Poor school performance • Low self-esteem • Post-traumatic stress disorder • Psychosomatic disorders • Suicidal behavior and self-harm
Other longer-term health issues	• Cancer • Chronic lung disease • Fibromyalgia • Irritable bowel syndrome • Ischemic heart disease • Liver disease

WHO (2002)

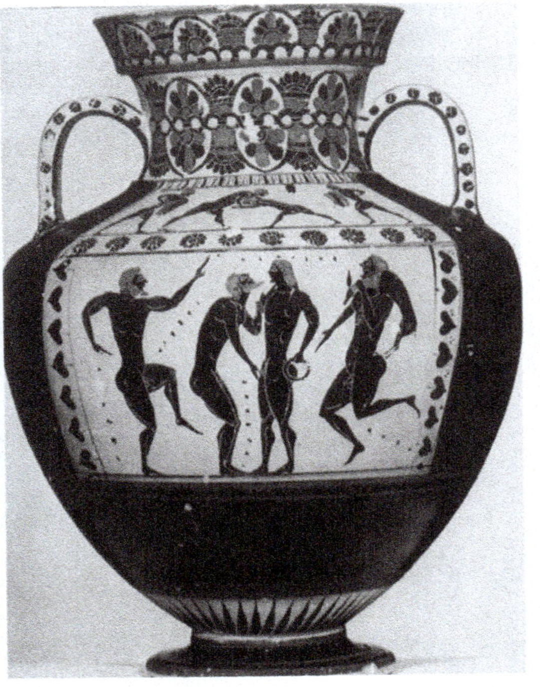

Fig. 1.9 An Athenian vase, depicting a sexual contact between an adult and a beardless boy

days. The negative effects of the behavior on children were not known or were denied.

Greek vases and other painted images, for example, depict sexual contacts between adults and male children (Figs. 1.9, 1.10, and 1.11) (Bilo et al. 2000). These contacts were accepted in the higher circles and considered to be healthy.

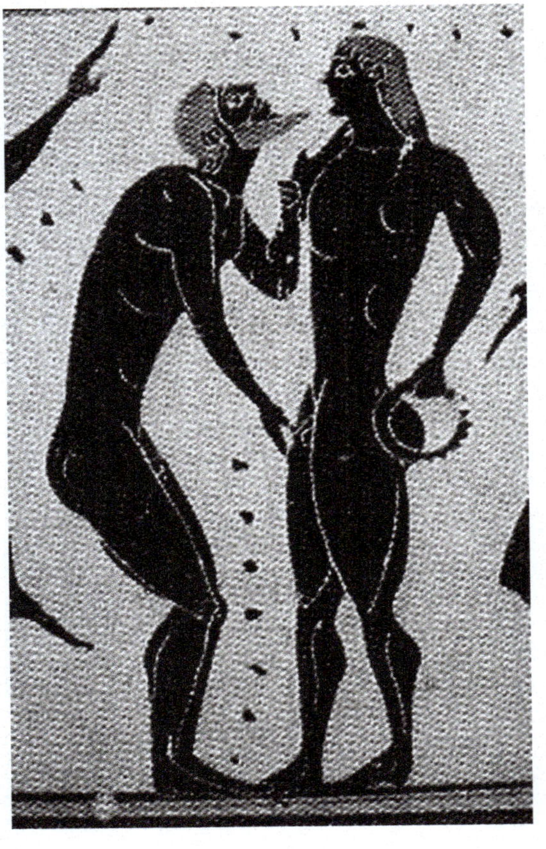

Fig. 1.10 Same vase as in Fig. 1.1 (detail): *"the boy usually looks as if he is solving some academic problem"*

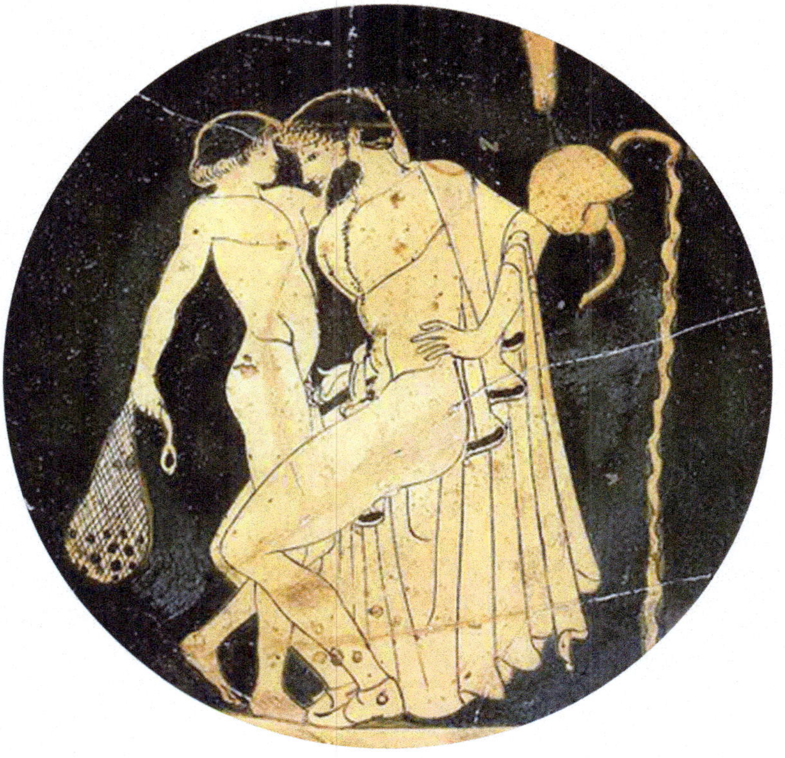

Fig. 1.11 Greek artwork, dated between 530 BC and 430 BC, depicting a sexual contact between an adult and a boy. The boy is holding a bag of nuts, probably a courting gift from or payment by the adult

The boys were rewarded for the contact materially and socially but were not expected to enjoy the contact (Isaacs 1993). Bremmer (1989) described this as follows: "The Athenian vases clearly show that only the adults were considered to derive satisfaction from pederastic intercourse; the boy usually looks as if he is solving some academic problem."

For a very long time, children had (or even still have) no rights of their own inside families and were (are) seen as personal property of their parents, especially their fathers, or the society. This principle became law in Roman times: the "patria potestas" (power of the father), which gave fathers the absolute and unrestricted authority to decide about the fate of their children. A father could, according to this law:

- Accept and raise the child as his child
- Reject and sell the child as a slave or sacrifice the child
- Decide that the child was not fit to live and to kill the child because of handicaps

1.4.1 The Nineteenth Century

In the nineteenth century, the society became aware for the first time that children should be protected against the harmful behavior of parents or carers. In fact, the child was "reinvented" as a person which had the right to be protected against maltreatment, including child abuse, child sexual exploitation, and child labor. Tardieu (1818–1879), a forensic pathologist and professor of the Sorbonne University in Paris, published a series of articles and books in which child abuse, including neglect, sexual abuse, and infanticide, was described and examples of physical findings in sexual abuse were depicted (Figs. 1.12, 1.13, 1.14, and 1.15) (Tardieu 1859, 1860, 1868).

The story of Mary Ellen Wilson is well known among people who are working in child protection (American Humane Association, not dated) (Figs. 1.16, 1.17, and 1.18). This case formed the immediate cause to create the first Society for the Prevention of Cruelty to Children in the

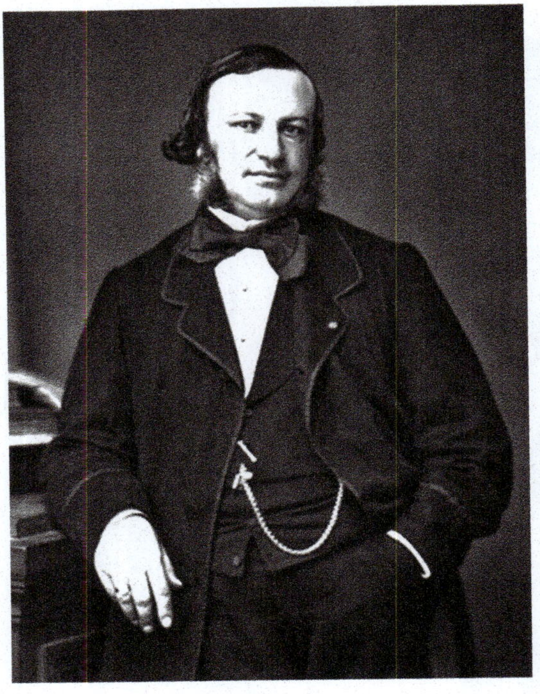

Fig. 1.12 Ambroise Tardieu

United States in the seventies of the nineteenth century (Fig. 1.19). On April 10, 1874, Mary Ellen herself testified before Judge Lawrence (cited from Watkins 1990): "…. Mamma has been in the habit of whipping and beating me almost every day. She used to whip me with a twisted whip – a raw hide. The whip always left a black and blue mark on my body. I have now the black and blue marks on my head which were made by mamma, and also a cut on the left side of my forehead which was made by a pair of scissors. She struck me with the scissors and cut me (figure 1.18); I have no recollection of ever having been kissed by any one – have never been kissed by mamma. I have never been taken on my mamma's lap and caressed or petted. I never dared to speak to anybody, because if I did I would get whipped…. I do not know for what I was whipped—mamma never said anything to me when she whipped me. I do not want to go back to live with mamma, because she beats me so. I have no recollection ever being on the street in my life."

The growing awareness about what could happen to children is also illustrated by the depiction of the maltreatment of children in *Illustrated Police News* in the seventies of the nineteenth century (Figs. 1.20, 1.21, 1.22, 1.23, 1.24, 1.25, and 1.26).

1.4.2 The Twentieth Century

The awareness increased further in the twentieth century and led to the conviction that children had rights of their own. It was no longer accepted that parents did have an absolute and unrestricted authority over their children, although abusive behavior sometimes was depicted as something "funny" (Fig. 1.27).

In 1961, Kempe and coworkers published their groundbreaking article on "the battered child syndrome," in which they described the effects of parental violence toward their children (Kempe et al. 1962). In fact, this article renewed the attention for child abuse, which started a century before with the work of Tardieu.

In 1989, the "Convention on the Rights of the Child" was adopted by the United Nations General Assembly, which confirmed these enormous societal changes. Health professionals, welfare agencies, and the civil/criminal justice system must act according to their national procedures within the legislative framework of that country when confronted with suspicions of child abuse. The position may vary from one based on good medical practice to one mandated by a legal obligation to report suspected child abuse. Considering the fact that almost all countries have their own legislation, which may differ in details or fundamentally from the legislation in other countries, this aspect will not be dealt with any further within the scope of this book. It would be impossible to show all types of legislation which vary from voluntary reporting, without any consequences for the non-reporting professional, to mandatory reporting with consequences for the non-reporting professional. Reporting is done within a large variety of reporting systems with or without involvement of governmental or non-governmental child protection services and with

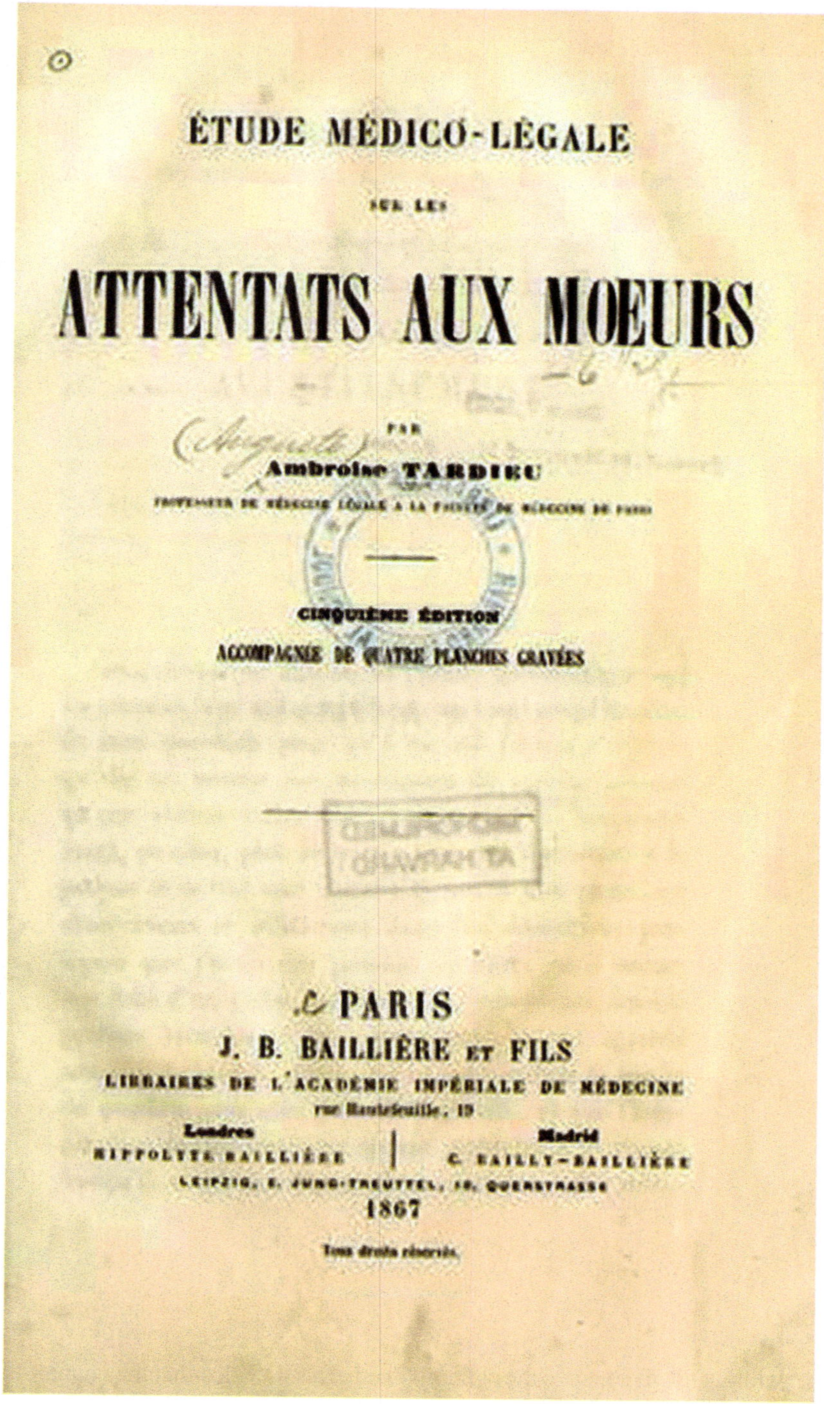

ÉTUDE MÉDICO-LÉGALE

SUR LES

ATTENTATS AUX MOEURS

PAR

Ambroise TARDIEU

PROFESSEUR DE MÉDECINE LÉGALE A LA FACULTÉ DE MÉDECINE DE PARIS

CINQUIÈME ÉDITION

ACCOMPAGNÉE DE QUATRE PLANCHES GRAVÉES

PARIS

J. B. BAILLIÈRE ET FILS

LIBRAIRES DE L'ACADÉMIE IMPÉRIALE DE MÉDECINE

rue Hautefeuille, 19

Londres	Madrid
HIPPOLYTE BAILLIÈRE	C. BAILLY-BAILLIÈRE

LEIPZIG, E. JUNG-TREUTTEL, 10, QUERSTRASSE

1867

Tous droits réservés.

Fig. 1.13 Frontpage of "Étude medico-legale sur les attentats aux moeurs"

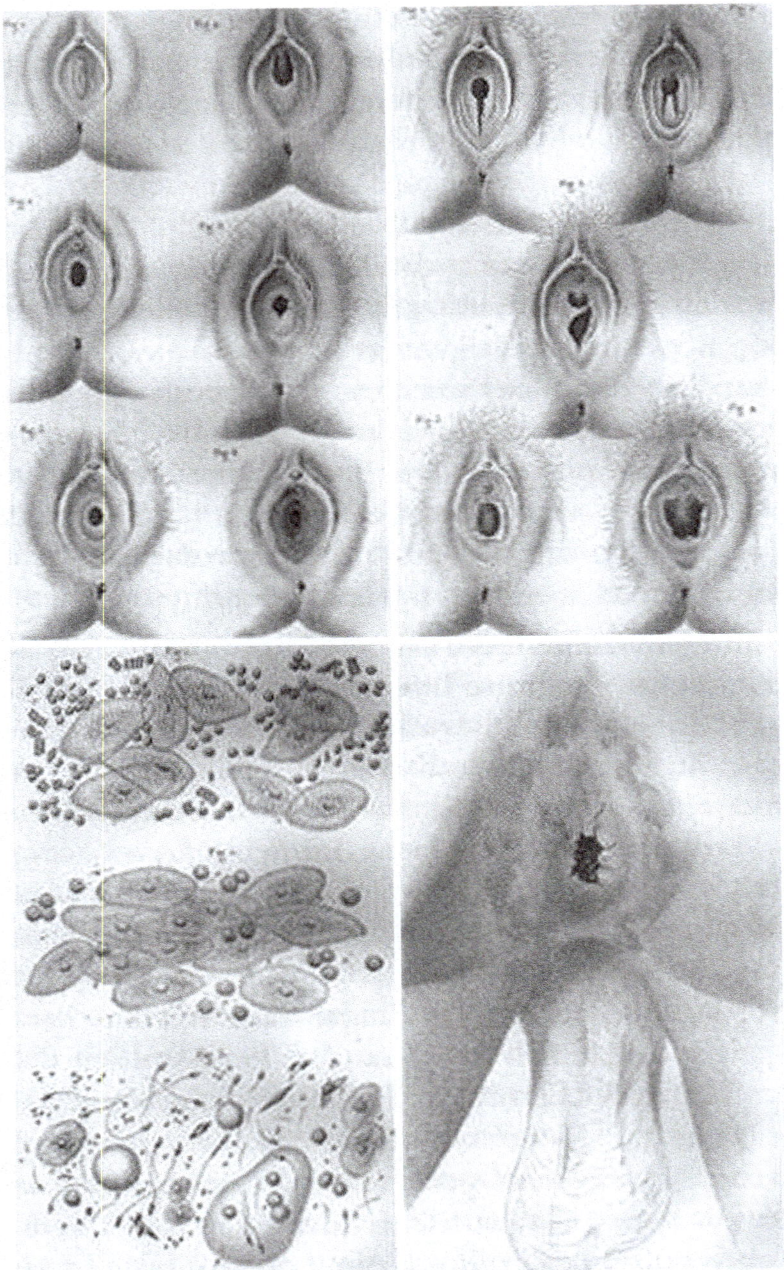

Fig. 1.14 One of the illustrations in "Attentats aux moeurs"

or without involvement of the police. Nonetheless, physicians and other professionals must realize that the "Convention on the Rights of the Child" provides an overarching framework for legislation applicable within a particular country, provided that the country has ratified the Convention (United Nations General Assembly 1989). When other national or international treaties or conventions are applicable, the most favorable regulation will apply to the child.

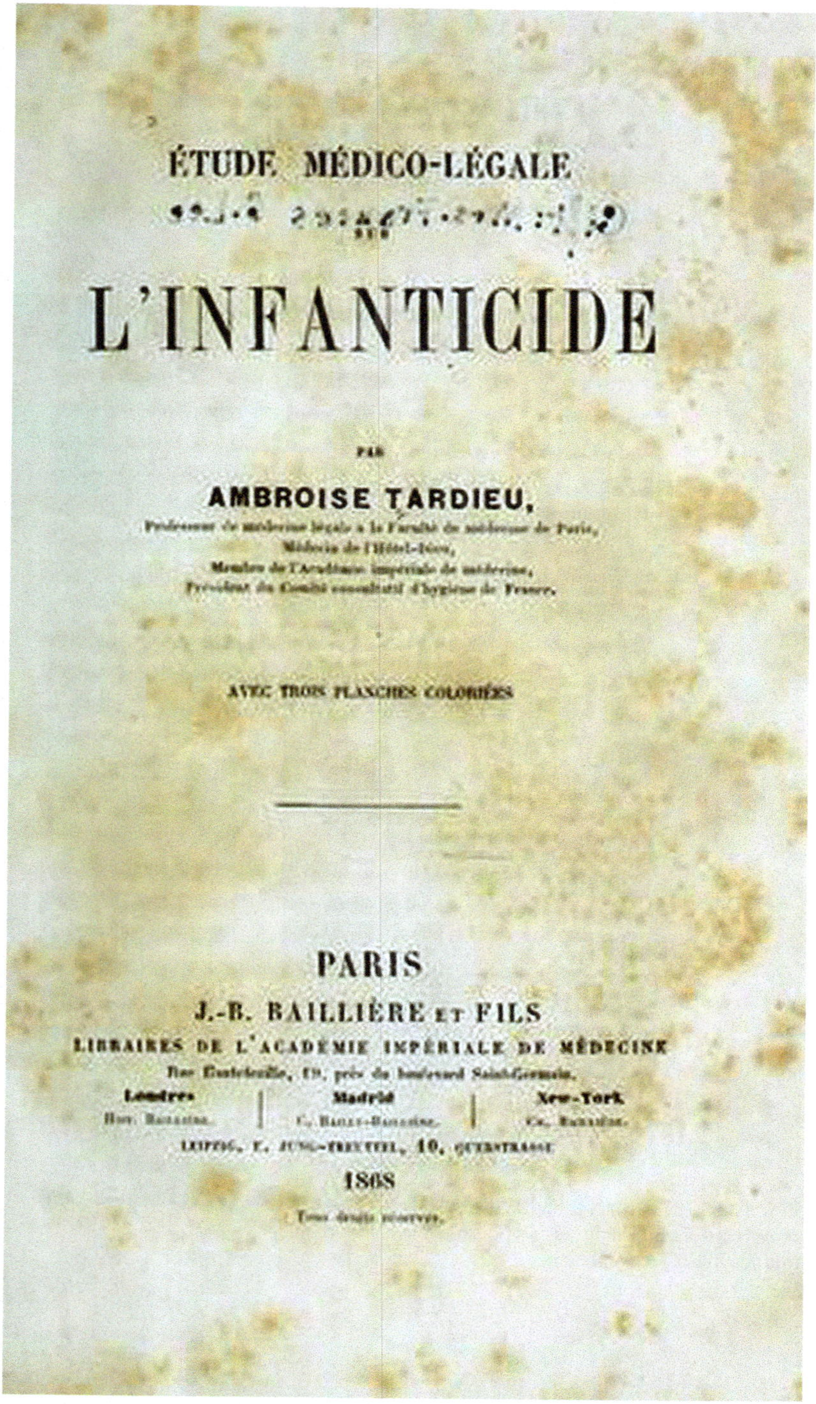

ÉTUDE MÉDICO-LÉGALE

SUR

L'INFANTICIDE

PAR

AMBROISE TARDIEU,

AVEC TROIS PLANCHES COLORIÉES

PARIS

J.-B. BAILLIÈRE ET FILS

LIBRAIRES DE L'ACADÉMIE IMPÉRIALE DE MÉDECINE

Londres | Madrid | New-York

1868

Fig. 1.15 Front page of "Étude médico-légale sur l'infanticide"

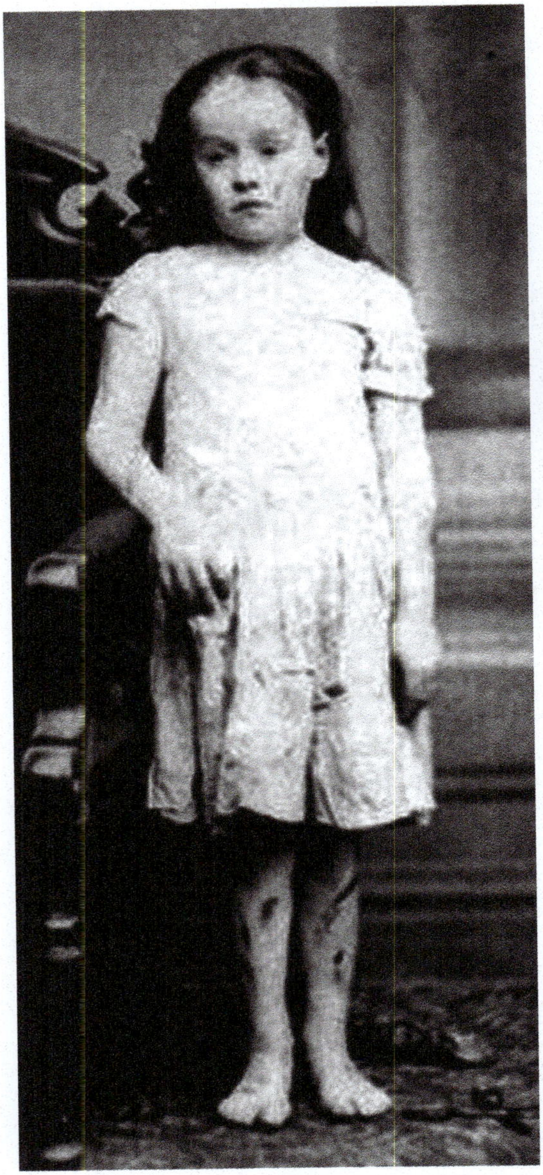

Fig. 1.16 1873: Mary Ellen Wilson, shortly after been removed from her stepmother's house with clearly visible injuries in her face and on her legs

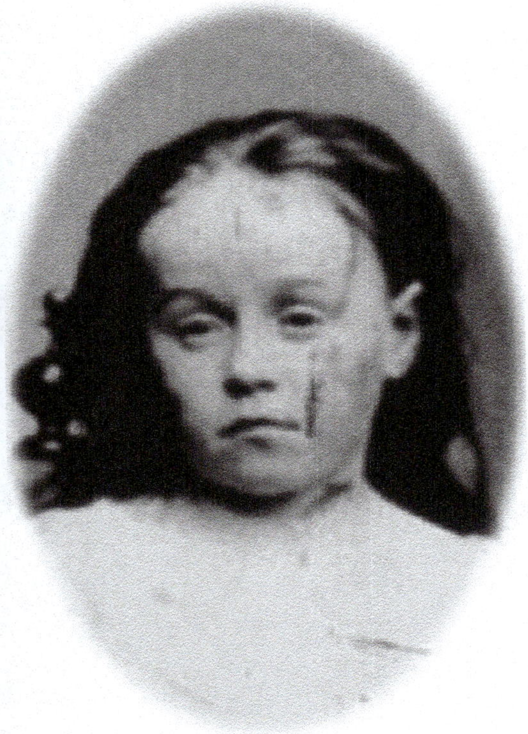

Fig. 1.17 1873: The facial injuries of Mary Ellen, caused by the scissors

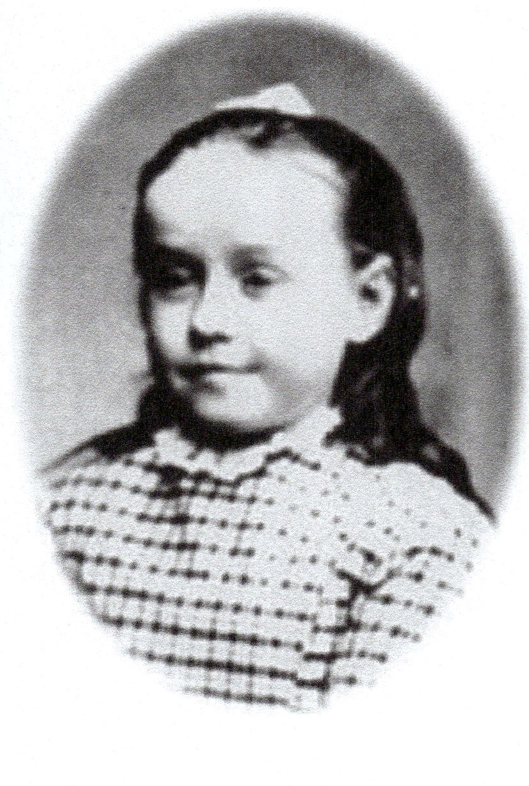

Fig. 1 18 1874: Mary Ellen, 1 year later

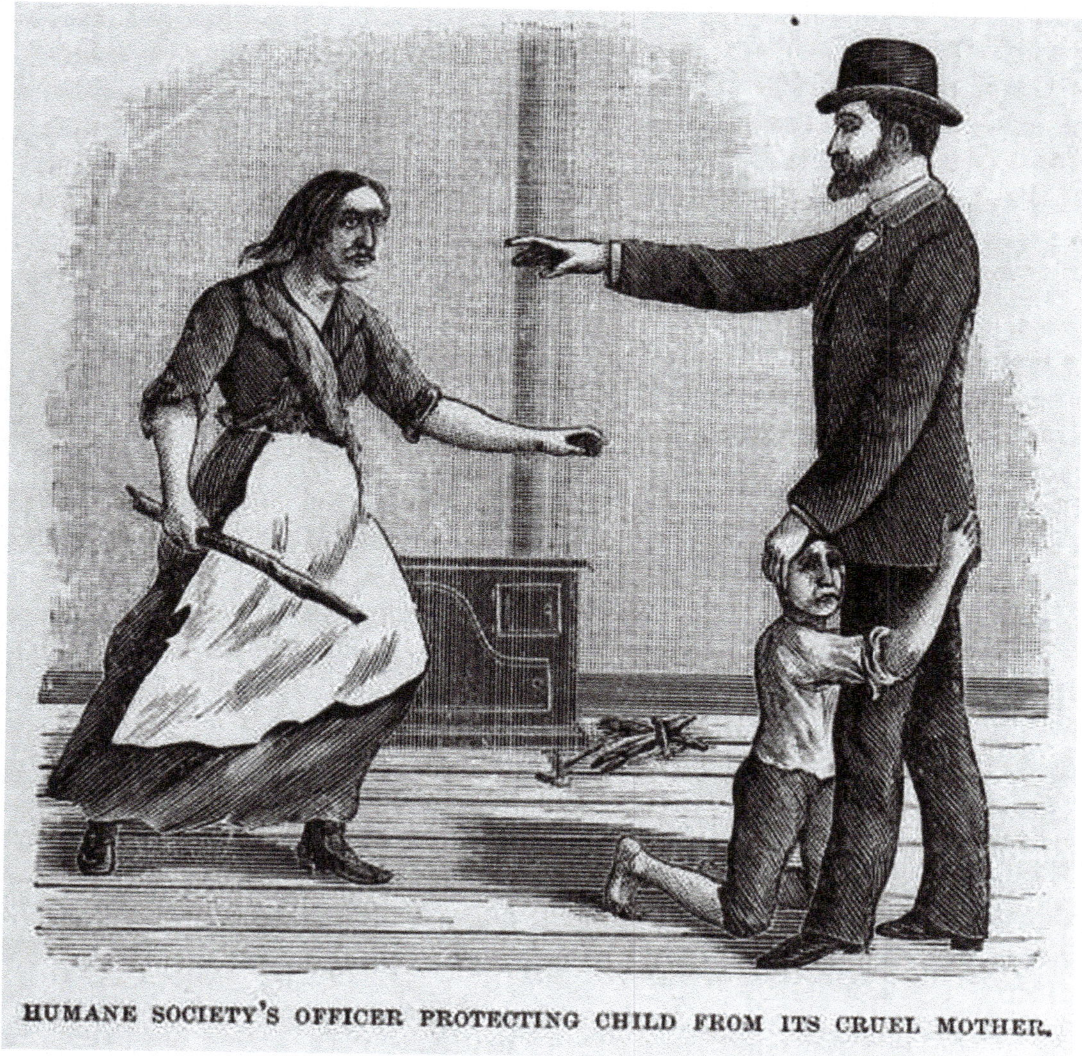

Fig. 1.19 Humane society's officer protecting a child from its cruel mother

1.4.3 The Convention on the Rights of the Child

1.4.3.1 Article 19

1. States parties shall take all appropriate legislative, administrative, social, and educational measures to protect the child from all forms of physical or mental violence, injury or abuse, neglect or negligent treatment, maltreatment or exploitation, including sexual abuse, while in the care of parent(s), legal guardian(s), or any other person who has the care of the child.
2. Such protective measures should, as appropriate, include effective procedures for the establishment of social programs to provide necessary support for the child and for those who have the care of the child, as well as for other forms of prevention and for identification, reporting, referral, investigation, treatment and follow-up of instances of child maltreatment

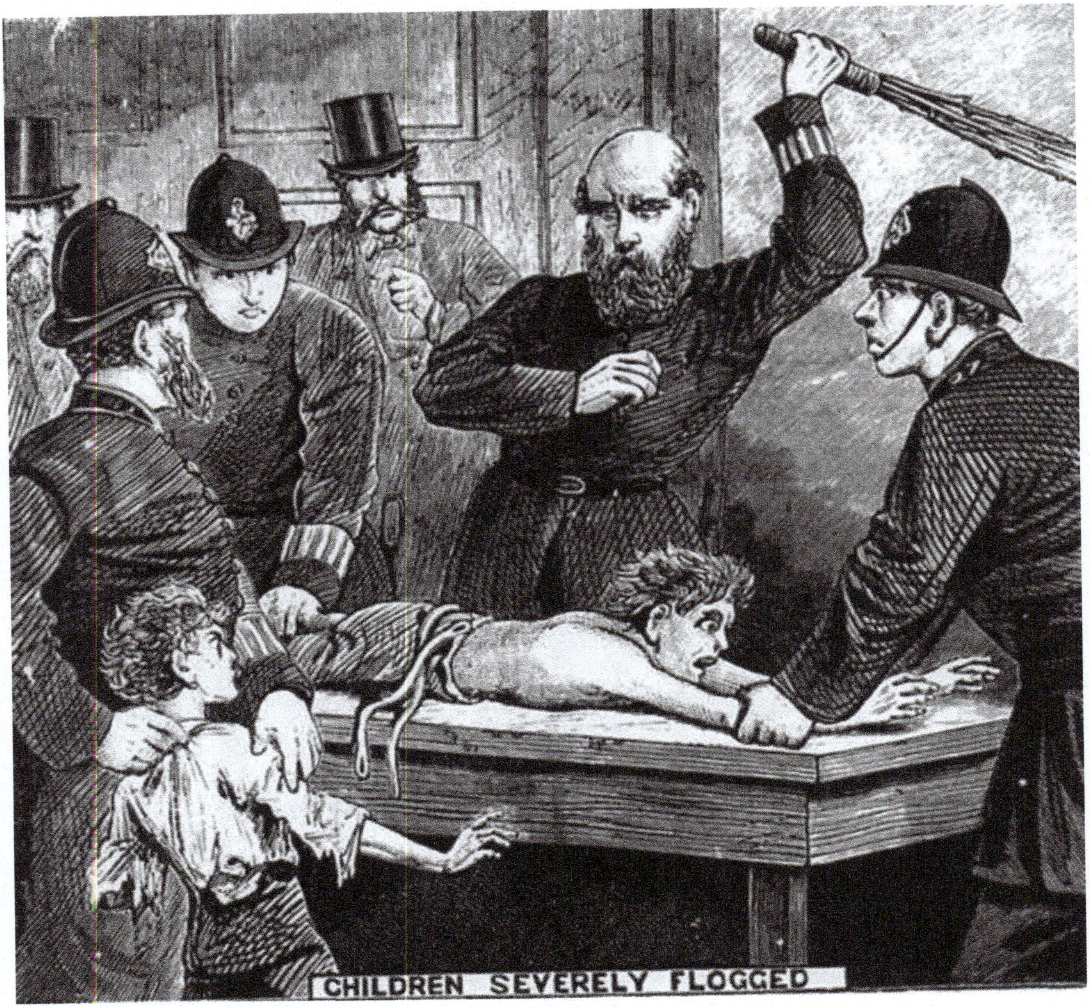

Fig. 1.20 *Illustrated Police News*: punishment by police officers

described heretofore, and, as appropriate, for judicial involvement.

1.4.3.2 Article 39

States parties shall take all appropriate measures to promote physical and psychological recovery and social reintegration of a child victim of any form of neglect, exploitation, or abuse; torture or any other form of cruel, inhuman, or degrading treatment or punishment; or armed conflicts. Such recovery and reintegration shall take place in an environment which fosters the health, self-respect, and dignity of the child.

1.4.3.3 Article 41

Nothing in the present Convention shall affect any provisions which are more conducive to the realization of the rights of the child and which may be contained in:

- The law of a State party
- International law in force for that State

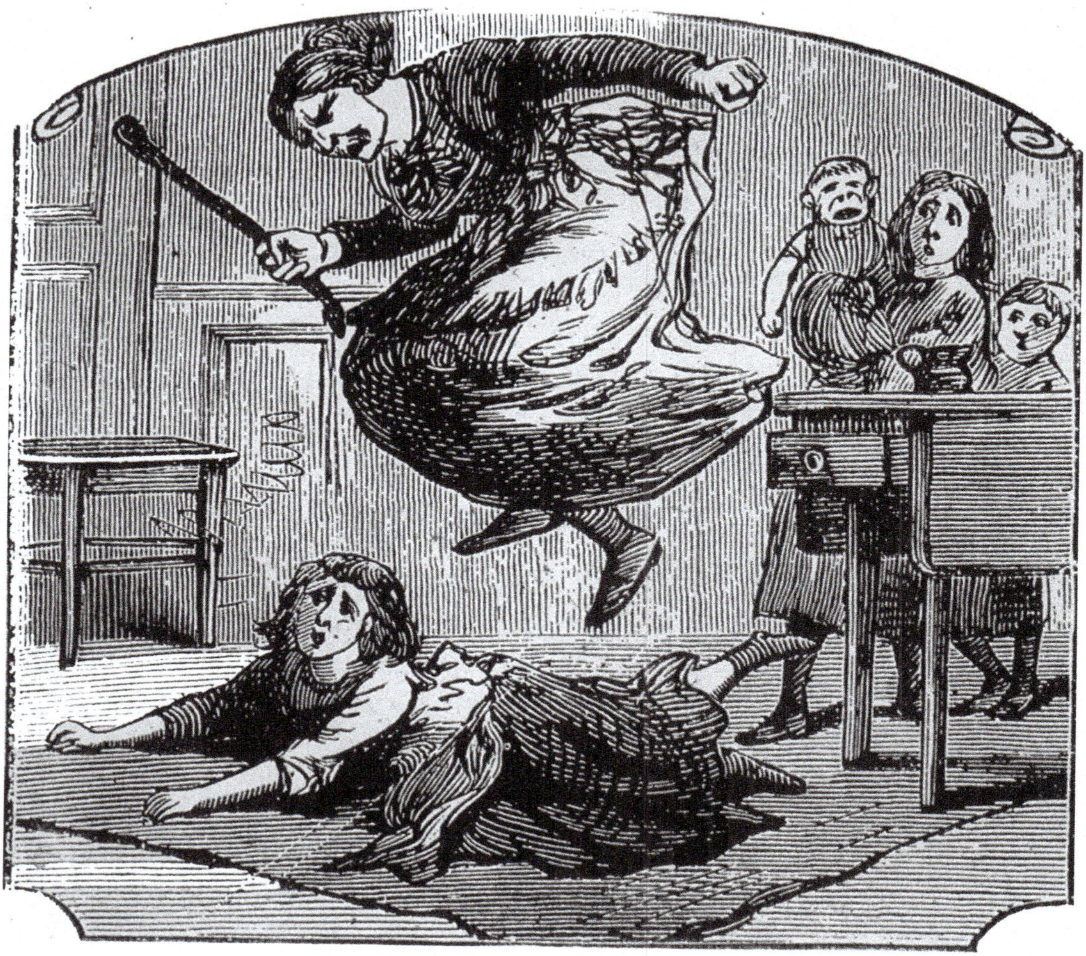

Fig. 1.21 *Illustrated Police News*: physical assault by a teacher

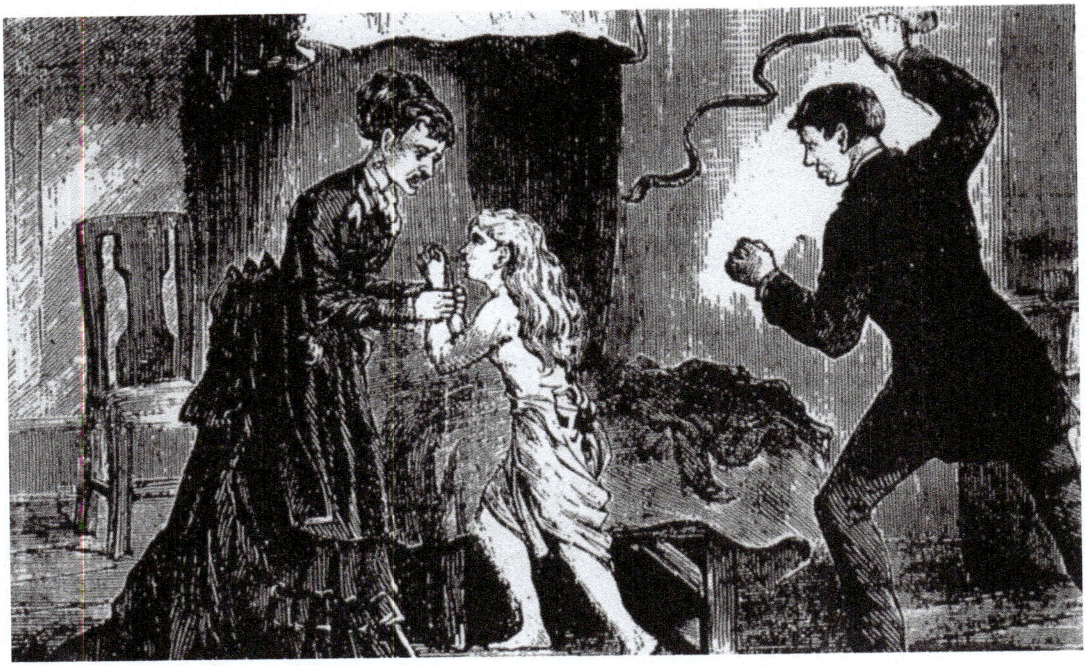

Fig. 1.22 *Illustrated Police News*: whipping with a belt

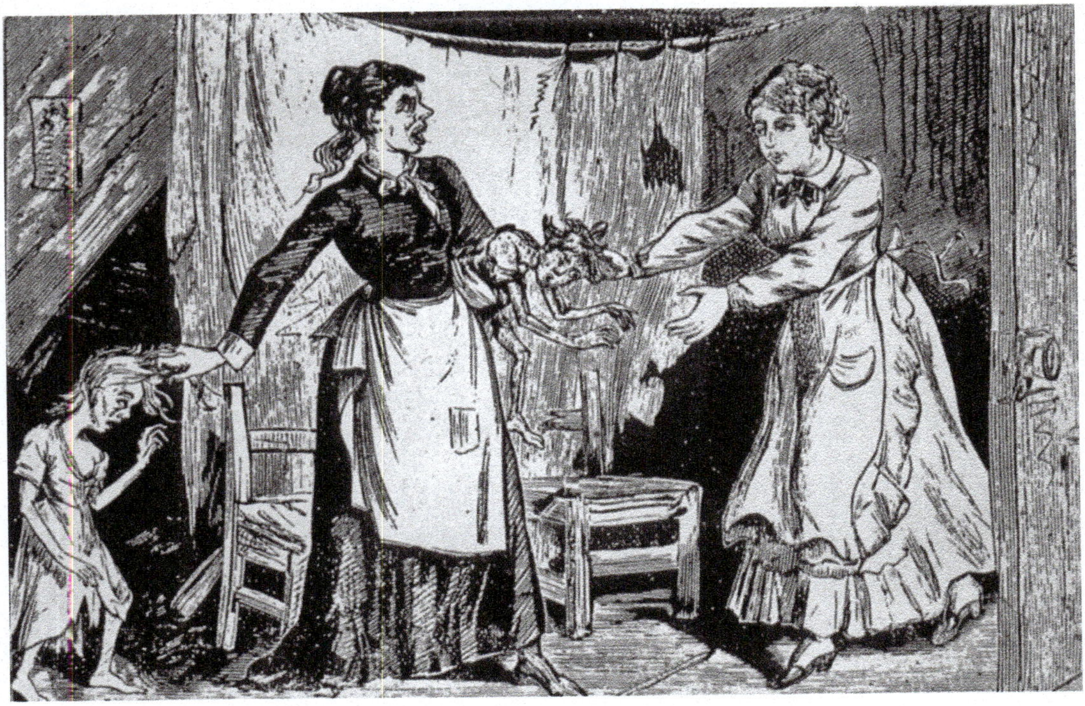

Fig. 1.23 *Illustrated Police News*: severe neglect

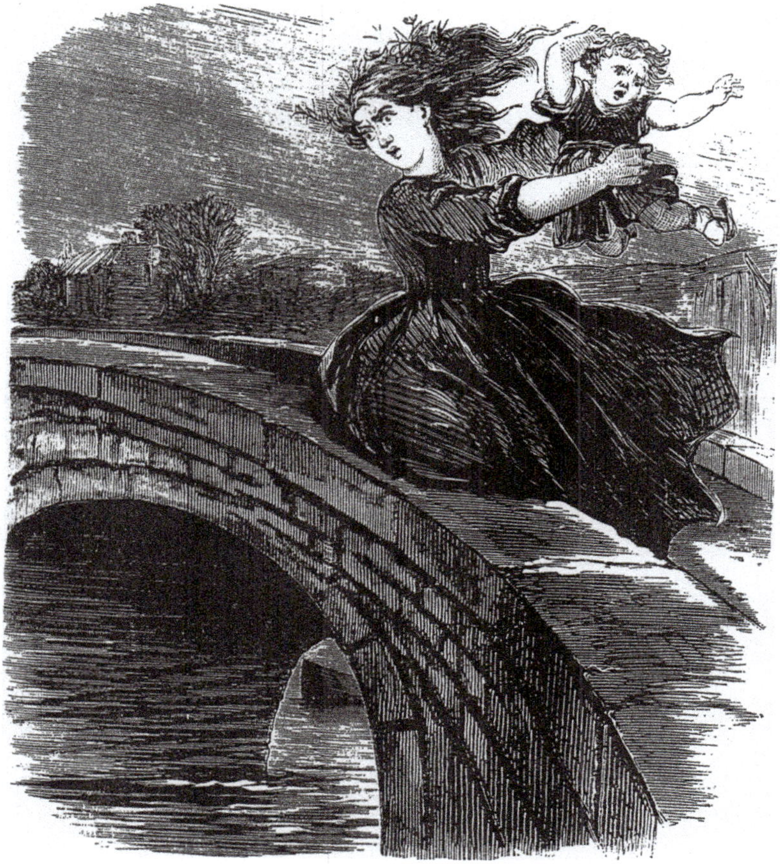

Fig. 1.24 *Illustrated Police News*: filicide

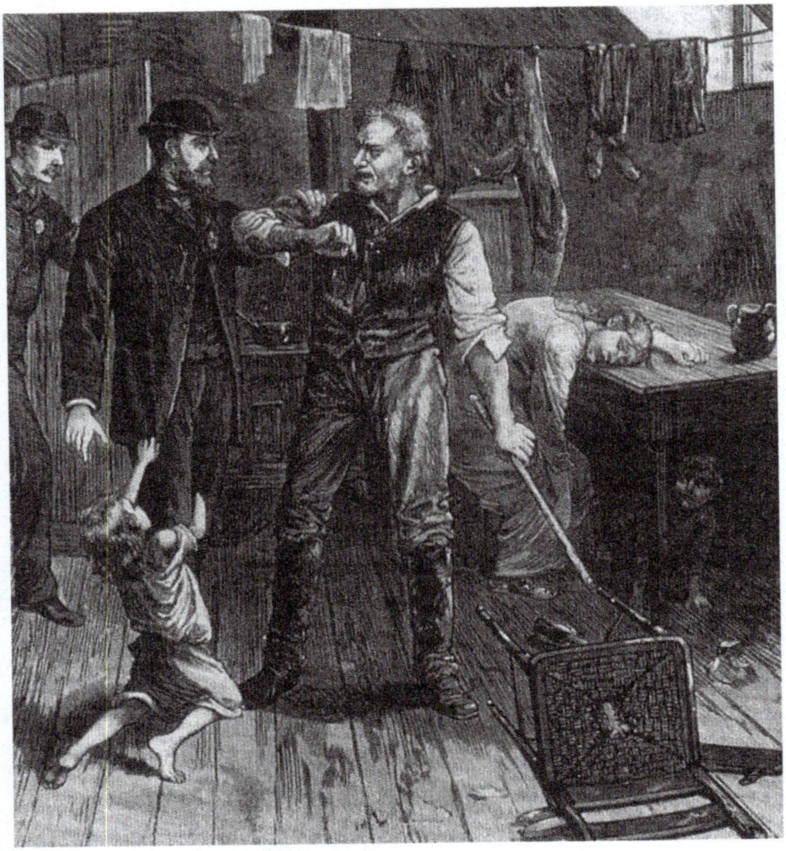

Fig. 1.25 *Illustrated Police News*: intervention by police officers

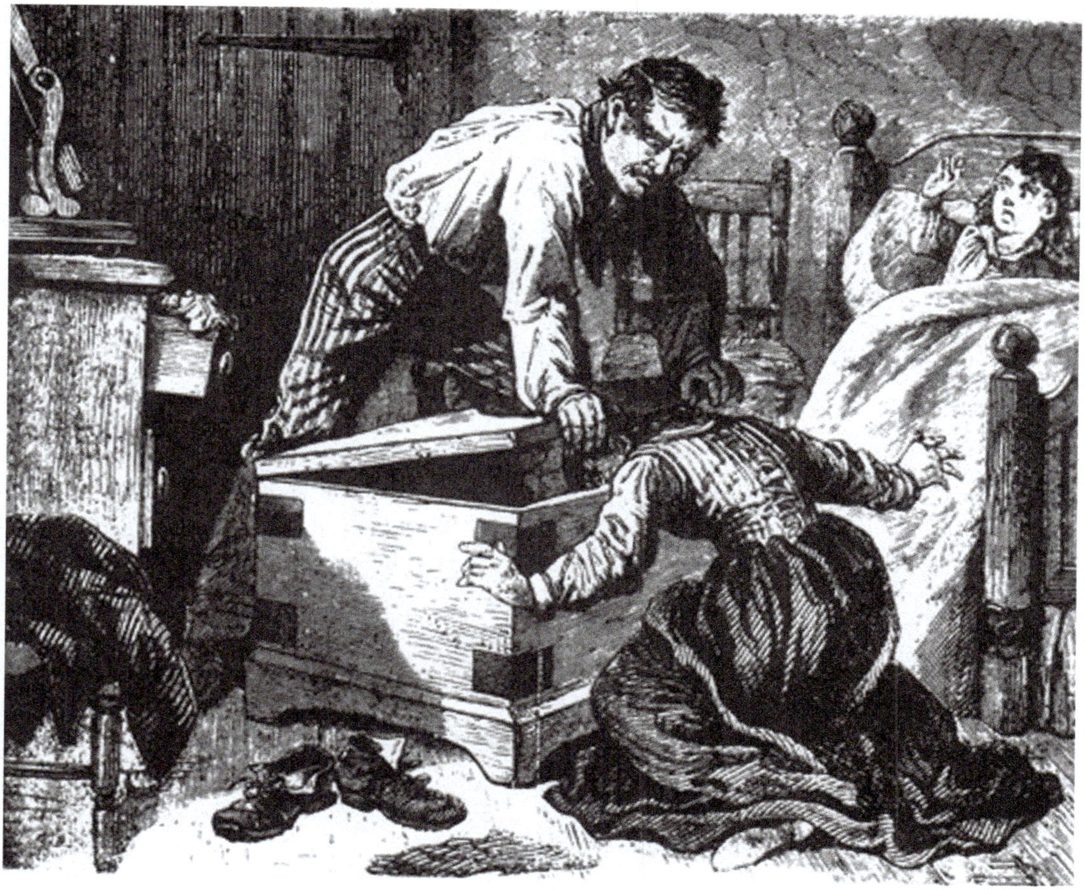

Fig. 1.26 *Illustrated Police News*: witnessing domestic violence

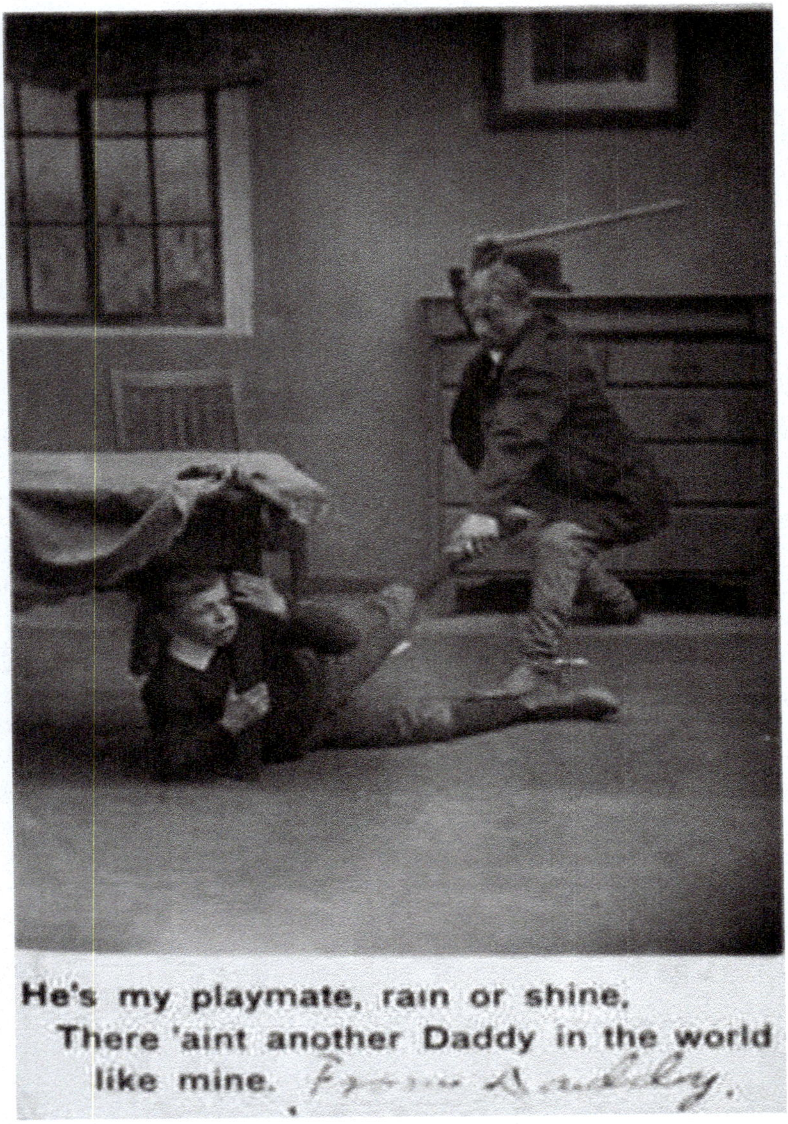
He's my playmate, rain or shine.
There 'aint another Daddy in the world like mine.

Fig. 1.27 Something "funny"?

References

Alink L, van IJzendoorn R, Bakermans-Kranenburg M et al (2011) Leiden attachment research program, TNO Child Health. Kindermishandeling 2010 (NPM-2010) [Child abuse, 2010]. Casimir Publishers, Leiden

American Humane Association (2000) Department of Health and Human Services Releases 2000 Child Abuse Report Data. AHA Legislative Activities. American Humane Association, http://www.americanhumane.org/actnoww/2000.abuse.data.htm. Accessed on 2010

American Humane Association. Mary Ellen Wilson. Not dated. http://www.americanhumane.org/about-us/who-we-are/history/mary-ellen-wilson.html

American Humane Association. The story of Mary Ellen. Not dated. http://www.americanhumane.org/about-us/who-we-are/history/story-of-mary-ellen.html

Andronicus M, Oates RK, Peat J et al (1998) Non-accidental burns in children. Burns 24(6):552–558

Bilo RAC, Beekwilder FM, van Wijk P, Houtman AJ (2000) Kinderpornografie – de stand van zaken.Gemeenschappelijk Voorziening Aanpak Kinderpornografie [in Dutch]. Child pornography in the Netherlands - 2000. Isala series, (30)

Bremmer J (1989) Greek pederasty and modern homosexuality. In: Bremmer J (ed) From Sappho to De Sade. Routledge, London, pp 1–14

Cawson P, Wattam C, Brooker S et al (2000) Child maltreatment in the United Kingdom. A study of the prevalence of child abuse and neglect. NSPCC, London

CDC (Centers for Disease Control and Prevention) (2008) Nonfatal maltreatment of infants – United States, October, 2005-September 2006. MMWR 57(13):336–339

Cramer KE (1996) Orthopedic aspects of child abuse. Pediatr Clin North Am 43(5):1035–1051

Deitch EA, Staats J (1982) Child abuse through burning. J Burn Care Rehabil 3(2):89–94

Felitti VJ, Anda RF, Nordenberg D (1998) Relationship of child abuse and household dysfunction to many of the leading causes of death in adults. The Adverse Childhood Experiences (ACE) Study. Am J Prev Med 14(4):245–258

Hight DW, Bakalar HR, Lloyd JR (1979) Inflicted burns in children. JAMA 242(6):517–520

Hobbs CJ, Hanks HGI, Wynne JM (1999) Chapter 4. Physical abuse. In: Hobbs CJ, Hanks HGI, Wynne JM (eds) Child abuse and neglect – a clinician's handbook, 2nd edn. Churchill Livingstone, London, pp 63–104

Hobbs C, Childs AM, Wynne J et al (2005) Subdural haematoma and effusion in infancy: an epidemiological study. Arch Dis Child 90(9):952–955

Holter JC, Friedman SB (1968) Child abuse: early case finding in the emergency department. Pediatrics 42(1):128–138

Hyden PW, Gallagher TA (1992) Child abuse intervention in the emergency room. Pediatr Clin North Am 39(5):1053–1081

Isaacs A (1993) Cassell sex and sexuality – a thematic dictionary of quotations. Market House Books, London, 41

Jones DN, Pickett J (1987) Understanding child abuse. Macmillan Education, Basingstoke, pp 74–75

Keenan HT, Leventhal JM (2009) The evolution of child abuse research. In: Reece RM, Christian CW (eds) Child abuse, medical diagnosis and management, 3rd edn. American Academy of Pediatrics, Elk Grove Village, pp 1–18

Kempe CH, Silverman FN, Steele BF et al (1962) The battered child syndrome. JAMA 181(1):17–24

King J, Diefendorf D, Apthorp J et al (1988) Analysis of 429 fractures in 189 battered children. J Pediatr Orthop 8(5):585–589

Lamers-Winkelman F, Slot NW, Bijl B et al (2007) Pupils on abuse. [Scholieren over mishandeling: resultaten van een landelijk onderzoek naar de omvang van kindermishandeling onder leerlingen van het voortgezet onderwijs.] Vrij Universiteit Amsterdam/PI Research [In Dutch]

Laming H (2003) The Victoria Climbié inquiry. Report of an inquiry. Presented to parliament by the secretary of state for health and the secretary of state for the home department by command of Her Majesty, http://www.victoria-climbie-inquiry.org.uk/. Accessed on 2009

Leventhal JM, Thomas SA, Rosenfield NS et al (1993) Fractures in young children. Distinguishing child abuse from unintentional injuries. Am J Dis Child 147(1):87–92

McMahon P, Grossman W, Gaffney M et al (1995) Soft tissue injury as an indication of child abuse. J Bone Joint Surg 77(8):1179–1183

National Committee to Prevent Child Abuse (1998) Child abuse and neglect statistics http://web.archive.org/web/19980515052303/http://childabuse.org/facts97.html. Accessed on 2009

Oosterlee A, Vink RM, Smit F (2009) Prevalence of family violence in adults and children: estimates using the capture-recapture method. Eur J Public Health 19(6):586–591

Purdue GF, Hunt JL, Prescott PR (1988) Child abuse by burning: an index of suspicion. J Trauma 28(2):221–224

Reijneveld SA, van de Wal MF, Brugman E et al (2004) Infant crying and abuse. Lancet 364(9442):1340–1342

Sinal SH, Stewart CD (1998) Physical abuse of children: a review for orthopedic surgeons. J South Orthop Assoc 7(4):264–276

Smith M, Bee P, Heverin A (1995) Parental control within the family: the nature and extent of parental violence to children. Thomas Coram Research Unit, London

Straus MA, Hamby SL, Finkelhor D et al (1998) Identification of child maltreatment with the parent–child conflict tactics scales: development and psychometric data for a national sample of American parents. Child Abuse Negl 22(4):249–270

Sullivan PM, Knutson JF (2000) Maltreatment and disabilities: a population based epidemiological study. Child Ab Negl 24(10):1257–1273

Tardieu A (1859) Étude medico-legale sur les attentats aux moeurs. JB Baillière, Paris

Tardieu A (1860) Étude médico-légale sur les sévices et mauvais traitements exercées sur des enfants. Annales d'Hygiène Publique et de Medecine Légale 13:361–398

Tardieu A (1868) Étude médico-légale sur l'infanticide. JB Baillière, Paris

UNICEF (2007) Child poverty in perspective: an overview of child well-being in rich countries. UNICEF Innocenti Research Centre, Florence. Innocenti Report Card 7

United Nations General Assembly (1989) Convention on the rights of the child. UN, http://www.unhchr.ch/html/menu3/b/k2crc.htm. Accessed on 2009

van IJzendoorn MH, Prinzie P, Euser EM et al (2007) Kindermishandeling in Nederland anno 2005: de nationale prevalentiestudie mishandeling van kinderen en jeugdigen (NPM-2005). Leiden University

Watkins SA (1990) The Mary Ellen myth: correcting child welfare history. Social Work 35(6):500–503

WHO (World Health Organization) (2002) Chapter 3. Child abuse and neglect by parents and other caregivers. World Report on Violence and Health, Geneva

WHO (World Health Organization) (2006a) Preventing child maltreatment: a guide to taking action and generating evidence. World Health Organization and International Society for Prevention of Child Abuse and Neglect, Geneva

WHO (World Health Organization) (2006b) Regional Office for Europe. Unintentional child injuries in the WHO European Region. World Health Organization, Geneva

Evaluating Suspicious Skin Findings in Children

2

If there is a discrepancy between the injury and the history, one should trust the injury and not the history!

2.1 Introduction

The skin is one of the largest organs of the human body (Goldsmith 1990). The total body surface of the skin varies from 0.2 m^2 in a full-term newborn to around 2 m^2 in an adult (Patient.co.uk 2007). The skin weighs about 15% of the total body weight. It is also the most accessible organ of the human being and plays an important role in the communication between human beings. Skin irregularities and abnormalities can be seen by everybody. Because of its easy accessibility, it is the most frequently damaged organ in accidents as well as in child abuse or physical assaults.

The skin has three major functions: protection against external influences, regulation (thermoregulation, osmoregulation, excretion, and secretion), and sensory perception (touch, temperature, kinesthetic sense, pain). In forensic terms, the most important function of the skin is protection. The skin forms a barrier between the environment and the organism and protects the organism against injuries caused by mechanical (static and dynamic loading; Sect. 2.5) and nonmechanical or physical (thermal, chemical, electrical, and radiation trauma; Sect. 2.6) agents.

The skin consists of three layers, namely, the epidermis, the dermis, and the hypodermis. These layers form together a smooth and supple protective shield, which protects the body against injuries.

The epidermis is the compact, firm, and elastic outer layer of the skin. The epidermis protects the body against external influences. Because of its elasticity, the epidermis is not easily damaged in blunt-force trauma or crushing (Langlois and Gresham 1991).

The second layer is the dermis which is composed of three types of tissue that are present throughout the dermis: collagen, elastic tissue, and reticular fibers (Brannon 2007). Because of this composition, the dermis is capable of stretching under force and returning to its original form without damage (Kaczor et al. 2006). The dermis is the second skin layer to absorb the energy which is transferred during blunt-force trauma. The dermis is very well vascularized and has an extensive superficial capillary network. In adults, up to 4.5% of total blood volume is found in the dermis (Coleman 2001).

The hypodermis consists of connective tissue and fat. It is richly vascularized, just like the dermis. Because of the elasticity of the hypodermis, this layer will easily deform and will function as a shock absorber for the underlying structures, such as bones. The fat tissue in the hypodermis functions not only as a shock absorber but also as a thermal insulator. The fat protects the body against cold and defines the body's contours.

One square centimeter of the dermis and hypodermis may contain up to 70 cm of blood vessels (Fridman 2001). During blunt-force trauma, these

R.A.C. Bilo et al., *Cutaneous Manifestations of Child Abuse and Their Differential Diagnosis*,
DOI 10.1007/978-3-642-29287-3_2, © Springer-Verlag Berlin Heidelberg 2013

vessels are the most vulnerable structures with the majority of bleeding occurring from the capillaries and venules in the subcutaneous tissue (Langlois and Gresham 1991). The injury threshold of these vessels is lower than that of the epidermis or other parts of the dermis or hypodermis. Blood will leak into the perivascular tissues when damage occurs (Kaczor et al. 2006). The extravasated blood will spread along any line of cleavage in the tissue producing a visible discolored area – a bruise (Langlois and Gresham 1991). The blunt-force trauma will in most cases not lead to loss of the integrity of the epidermis or the superficial layers of the dermis, as happens in a laceration.

According to Kaczor et al. (2006), the skin varies in relative tissue composition and thickness throughout the body to meet the functional requirements of the different body parts. The thickness of the epidermis and dermis together varies in thickness from less than 0.5 mm on the eyelids to 4 mm or more on the palms and soles (Fridman 2001). The epidermis itself is the thinnest on the eyelids (0.05 mm) and the thickest on the palms and soles (1.5 mm). The thickness of the dermis also varies depending on location, for example, 0.3 mm on the eyelid and 3.0 mm on the back. The size of the hypodermis varies throughout the body and from person to person (Brannon 2007).

As a consequence of these structural differences of the skin between body regions, some parts of the body will bruise or be injured in another way more easily, while other parts of the body require more loading. One will see increasing extravasation of blood in areas with increasing laxity and loose subcutaneous elements in the tissues, for example, bruising around the eyes is more obvious than bruising of the hand palm (Langlois and Gresham 1991).

A superficial bruise may be visible as a discoloration immediately, while deep bruises may take hours to days before becoming visible (Wilson 1977; Langlois and Gresham 1991). Deeper bruising sometimes will not become visible, except when the skin is incised, for example, during a forensic autopsy (Langlois and Gresham 1991).

2.2 Evaluating Skin Injuries: "The Kipling Principle"

> I Keep six honest serving-men
> (They taught me all I knew);
> Their names are What and Why and When
> And How and Where and Who. (Kipling 1902)

In 1990, Johnson stated: "Physicians must approach an injury as a symptom requiring a diagnosis of cause. This is best accomplished by careful examination and documentation of each injury." In other words, evaluating an injury in a child should be done in a standardized way, and findings should be described in a standardized and well-defined terminology. Only then the findings can be understood correctly and used properly by others if a child needs protection.

In 1902, Rudyard Kipling (1865–1936) published the "Just So Stories" (Fig. 2.1). He ended one of the stories in this book, "the Elephant's Child," with a poem in which he described the questions a child has to answer to find solutions for daily problems. These questions are also the questions to be asked and answered by doctors in a standardized forensic evaluation of suspicious physical findings in a child: "What and Why and When and How and Where and Who."

2.3 What: Defining Injury and Types of Skin Injuries

2.3.1 Defining Injury

The first question to be answered in a forensic medical evaluation of a suspicious physical finding is what do I see? In other words, whether the finding is an injury or something else, for example, a normal variant or a disorder. Sometimes, the answer to this question can only be formulated after a comprehensive evaluation and differential diagnosis.

An injury (bodily injury, physical injury) is defined as any wounding or physical damage that results from the (sudden) subjection of the body or parts of the body to amounts of energy that exceed the threshold of physiological tolerance or, in other words, that are beyond the body's

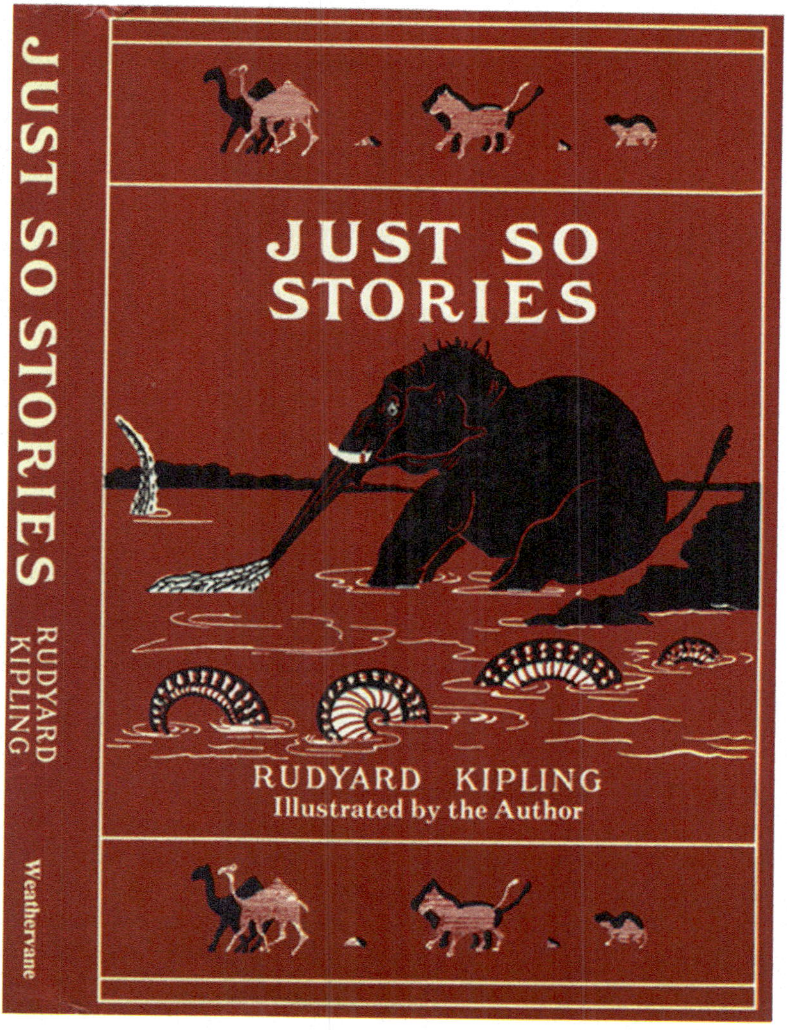

Fig. 2.1 Rudyard Kipling: Just So Stories (the elephant's child)

ability to absorb (Health Canada 2003; WHO 2006),

- Without or with externally visible damage to the skin or the mucous membranes and/or.
- Without or with externally visible signs of damage to the skeleton or internal organs.

Physical injury can also be the result of lack of one of the vital elements (e.g., oxygen, trace elements, vitamins, water, or warmth) (Health Canada 2003; WHO 2006). Although not mentioned by Health Canada or the WHO, an excess of one of the vital elements can also result in physical injuries of all body parts (including the skin) or even death as can be seen, for example, in salt poisoning, hypervitaminosis, water poisoning (hyperhydration), or overheating (hyperthermia, heat stroke) (el Awad 1994; Meyer-Heim et al. 2002; Zhu et al. 1998; Arieff and Kronlund 1999; Martos Sánchez et al. 2000; Quereshi et al. 2010).

During a forensic medical evaluation (including a forensic autopsy), all physical findings are important, irrespective of how trivial they may seem to be from a clinical and medical point of view. Even the combination of injuries on certain parts of the body and the absence of injuries on other parts of the body is forensically relevant because this may help to determine what happened. Therefore, a correct and complete description and registration of all medical findings (with the standardized description of anatomical

Table 2.1 Types of skin injuries in mechanical trauma: closed injuries

Bruise (Chap. 3)	Bleeding, due to the rupture of blood vessels, generally located superficially in the skin and subcutaneous tissues with usually externally visible surface discoloration Caused by blunt-force trauma (collision/compression or stretching) Will not blanch under diascopy (Figs. 2.2 and 2.3) Synonyms (sometimes used for specific types of bruising and bleeding): contusion, hematoma, purpura, and ecchymosis
Petechia (Chap. 3)	Small red, purple, or brown spot caused by minor bleeding (0.1–2 mm – pinpoint to pinhead) in the skin, the mucous membranes, and/or the serosal surfaces, due to leakage of blood from the postcapillary venules (Fig. 2.4) Caused by a sudden rise of the venous pressure in the postcapillary venules Will not blanch under diascopy Synonym: pinpoint bleeding
Erythema (Chap. 7)	Redness of the skin, due to cutaneous vasodilatation Caused by a local reaction to physical agents (e.g., friction, rubbing, or pressure) or application of irritating chemical substances Will blanch under diascopy (Figs. 2.5 and 2.6)

locations and injuries – mechanical trauma, see Tables 2.1 and 2.2 and Sect. 2.5; nonmechanical trauma, see Table 2.5 and Sect. 2.6), including the description and registration of absence of findings, is imperative.

2.3.2 Injury Classifications

Injuries can be classified in many other ways than purely on the type of injury (Tables 2.1 and 2.2). An overview of examples of injury classifications is given in Table 2.3 by using the "Kipling principle."

2.4 How and Why: Cause and Manner of Skin Injuries

The cause (or mechanism) of injury refers to the way the skin, the mucosa, or any other tissue (muscles, organs, and bones) is damaged; in other words, how skin injury occurred (what caused the injury). The manner (or mode) of injury describes the circumstances under which the injury was sustained or the injury event happened; in other words, why (under which circumstances) the injury occurred.

In general, injuries to the skin are caused by the transfer of energy to the skin, in which the transferred energy exceeds the capacity of the skin (and/or the underlying tissues) to absorb the energy. Transfer of energy, leading to injuries, results from mechanical trauma (static and dynamic loading; Sect. 2.5) or nonmechanical trauma (contact or near contact with physical agents; Sect. 2.6).

While determining the cause of an injury, one should also differentiate between the underlying cause and the direct cause. According to the CDC (2007), the underlying cause is what starts the chain of events that leads to an injury. The direct cause is what produces the actual physical harm. In children and adults, the underlying and direct causes can be the same or different (CDC 2007).

If a child sustained bruising on the forehead after he or she stumbled while walking and hit his or her head on a coffee table, the fall, caused by the stumbling, is the underlying cause (the action that started the chain of events leading to the injury = stumbling and falling), leading to the contact with the table, which is the direct cause of the bruising (the action that caused the actual physical harm = impact trauma).

Determining the cause of injury does not say anything about the manner (mode) of injury. The cause of injury may indicate the circumstances in which the injury was sustained (manner of injury), but rarely ever will prove the exact manner. Determining that the child fell and hit the table (causing a bruise to the forehead) does not determine under which circumstances the tumbling

Table 2.2 Types of skin injuries in mechanical trauma: open injuries

Abrasion (Chap. 7)	Superficial injury to the skin, characterized by the traumatic removal, detachment, or destruction of the epidermis (Figs. 2.7 and 2.8) Caused by blunt-force trauma (collision/compression or stretching or friction/transverse motion during collision/compression/stretching – shearing force) Synonyms: scrape, graze, erosion, excoriation
Laceration (Chap. 7)	Full-thickness injury of the skin and subcutaneous tissues, characterized by tearing of tissue in a frayed and irregular pattern and often associated with abrasions, contusions, and crushing of the wound margins (Fig. 2.9) Caused by blunt-force trauma (collision/compression or stretching – shearing force) Synonyms: tear, tear wound
Avulsion (Chap. 7)	Laceration in which skin and subcutaneous tissues are not just separated but torn away from the underlying tissues Caused by blunt-force trauma (collision, compression, or stretching – shearing force)
Cut	Injury in which the integrity of the skin is compromised by blunt-force (laceration, avulsion) or sharp-force trauma (incision, stab wound)
Incision	Slicing injury with sharp edges (clean cut), which is longer than deep, varying from minimal as a paper cut to significant as a surgical incision, if caused by sharp-force trauma with a clean, sharp-edged object (e.g., a knife, a razor, or a glass splinter) (Figs. 2.10 – 2.13) Slicing injury with laceration-like edges, which is longer than deep, if caused by sharp-force trauma with a sharp serrated object (e.g., a bread knife) Synonym: incised wound
Stab wound	Deep, narrow injury, which is deeper than its length visible in the skin, caused by a sharp-pointed object puncturing the skin (e.g., nail, needle, knife, or broken glass). Usually sharp edged, except often in case of a sharp serrated object (Figs. 2.14 – 2.19) Synonyms: puncture wound, penetrating injury
Gunshot wound	Injury caused by an object entering and often leaving the body at a high speed, typically a bullet or similar projectile Often two wounds are found, one at the site of entry and one at the site of exit (through-and-through injury) (Fig. 2.20). Wound characteristics depend on size of projectile, speed, and distance between gun and target Synonyms: missile wound, velocity wound

Table 2.3 Classifications of injuries

	Classification based on	Example
What	Probability	No injury – inconclusive – possible – probable – reasonable medical certainty – injury proven
	Severity	Mild – moderate – severe – fatal
	Type	Closed and open (Tables 2.1 and 2.2) Blunt force versus sharp force (penetrating) Mechanical and nonmechanical
How	Cause/mechanism (biomechanics)	Mechanical (static and dynamic loading) and nonmechanical (physical agents) (Tables 2.4 and 2.5)
Why	Manner/mode (circumstances)	Accidental versus non-accidental Non-inflicted versus inflicted Non-intentional/unintentional versus intentional/deliberate Non-abusive versus abusive/negligent
Where	Anatomical location	Head/neck – trunk – extremities External (skin, mucosa) – internal (muscles, brain, abdomen)
	Tissue	Soft tissues (skin, mucosa, muscles, joints) – hard tissues (skeleton) – special tissues (brain, thoracic and abdominal organs, eyes)
When	Dating	Old – recent
Who		Person – object Self-harm – harm by others

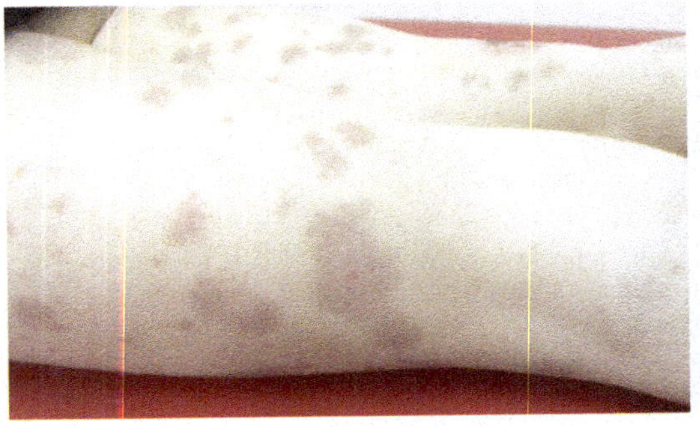

Fig. 2.2 Bruising

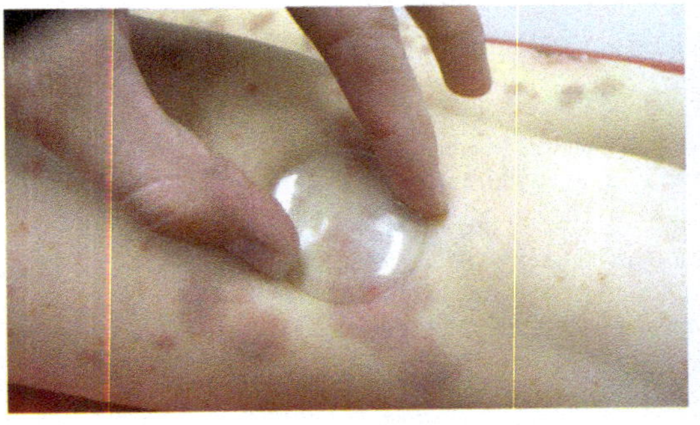

Fig. 2.3 Diascopy in bruising: no blanching

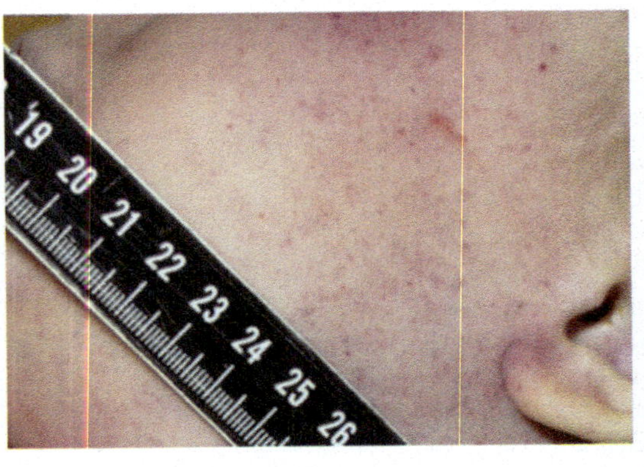

Fig. 2.4 Extensive petechiae in the face of a strangled child (= Fig. 3.95)

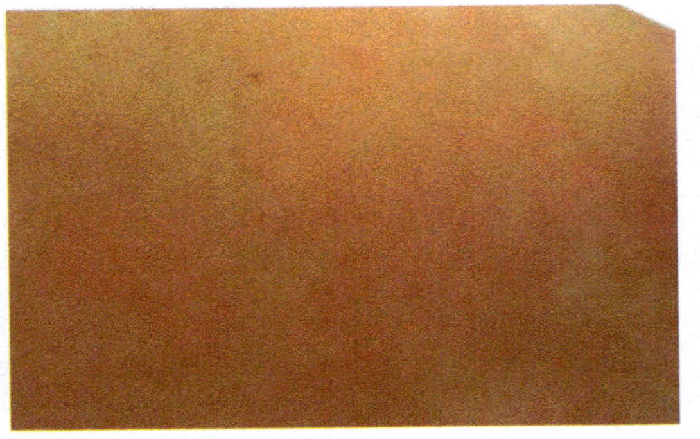

Fig. 2.5 Erythema

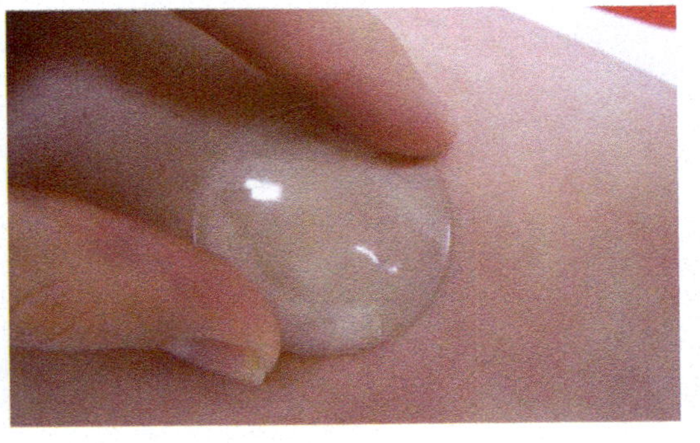

Fig. 2.6 Diascopy in erythema: blanching

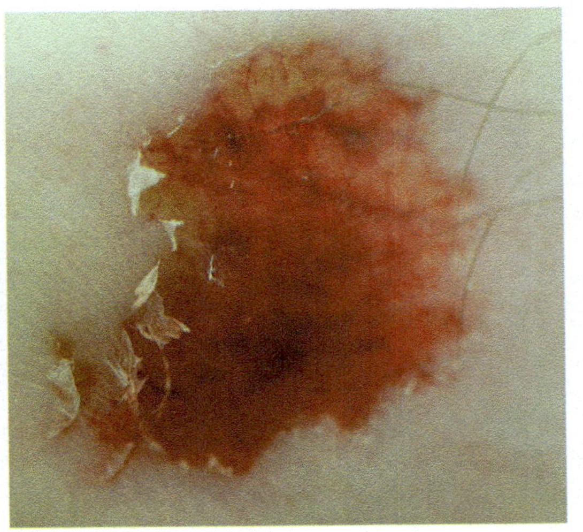

Fig. 2.7 Abrasion

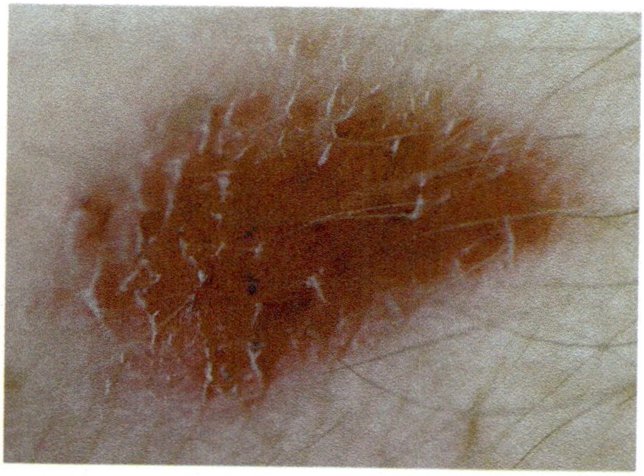

Fig. 2.8 Abrasion

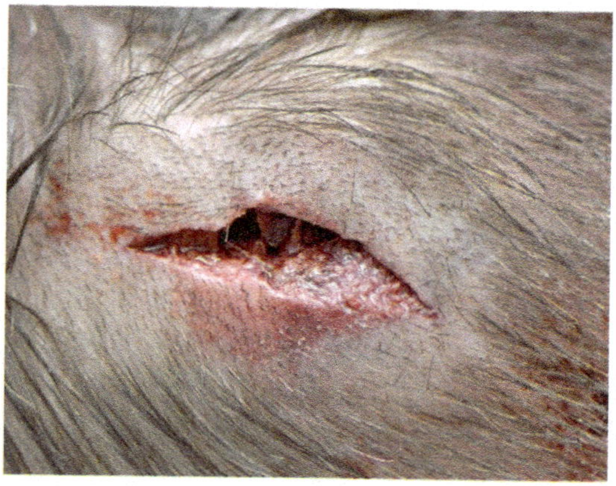

Fig. 2.9 Laceration of the scalp with tissue bridges of vessels and/or nerves within the tear (= Fig. 7.53)

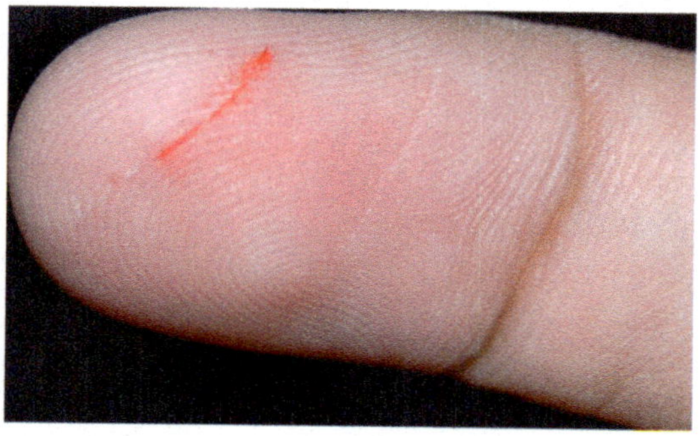

Fig. 2.10 A small paper cut wound (Laurence Facun 2008 from Wikimedia Commons 2011: Oww Papercut 14365.jpg)

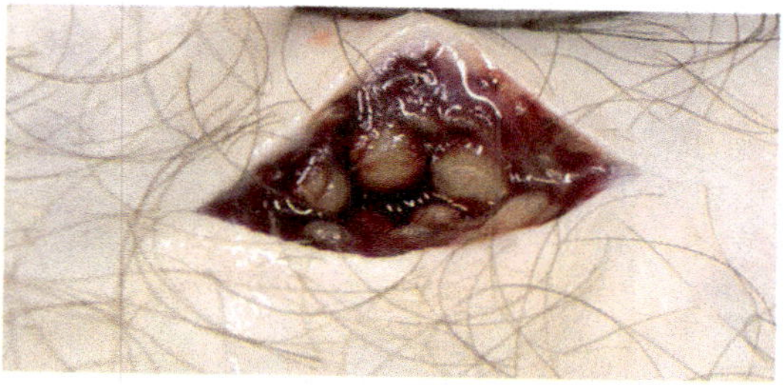

Fig. 2.11 Incision in a bruise: visible blood (= Fig. 3.86)

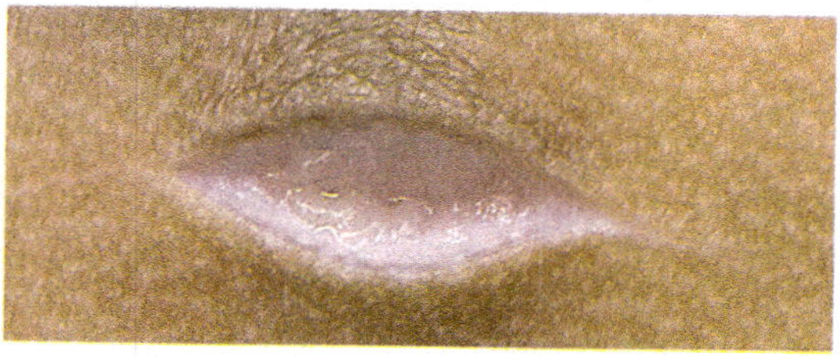

Fig. 2.12 Incision in a Mongolian spot: no visible blood (= Fig. 3.88)

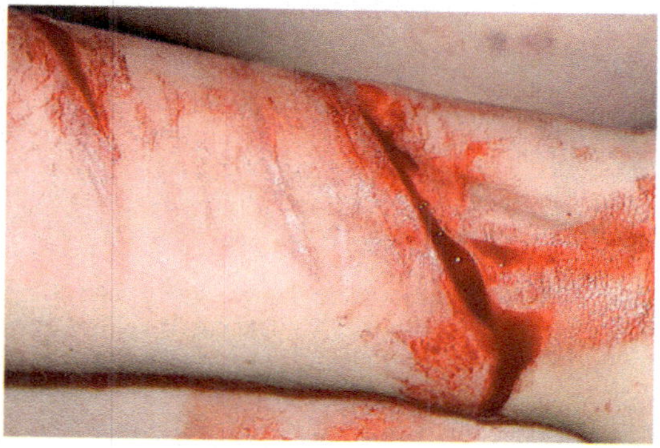

Fig. 2.13 Fresh incised wounds, next to scars in self-cutting (Hedwig Klawuttke 2009 from Wikimedia Commons 2011: Borderline.jpg)

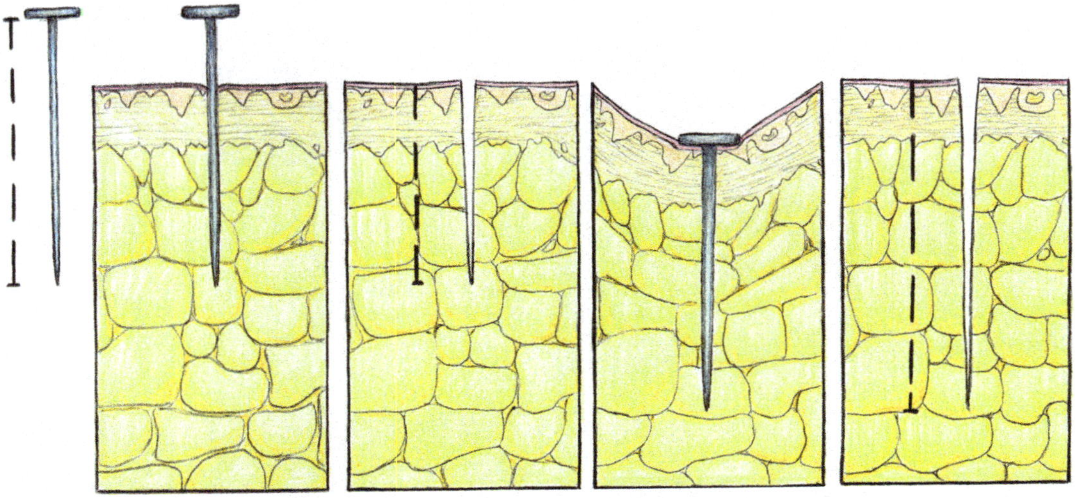

Fig. 2.14 Sharp penetrating trauma (puncture wound): deeper than its length visible in the skin and often deeper than the length of the penetrating object

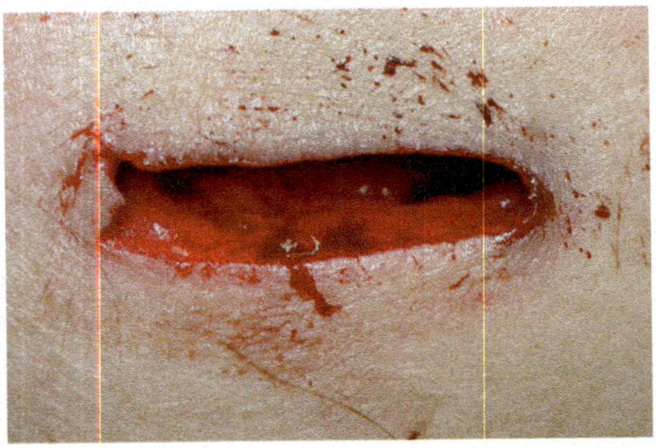

Fig. 2.15 Sharp penetrating trauma: stab wound with a sharp object, probably with a single-edged knife because of the fishtailing on one side of the wound (= Fig. 7.65)

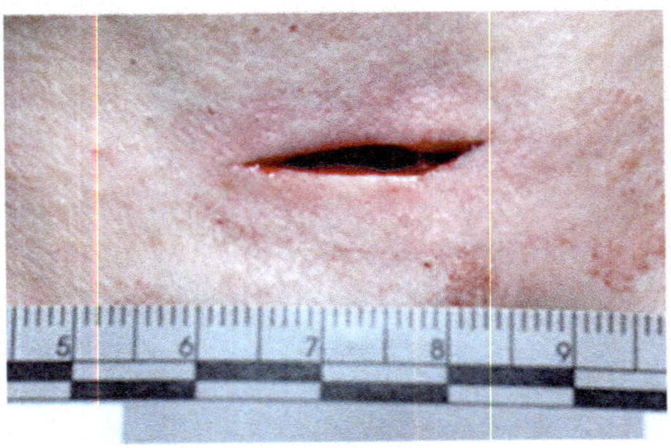

Fig. 2.16 Stab wound, probably with a double-edged knife because of the sharp angles on both sides of the wound

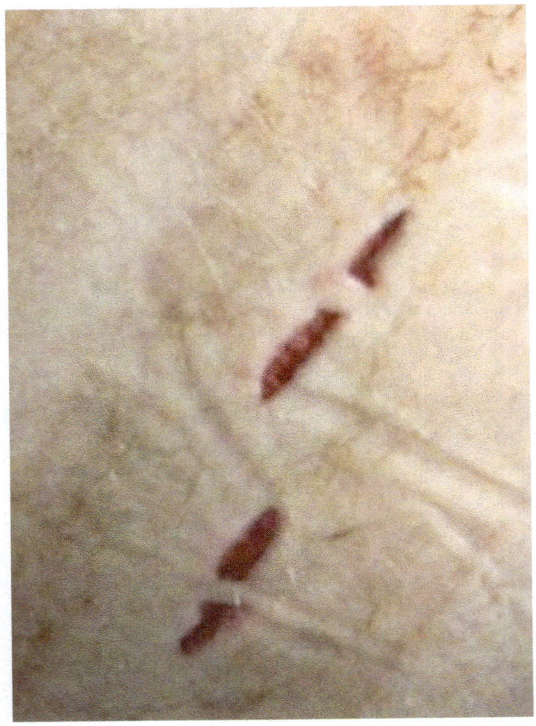

Fig. 2.17 Stab wounds: paired injuries

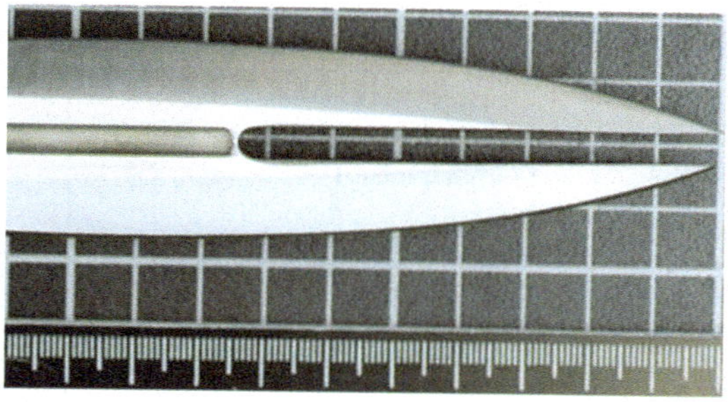

Fig. 2.18 Knife: paired blades

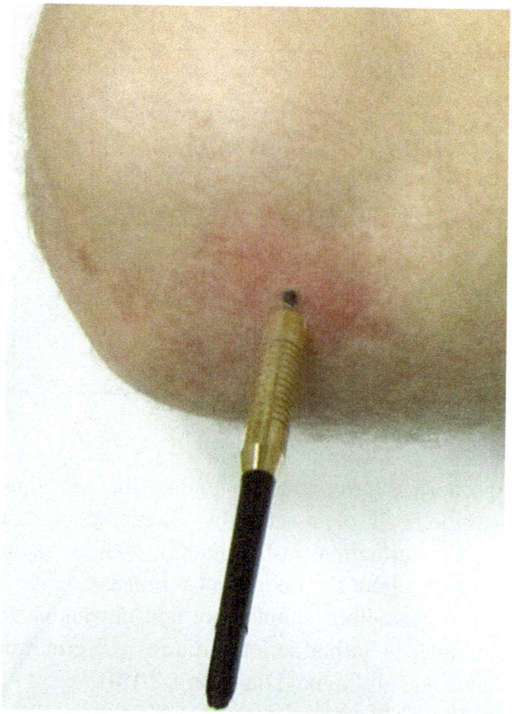

Fig. 2.19 A puncture wound from playing darts (James Heilman 2010 from Wikimedia Commons 2011: Knee puncture.JPG)

took place. The stumbling may have been caused, for example, by the unstable walking of the child (developmental level), just being wild during play, being pushed by another child during play or during a fight, or intentionally or unintentionally being pushed by an adult. The resulting injury may look the same, because it is caused by an impact trauma (cause of injury), despite the different circumstances (manner of injury).

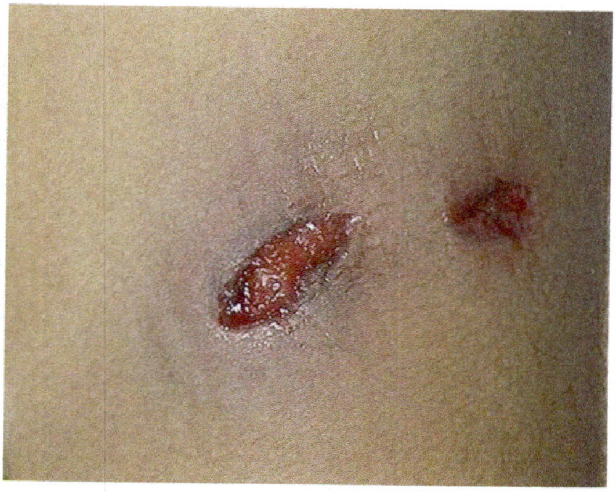

Fig. 2.20 Gunshot wound to the left thigh showing entry and exit wounds in 3-year-old girl (Bobjgalindo 2010 from Wikimedia Commons 2011: Gunshot wound to leg.jpg)

As stated before, the manner of injury describes the circumstances under which the injury was sustained or the injury event happened (NCECI 2007). The manner of injury can be divided in three types of circumstances. Terms used in the medical literature to describe the manner of (pediatric) physical trauma are:

- Accidental (often used synonyms: non-inflicted, non-intentional or unintentional, non-abusive)
- Non-accidental (often used synonyms: non-accidental, inflicted, intentional, deliberate, abusive/negligent)
- Unexplained (undetermined)

Using the term "accidental" is factually misleading. It implies that the events leading to the injury were inevitable and could not be avoided. In case of minors, especially younger children, most accidents (perhaps even almost all) are, at least in retrospect, preventable and sometimes even predictable (WHO 2006). Non-inflicted is a misleading term just like accidental: the use of this term implies that the injury was not inflicted and that nobody was involved in causing the injury, although, for example, in a motor vehicle accident, the driver is involved in causing the injury. "Non-intentional or unintentional" are more neutral terms: the injury event happened but there was no intention for it to happen, despite the fact that the incident could have been

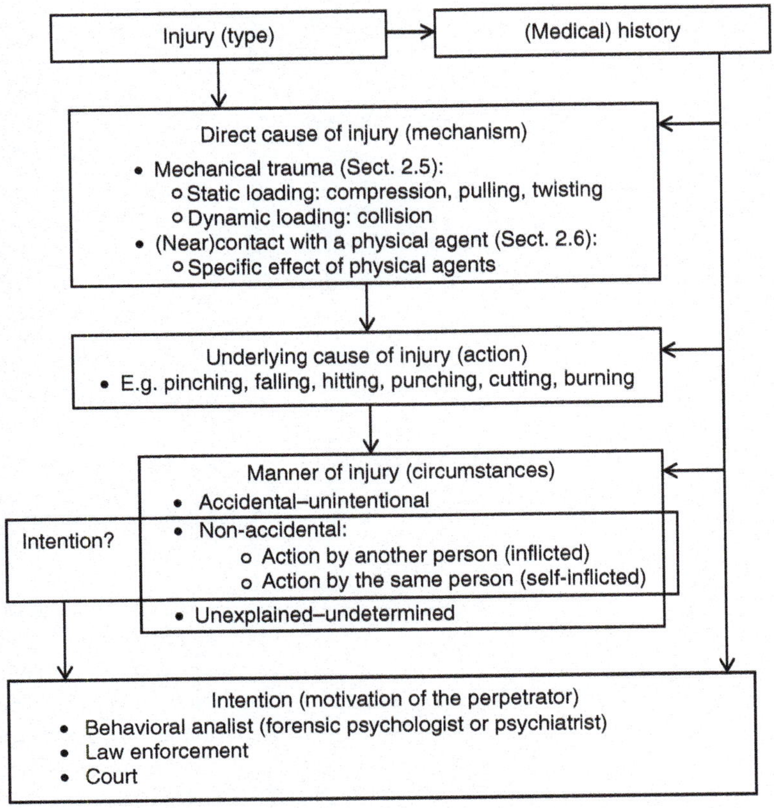

Scheme 2.1 Evaluation of suspicious injuries: the relation between injury and medical history, cause of injury, manner of injury, and the motivation of the perpetrator

prevented if the necessary precautions had been taken. Nevertheless, in this book, the terms "accidental" and "unintentional or unintended" will be used for injuries which are the result of an unintended non-abusive incident, despite all shortcomings of these terms.

Using the term "intentional" as synonymous for "non-accidental," "inflicted," or "abusive" in the medical evaluation of injuries is also misleading. It would mean that the motivation of the perpetrator (intentional: willingly, consciously, deliberately) to inflict an injury can be determined by using characteristics of the injury. This is almost never possible purely on the findings during the physical examination, except probably for pinch marks (Chap. 3), bitemarks (Chap. 8), or multiple stab wounds. In a physical assault, the action that led to an injury is almost always the result of a conscious decision and therefore intended, but it is almost never the intention of the perpetrator to inflict (serious) injuries. "Inflicted" is a more appropriate term, because it states that the injury was the result of an action by a human being (and perhaps an animal in bitemarks), without saying anything about the intention (to inflict = to give or impose something unpleasant and unwanted, for example, to inflict serious injuries – Kernerman English Multilingual Dictionary, 2010).

The evaluation of injuries is a (forensic) medical task, in which injury characteristics and the patient's or parent's (medical) history can be used to a certain extent to differentiate between inflicted, accidental, and unexplained injuries (Scheme 2.1). In each step, a carefully taken and comprehensive (medical) history may add information, which may enable differentiation.

The evaluation of the motivation (the intention) of the perpetrator is not a (forensic) medical task but is the task of the behavioral analyst (forensic psychologist or psychiatrist) or law enforcement. In this book, the terms "non-accidental" or "inflicted" will be used for the circumstances in which injuries resulted from an abusive incident (an injury event resulting from violent behavior of an adult toward a child).

The clinical assessment of the circumstances is based on a careful evaluation of the context, including:

- Data about the age and developmental level of the child
- Explanations given by the child (if possible), the parent(s), and others (people involved in the case, regardless of their background: professionally involved or not)
- Other (historical) physical signs and symptoms (e.g., stress-related physical signs or older bruises and/or other soft tissue injuries, fractures, head injury, and abdominal injury)
- Additional findings during physical examination/forensic medical examination
- Findings during laboratory examination: blood tests (e.g., blood clotting)
- Findings during imaging: skeletal survey, CT/MRI brain, abdomen, total body
- Assessment by social work/child protection service. Inquiry by the police
- Data from the clinical and forensic pediatric literature about the differential diagnosis of physical findings and the possibility and probability of injuries in certain circumstances
- In case of suspicions of fatal abuse, findings during a forensic autopsy

Even if all these data are used, it is not always possible to conclude whether the injury resulted from an abusive act or negligent behavior. For example, a young child (age 3) becomes a victim of a house fire (and dies). Cause of (injuries and) death: carbon monoxide intoxication and/or burn injuries. The house fire was not supposed to happen; the injuries (and death) were the result of the fire:

- The fire resulted from, for example, a malfunctioning electrical device and the parents tried everything to save the child: the manner of the injuries, resulting in death will be categorized as accidental and unintended.
- The child was left alone in house without any supervision, and the injuries, resulting in death, could have been prevented if the child had been taken care of in a proper way: the manner of death will be negligent and non-accidental.
- The fire was started deliberately. The manner of death will be manslaughter, if the death of the child was not intended to happen, or homicide, if the death of the child was intended to happen.

However, sometimes, medical findings will remain unexplained (by history) even after comprehensive investigations, including a clinical examination or forensic autopsy.

2.5 Mechanical Trauma

Mechanical trauma (Figs. 2.21 and 2.22) can lead to injuries caused by either static or dynamic loading. Skin injuries occur when the loading during the contact exceeds the capacity of the skin (and/or the underlying tissues) to absorb the transferred energy. Burton (2007) exemplifies

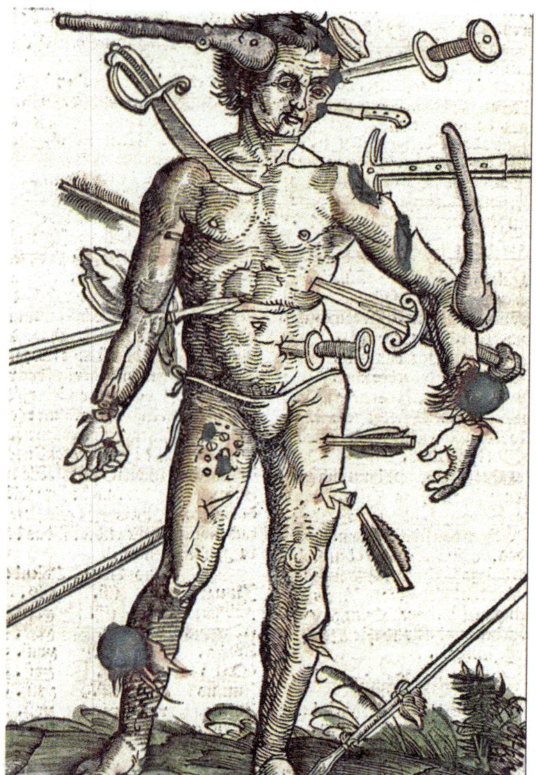

Fig. 2.21 Blunt- and sharp-force trauma: der verwundete Mann (the wound man) (Hans Gersdorff, Feldtbuch der Wundartzney 1517)

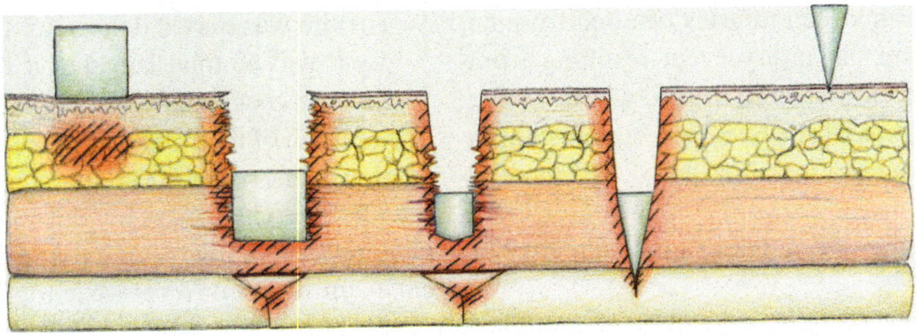

Fig. 2.22 Blunt- and sharp-force trauma (from *left* to *right*): (1) Superficial blunt force – bruising. (2) Blunt penetrating trauma – damage to subcutaneous tissue (e.g., bones). (3) Blunt penetrating trauma – damage to subcutaneous tissue (e.g., bones). (4) Sharp penetrating trauma – damage to subcutaneous tissue (e.g., bones). (5) Superficial sharp-force trauma – superficial incision or abrasion with or without damage to the underlying dermis and subdermis

Table 2.4 Injuries resulting from mechanical trauma (static or dynamic loading)

Blunt-force trauma	Erythema (Sect. 7.2) Bruising (Sect. 3.2) Abrasion (Sect. 7.3) Laceration (Sect. 7.4) Avulsion (Sect. 7.4) Blunt penetrating trauma (Sect. 7.4.5)
Sharp-force trauma	Incision/incised wound Puncture wound/stab wound/ penetrating injury Gunshot wound/missile wound/ velocity wound

the difference between static and dynamic loading: "Consider the effect of a stationary bullet resting on your chest, compared to the effect of a moving bullet striking your chest. The stationary bullet exerts a static load on your chest. A moving bullet exerts a dynamic load" (Burton 2007).

An overview of injuries resulting from mechanical trauma is given in Table 2.4.

2.5.1 Static Loading and Injuries

In mechanics, a static load is defined as a nonvarying load, for example, a nonvarying force exerted on a surface by the weight of a mass at rest. In everyday language, the mass of an object equals the weight of the object. In mechanics, however, mass and weight are defined differently (NYU 2003; Wikipedia 2011):

- Mass is a measurement of the amount of matter in an object by using a balance comparing a known amount of matter to an unknown amount of matter (unit of mass: kilograms or pounds).
- Weight is the measurement of the force experienced by an object due to gravity or the force exerted on a surface by the object. Weight is measured on a scale (unit of force: Newton). Weight is calculated as followed: Force (weight) = mass × (gravitational) acceleration (F = ma or W = mg). In other words, an object with a mass of 1.0 kg will weigh 9.8 N.
- The mass of an object does not change when an object's location changes. Weight, on the other hand, does change with location, if the gravity changes.

In static loading, an object does not change direction, level of exerted force (except when the gravity changes), and position during the time of exposure of the surface. In other words, there is neither a change in loading nor a gradual buildup of loading, and the transferred energy stays the same during the contact. For that reason, a static load in mechanics is also known as a dead load.

In the biomechanics of skin injuries, static load and static loading are used slightly different than in mechanics in general. The type, severity, dimensions, and appearance of skin injuries (and injuries of the underlying tissues), caused by static loading, are not only determined by mass, weight, gravity, or force but also by:

- The surface of the compressing object (flat, curved, patterned, blunt, sharp, more or less flexible) and of the compressed skin (flat,

curved, underlying tissues – connective tissue, fat, bone)
- The size of the contact surface between the compressing object and of the compressed skin
- The source that determines the mass of the object (gravity, human behavior, accidental wedging)
- The force exerted on the skin (the level of loading). Gradual or repetitive buildup of loading or changes in loading of the skin during the time of exposure may happen, because the force that is exerted is not only determined by gravity but also by the amount of changes in pressure actively exerted on the skin, for example, if a person is grabbed by another person, or if a person is overrun by a very slow driving car, or by movements of the person who is subjected to the load and actively resist the loading or passively changes position. This will lead to changes in the energy that is transferred from the compressing object to skin during the time of exposure (contact time) and will influence the final effect of the static load on the skin.

In physical assaults, static loading mostly will be caused by blunt-force trauma due to compression, but loading of the skin may also be caused by pulling or twisting the skin. Static loading may happen in sharp-force trauma, when a sharp-pointed object (e.g., a needle) is first held and then pressed against the skin (often leading to a penetrating trauma).

If static loading in blunt-force trauma leads to injuries of the skin and underlying tissues, including the vessels (subcutaneous veins or capillaries), the injuries are the result of direct damage by the distorting force (compressing, pulling, twisting) at the site of the distortion. The integrity of the skin (and/or the underlying tissues) may or may not be compromised during static loading.

Static loading varies from low- to high-pressure loading. The amount of pressure loading is mainly determined by the ratio between the exerted force and the surface exposed to the loading (the distribution of force per square centimeter). The difference between low- and high-pressure static loading can be exemplified as the difference between a stationary object of a certain weight passively resting on an extended surface of the skin (e.g., the back) (distribution of the exerted force over a larger area) and a stationary object with the same weight and a small surface being pressed against a small surface of the skin (concentration of the exerted force on a smaller area).

The risk of injuries to the skin and the underlying tissues, for example, bones or visceral organs, will be much higher in high-pressure loading than in low-pressure loading.

In case of low-pressure static loading, for example, in normal daily activities like holding the child, the loading caused by the holding of the child will not result in bruising or other skin injuries. However, this accounts only if there are no complicating factors added to the low-pressure loading, which decrease the capacity of the skin and the underlying tissues to absorb the transferred energy, for example, a coagulation disorder, other medical conditions, like vascular disorders or disorders of the connective tissue, or the use of medication, for example, corticosteroids and anticoagulants. Also prolonged exposure to low-pressure loading as sometimes can be seen in tight clothing may lead to superficial skin injuries, like bruises (if only compression takes places) and superficial abrasions (if there is some degree or friction between the tight clothing and the skin).

In case of high-pressure static loading, as can be seen in accidents (e.g., resulting from prolonged wedging in motor vehicle accidents) or in child abuse (e.g., in pinching, grabbing, or tying) (Sect. 3.2.5), it may result in more extensive bruising or other injuries of the skin or underlying tissues.

2.5.2 Dynamic Loading and Injuries

2.5.2.1 Defining Dynamic Loading

Dynamic (or rapid) loading can be divided in dynamic impulse and dynamic impact loading. Dynamic impulse loading is the result of rapid (often repetitive) movements without (external) impact (inertia effect), as can be seen in, for example, abusive head trauma due to shaking or some abdominal injuries. Dynamic impulse loading has never been described as the cause of skin injuries in child abuse. If dynamic loading leads to skin injuries, these are always caused by dynamic impact loading: the application of an external force with a certain mass and velocity during a relatively short period of contact between the object and the skin/body.

An injury caused by dynamic loading is also referred to as a kinetic injury. A kinetic injury in impact loading is an injury caused by the exchange of energy during motion, leading to a transfer of energy during collision as long as the contact continues between the human body and the colliding object, for example, an object or (parts of) another human body (mechanical trauma). Kinetic energy is the energy contained in a moving object or body.

2.5.2.2 The Occurrence of Injuries in Dynamic Impact Loading

During a collision, the energy of a moving body/object (bodies/objects) is transferred. Whether an injury does occur in dynamic impact loading is mainly determined by the amount of kinetic energy, which is transferred during the collision plus the total contact area during the collision. The amount of the transferred kinetic energy (KE) can be calculated and is determined by the mass and velocity of the moving body/object: $KE = (mass \times velocity^2)/2$. The formula shows that velocity is a more important determinant of the amount of kinetic energy than mass. If the velocity doubles, the kinetic energy quadruples. If the mass doubles, the kinetic energy doubles.

Depending on the difference in velocity between the colliding body and object, the effects of dynamic impact loading can be divided in low- and high-velocity impact loading or low- and high-velocity impact trauma. Although the defining of an injury, caused by blunt-force trauma, as a low- or high-velocity injury does suggest a clear dividing line between high- and low-velocity impact trauma, this is not true. There is a continuum in the effects of the impact velocity, in which injuries show more or less typical characteristics that fit to a high-velocity or a low-velocity impact trauma. The difference between low- and high-velocity loading is best illustrated by comparing the effects of a bullet thrown at a person and hitting the person (low-velocity dynamic impact loading – not penetrating or even bouncing back) to the effects of a bullet fired at a person and hitting the person (high-velocity dynamic impact loading – penetrating). The risk of injuries to the skin and the underlying tissues, for example, bones or visceral organs, will be much lower when the bullet is thrown at the person than when the bullet is fired at the person, because during the collision with the fired bullet, much more kinetic energy is transferred than during the collision with the thrown bullet.

In case of low-velocity impact loading, for example, in normal daily activities, during play or sports or in short-distance falls, injuries may occur but will be less serious or extensive (because of the lower amount of transfer of kinetic energy) than in high-velocity impact loading. The loading in low-velocity impact does not exceed the capacity of the skin to absorb the energy as much as it does in high-velocity impact. However, this accounts only if there are no complicating factors added to the low-velocity loading that decrease the capacity of the skin and underlying tissues to absorb the transferred energy. These factors are the same as in static loading: medical conditions or the use of medication. More complicated injuries may also occur in short-distance falls, in which the child falls on an object (Wheeler and Shope 1997).

High-velocity impact loading may happen in accidents (e.g., resulting from pedestrian versus motor vehicle accidents or long-distance falls) or in child abuse (e.g., in hitting or kicking) (Sect. 3.2.5). The high-velocity loading of the skin during the collision may result in more extensive bruising or other more serious skin injuries than in low-velocity impact loading.

2.5.2.3 The Type of Injuries in Dynamic Impact Loading

What type of injury does occur depends not only on mass and velocity during collision but also on the specific characteristics of the collision, the impacting and the impacted object/body:

- Type of mechanical trauma
- Type of collision
- Angle of collision
- The amount of the absorbed and returned (=transferred) kinetic energy
- The type of object used as "weapon" and the impact site on the body
- The structures underneath the skin

2.5.2.4 Type of Mechanical Trauma

Dynamic impact loading of the skin is mainly caused by two types of mechanical trauma, namely, blunt-force trauma and sharp-force trauma. During blunt-force trauma, the energy, which is transferred during the collision between a blunt object and the body, is distributed over a relatively large body area. For that reason, the integrity of the surface of the skin will not be broken in most cases of blunt-force trauma, even if underlying structures, like vessels, are damaged. This damage will result in bruising.

In sharp-force trauma, the kinetic energy of the colliding object, for example, a more or less sharp object like a knife (sharp penetrating trauma) or a bullet (gunshot wounds), is concentrated on a small body area. This will lead to piercing of the skin and underlying structures, which can result in complete perforation of a body part, for example, an extremity, or the whole body.

Blast injuries are also the result of dynamic loading caused by extreme differences in pressure (the transfer of kinetic energy, resulting from the impact caused by a shock wave). This type of trauma is rare in childhood, except, for example, in case of war or terrorism. It has never been described in suspected child abuse and will therefore not be discussed in this book.

2.5.2.5 The Type of Collision

In dynamic impact loading, there are three possible types of collision:

- An object impacting a static body
- The body impacting a static object
- The body and the object both moving during the impact

During the collision, the energy of a moving body/object (bodies/objects) is transferred (see before). If the colliding objects are both moving in the same direction, the transferred energy equals the KE of the fastest moving objects minus the KE of the slowest moving object (front to back collision). If both objects continue to move in the same direction after the collision, less energy will be transferred than in a situation in which the colliding object stops moving after the colliding and the object that was hit "shoots away."

If the objects are moving in an opposite direction, the kinetic energy of both moving objects will be combined (front to front collision, in which both objects/bodies may stop moving after the collision), leading to deformation of one object or both objects (= injury).

In general, collision while moving in the same direction will result in less serious injuries than collision while moving in opposite directions at the same speeds. In other words, the amount of transferred depends on the relative speed of objects compared to each other.

When a child is beaten and the child's momentum is away from the blow (moving in the same direction before or during the collision), the difference in velocity between the colliding object and the child is less than when the child remains stationary or is leaning into the blow (moving object against static body or moving in opposite directions). If the child's momentum is away, the duration of the contact (the moment of transfer of energy) between the object and the body is generally more protracted. This will lead to less severe injuries than when the child remains stationary or is leaning into the blow, in which more kinetic energy is transferred. However, if the child is falling away from the blow, this may lead to double impact, namely, first the impact of the object and second the impact against another object such as a table or a wall, in which case the overall severity of the injury increases.

2.5.2.6 The Angle of Collision

The angle between the object and the body during collision in blunt-force trauma will also influence the resulting type of injury. The angle of contact may vary from almost parallel to the skin surface (0°) to perpendicular (90°) in a collision between a moving and a static object.

The angle of contact during moving of the colliding objects/bodies may vary from almost zero to almost 180°: in other words, from an impact while moving in the same direction to a frontal collision while moving in the opposite direction and all impact angles in between. The angle may increase the type and degree of distortion of the skin (and underlying structures) and, because of the distortion, the chance of compromising the integrity of the skin, resulting in injuries varying from erythema and bruises in perpendicular loading without much distortion to abrasions, lacerations, and avulsions in tangential and distorting loading.

2.5.2.7 The Amount of Transferred Kinetic Energy

The degree of force used during the incident will determine the amount of energy that will be transferred upon contact with the skin. If the object used in, for example, beating, deforms or breaks upon impact, less energy will be exchanged between the object and the body and finally transferred on the body because part of the energy will be absorbed by the deformation or breaking of the object. Consequently, this will lead to a less severe and/or less extensive injury than when the object had remained intact.

2.5.2.8 The Type of Object Used as "Weapon" and the Impact Site on the Body

The severity of an injury decreases as the area of the contact surface increases. When a child is beaten with a flat object, for example, a shoe or slipper, the energy will spread over the entire surface of the impact area and as such will lead to less severe injuries than when a child is beaten with equal force but with a small object, for example, a cane.

If a child is beaten with a flat, rigid object, the damage caused by beating on a curved, relatively rigid body surface such as the head will be more serious than when the beating takes place on a flat, reasonably flexible surface such as the back. Because on the back the contact area between the object and the body is larger, the energy is spread over a wider surface. When the beating is on the head, the energy will spread in such a manner that it will lead to deformation of the skull and to fractures at the point of maximal deformation. This may be the site of impact, but depending on the deformation, it can also be found in other sites on the skull.

If the object is rounded, the chance of rupturing the skin is less than if the object has a more or less angular form.

2.5.2.9 The Structures Underneath the Skin

Usually there will be no damage to internal organs or bony structures in abusive blunt-force trauma to the skin. The damage will be inflicted predominantly to the venules and capillaries in the dermis and hypodermis, while the epidermis and the underlying organs stay undamaged. However, skin lesions such as bruises and abrasions may be the first indications of damage to the underlying structures, such as intra-abdominal organs or bones (Johnson 1990).

Bruising of the abdominal wall may indicate trauma to intra-abdominal organs. However, in physically abused children with intra-abdominal injuries, bruising is absent in a considerable percentage of the children. Barnes et al. (2005) reported the absence of abdominal wall bruising in about 25%, while others report absence of bruises in as much as 80% or more of the children with abdominal trauma (Ledbetter et al. 1988; Bowkett and Kolbe 1998; Gaines et al. 2004). Bruising of the abdominal wall is also not necessarily instantly visible at the location of the impact. Traumatically extravasated blood can migrate through the surrounding connective tissues and only become visible after a number of days at a different location than the impact area, for example, bruising caused by blunt-force trauma to the upper abdomen may be visible after a number of days as a hematoma in the groin (Herr and Fallat 2006).

There is also a widespread misconception that the force required to cause traumatic fractures (either intentional or non-intentional) will generally also cause bruising. Others believe that, according to the opposing premise, the absence of bruises would indicate that only minimal force was required to cause the bone to fracture and that the fracture should not be explained as a result of trauma but as the consequence of metabolic disease or osteogenesis imperfecta (Paterson 1987; Taitz 1991a, b). Mathew et al. (1998) and Starling et al. (2007) showed that bruising is seen in only a minority of fractures (<10–30%, excluding skull fractures) regardless of their etiology. According to Mathew et al. (1998), one cannot differentiate between abusive and non-abusive fractures based on the presence or absence of bruising. Cutaneous bruising is seen in less than 10% of the children with fractures immediately after the fracture occurred. When bruising arises, it becomes visible within 1 week in 30% of the cases (Mathew et al. 1998).

2.5.3 Telltale Injuries in Static or Dynamic Loading

Skin injuries, resulting from static or dynamic loading, may show a recognizable grouping or a specific shape. In that way, these injuries may suggest what happened (or what did not happen) and what caused the injury (or what did not cause the injury). These injuries are called telltale injuries, pattern injuries, shaped injuries, or mirror injuries. Telltale injuries may occur in accidental or non-accidental circumstances (Fig. 2.23). Recognition of a pattern injury without a clear history, however, may indicate that the injury was inflicted. Another example of a "telltale" in an injury in a young child is a pattern or shape and location of an injury that cannot be explained through play or normal interactions with other children or adults and therefore indicates that it was inflicted.

Through careful examination of a patterned injury, it is often possible to identify which object caused the injury, especially within the first 24 h. Sometimes, it will take longer to recognize the implement in question, for example, in bitemarks. For that reason, it is advised to photograph this kind of injury at regular time intervals, for example, every 6 h (see Chaps. 8 and 9).

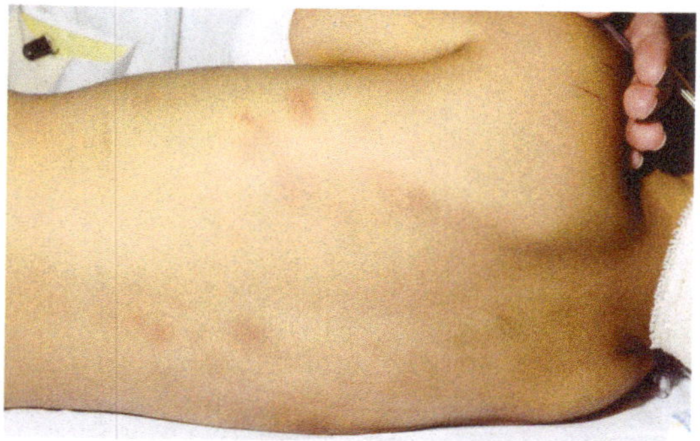

Fig. 2.23 Pattern injury in static (and dynamic impact) loading: extensive bruising on the trunk of an abused child (suggestive for gripping, punching, and prodding) (= Fig. 3.69)

2.5.3.1 Telltale Injuries in Static Loading

As stated before, in static loading, the skin and subcutaneous tissues, including the vessels (subcutaneous veins or capillaries), are damaged directly by the distorting (compressing, pulling, twisting) force at the site of the compression. This may lead, especially in high-pressure loading, to a recognizable pattern, caused by grouping of bruises (e.g., in fingertip bruising or in a grip mark) (Fig. 2.23) or recognizable compressive bruising, for example, in more complex "imprints" such as a car tire (accidental: pedestrian overrun by motor vehicle) or a shoe sole (accidental during a stampede; non-accidental when a perpetrator is standing on the victim).

2.5.3.2 Telltale Injuries in Dynamic Impact Loading

Skin injuries in dynamic loading result from impact with velocities, varying from low to high. High-velocity blunt-force trauma may lead to injuries with a pattern or imprint, especially if the impact is in a location with soft tissues and no bone underlying the skin (e.g., cheeks and thighs) and if the applied force is spread over a small area, for example, by using a small implement such as a stick or a cord. The object causing the

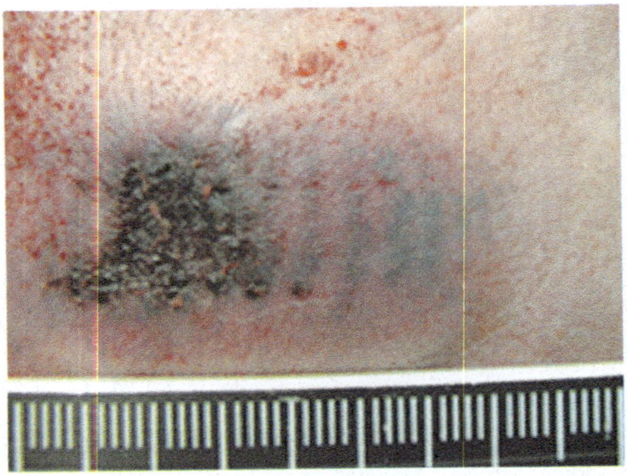

Fig. 2.24 Pattern injury in dynamic impact loading: repeating pattern in the injury – ca. 4 per 1 cm

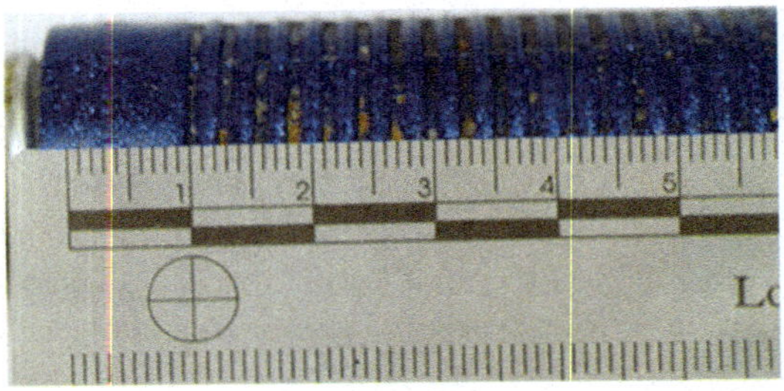

Fig. 2.25 The object, which probably caused the pattern in Fig. 2.24: repeating pattern in the object – ca. 4 per 1 cm – possible match

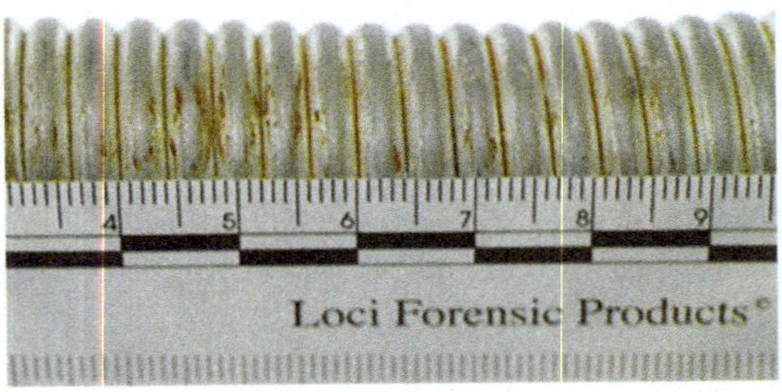

Fig. 2.26 An example of an object which resembles the object in Fig. 2.25: repeating pattern in the object – ca. 2.5 per 1 cm – no match

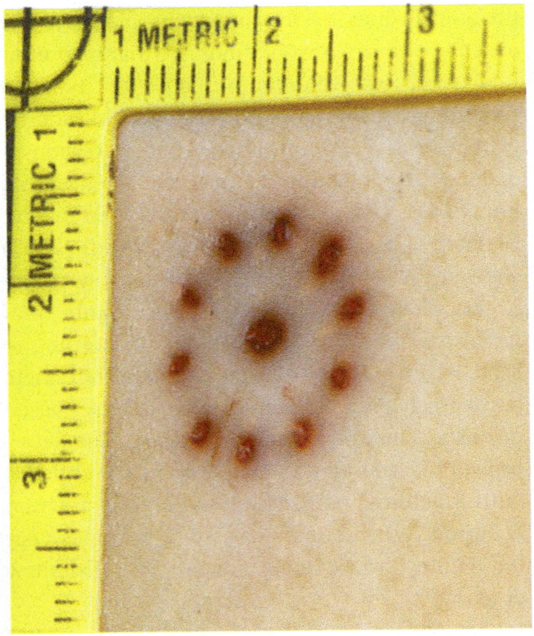

Fig. 2.27 Pattern injury, caused by a bone injection gun

injury, mostly bruising, is mirrored by the pattern: a silhouette or outline of the implement on the skin (Figs. 2.24, 2.25, 2.26, and 2.27). The kinetic energy transferred on impact is absorbed mostly by the skin at the periphery of the object. The impact caused by the blow with the object will distort and crush the skin and underlying tissues and rupture subcutaneous vessels (venules and capillaries) in contact with the edges of the object. According to Williams (2003), whip injuries (caused by a rope, belt, or electrical cord) show a recognizable pattern injury with a uniform depth which follows the body curvatures, reflecting the object used. These injuries may be deeper at their distal end or at the body curvatures, because of the higher distortion and crushing of the skin and underlying tissues at these sites, sometimes leading to an abrasion or even laceration at these sites. These injuries may result in hypopigmented scarring. In an infant or a young child, an injury with the characteristics of a high-velocity impacttrauma usually will be inflicted, although accidental circumstances cannot be excluded automatically.

It will be more difficult to recognize the pattern (or the object) if the high-velocity impact loading is spread over a broader area, for example, in slapping with an object, like a slipper, with flexible, broad, and flat surface.

Injuries caused by low-velocity impact loading usually do not show recognizable patterns or shapes. These injuries usually result from accidents during daily activities, like collisions during play or short-distance falls. If present, these skin injuries are usually located at places where the skin is more at risk of diffuse "crushing" between the impacting object and underlying bone (e.g., knees, shins, or elbows). The resulting injuries may resemble the more diffuse injuries caused by static loading.

2.6 (Near) Contact with Physical Agents and Injuries

The transfer of energy during a direct contact or near contact of the skin with a physical agent (thermal, chemical, electrical, electromagnetical, and ionizing trauma) may lead to a nonmechanical trauma. Most important injuries caused by a nonmechanical trauma are burns (Table 2.5). Burns are not only caused by exposure of skin to heat but also by the effect of chemical or physical agents (acidic and alkaline chemicals, electricity, microwaves, and radiation), which may have a similar effect on the skin and the subcutaneous tissues as heat, or may create heat at the moment of contact with the skin (Panke and McLeod 1985; Richardson 1994; Pounder 2000). Besides external burns, internal burns may arise due to electrocution or swallowing and inhalation of chemicals.

2.6.1 Thermal Trauma

In a thermal skin trauma, the damage to cells is caused by the direct transfer of thermal energy to the skin and/or the subcutaneous tissues, as a result of the exposure of tissue to high and low temperatures. The extent of the damage is determined both by the temperature and the duration of exposure. Thermal trauma may result from:

- Direct contact (transfer of energy by conduction) with a solid heat source (dry burns – Fig. 2.28), hot liquids, vapors, or gases (scalds or wet burns – Figs. 2.29 – 2.34), and open fires (cigarette burns, fire and flame burns – Figs. 2.35 – 2.40)
- Exposure of the skin and the subcutaneous tissues to the radiant heat of an object, for example, the close proximity to a radiant fire or electrical heater (Fig. 2.41)

Thermal trauma can also be caused by low or freezing temperatures (cold-related injuries) (Figs. 2.42 and 2.43).

Table 2.5 Injuries caused by nonmechanical trauma

Thermal injuries	Heat: burns and scalds Cold: chilblains and frostbite (Sect. 6.5)
Chemical injuries	Burns Allergic reactions (topical and generalized) Generalized poisoning manifestations
Electrical injuries	Burns High- and low-voltage injuries
Radiation injuries	Burns

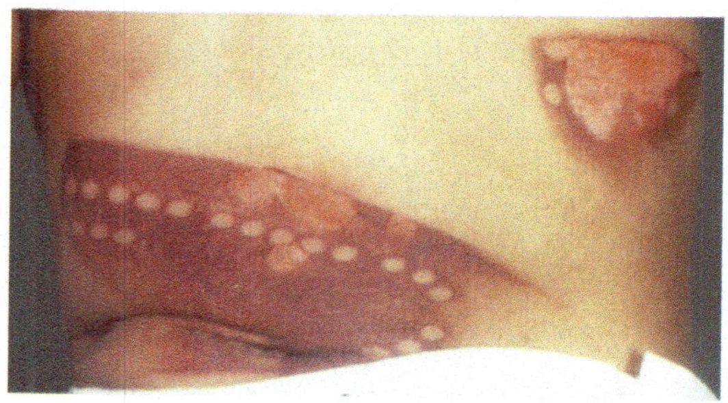

Fig. 2.28 Dry contact burn: steam iron (= Fig. 8.10)

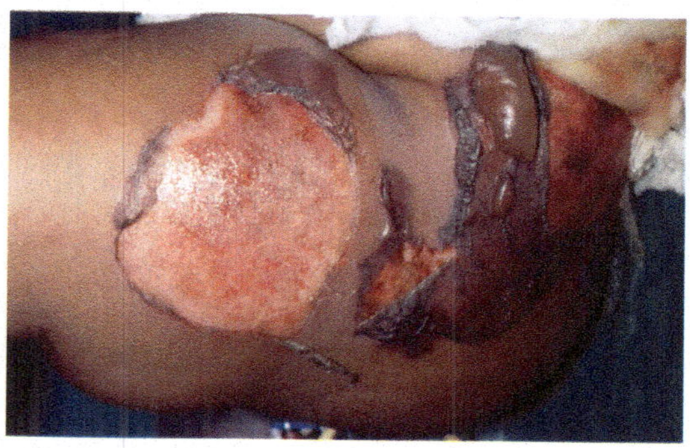

Fig. 2.29 Inflicted hot water burn

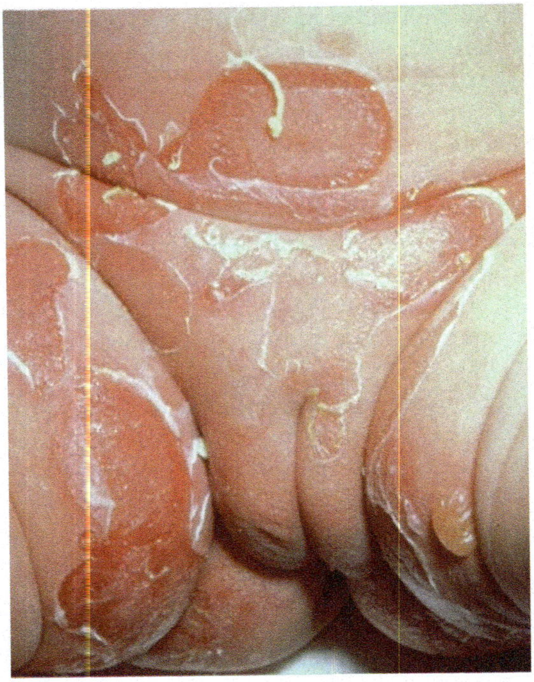

Fig. 2.30 Bullous impetigo in the differential diagnosis of hot water burns in the diaper area

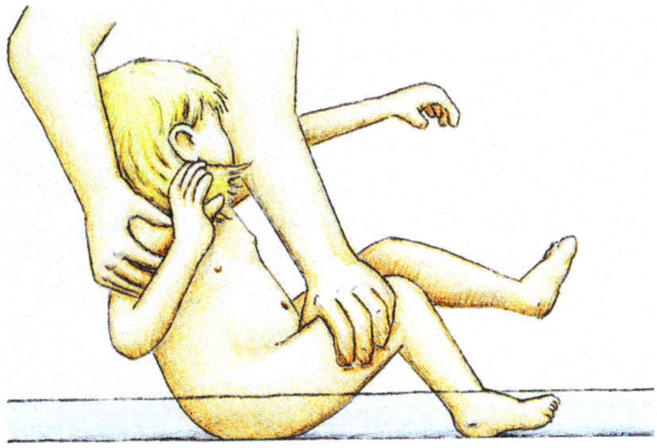

Fig. 2.31 Forced immersion in hot water (low level)

Friction burns do not occur because of heat transfer through direct contact or radiation but occur because of the development of high temperatures caused by the friction generated between the skin and a surface (generally with a normal temperature) over which the body moves (Fig. 2.44).

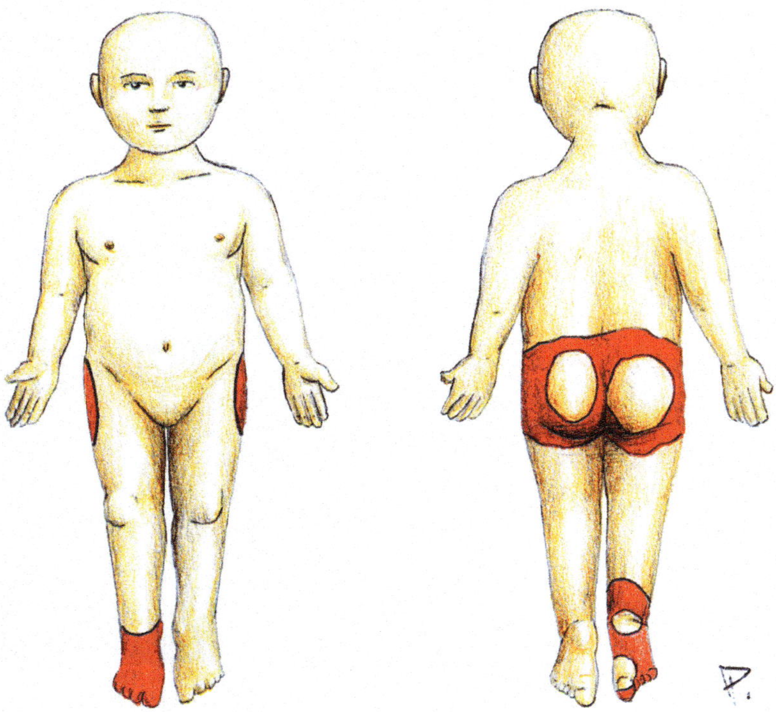

Fig. 2.32 Burn pattern due to immersion, as seen in Fig. 2.31: hole in the donut phenomenon on the buttocks

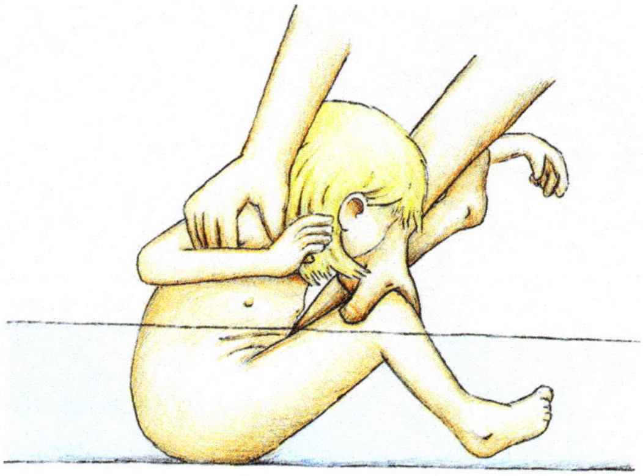

Fig. 2.33 Forced immersion in hot water (higher level)

2.6.2 Chemical Trauma

In chemical injuries, the damage to tissues is determined by many more variables than in thermal injuries, for example, the acidity and amount of the agent, the level to which the agent penetrates the skin, and the contact site and manner of contact. The harmful effect of the agent continues until the agent is neutralized by another chemical agent or is inactivated as a result of tissue reaction (Pounder 2000) (Figs. 2.45 – 2.50).

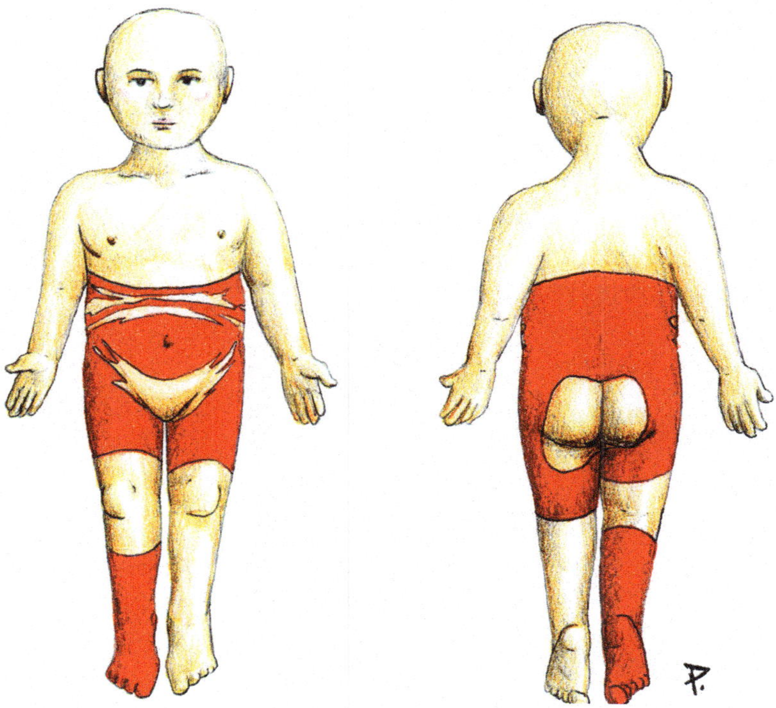

Fig. 2.34 Burn pattern due to immersion, as seen in Fig. 2.33: hole in the donut phenomenon on the buttocks and zebra distribution on the abdomen

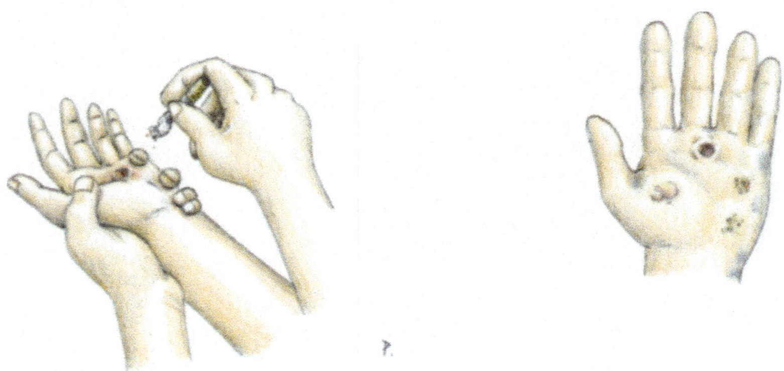

Fig. 2.35 Thermal trauma: cigarette burns

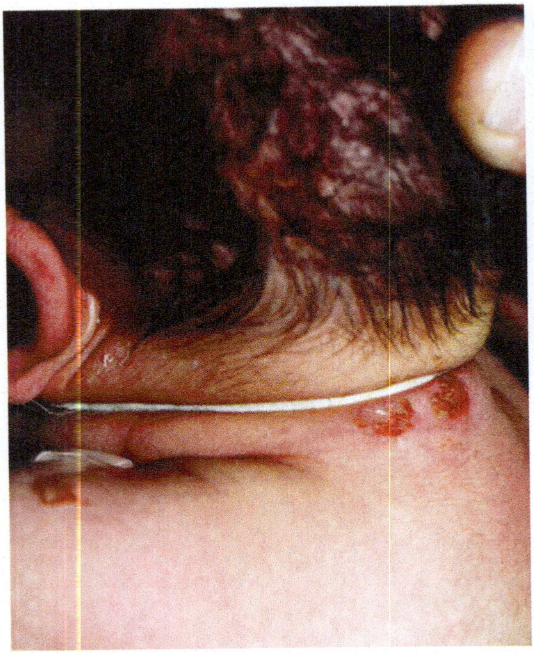

Fig. 2.36 Thermal trauma: cigarette burns

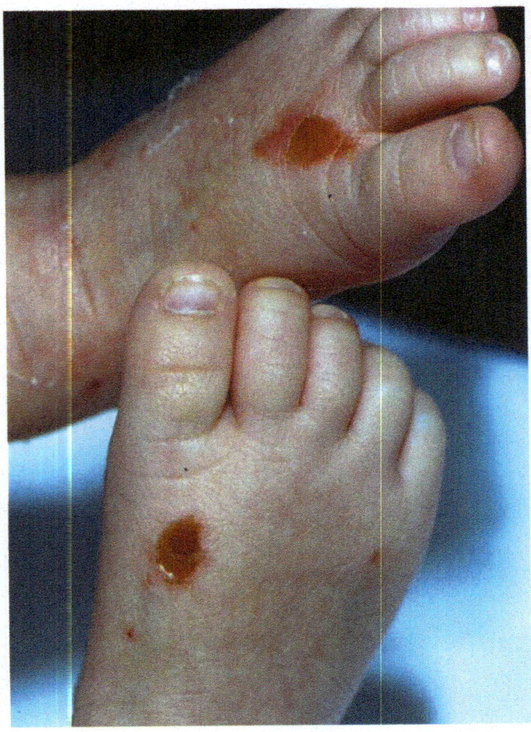

Fig. 2.37 Same child as in Fig. 2.36: superficial cigarette burns

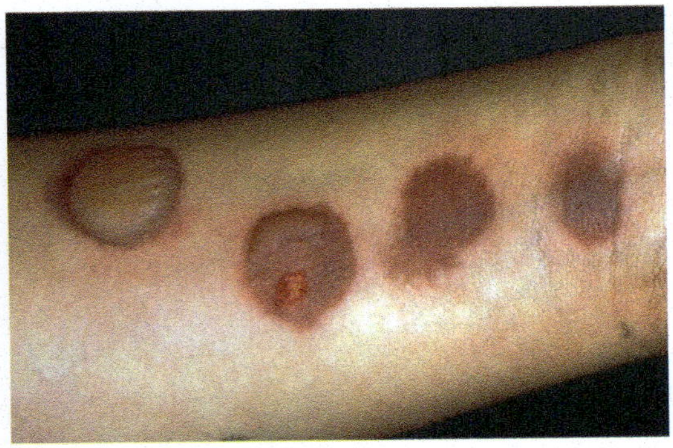

Fig. 2.38 Thermal trauma: cigarette burns, due to self-mutilation (= Fig. 1.1)

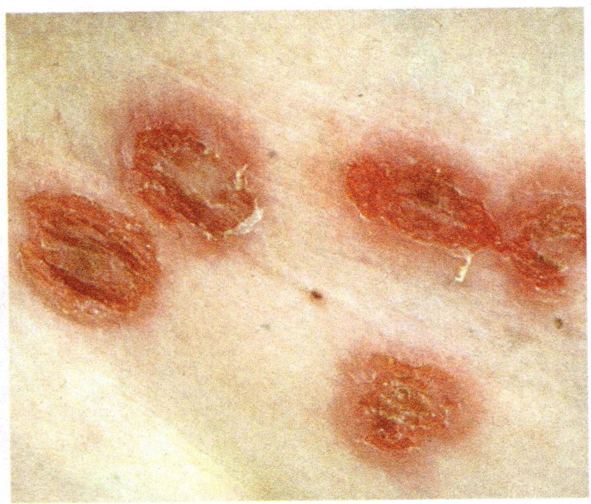

Fig. 2.39 Impetigo in the differential diagnosis of cigarette burns

2.6.3 Electrical Trauma

Electrical injuries are caused by a combination of heat (leading to burns) and a direct effect of electricity (electrical forces) on polarized molecules in the skin, the subcutaneous tissues, and the organs. The extent of the damage generally depends on the amount of heat that is generated during the incident. According to Koumbourlis (2002) and Hettiaratchy and Dziewulski (2004), voltage is a more important

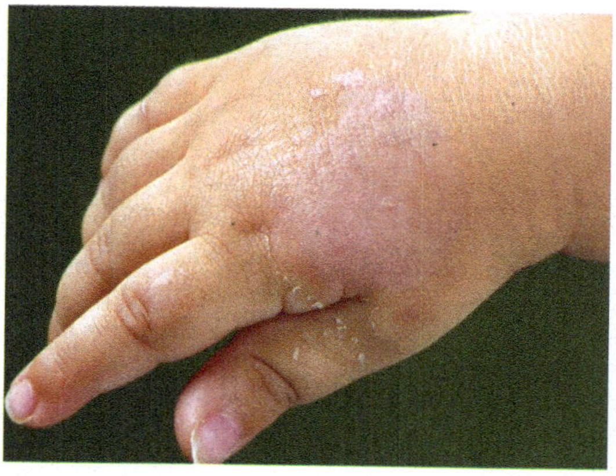

Fig. 2.40 Depigmentation as a result of an inflicted burn

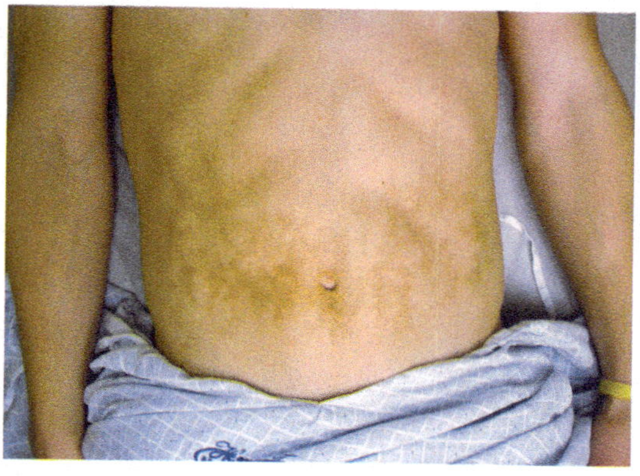

Fig. 2.41 Erythema ab igne on trunk (= Fig. 6.23)

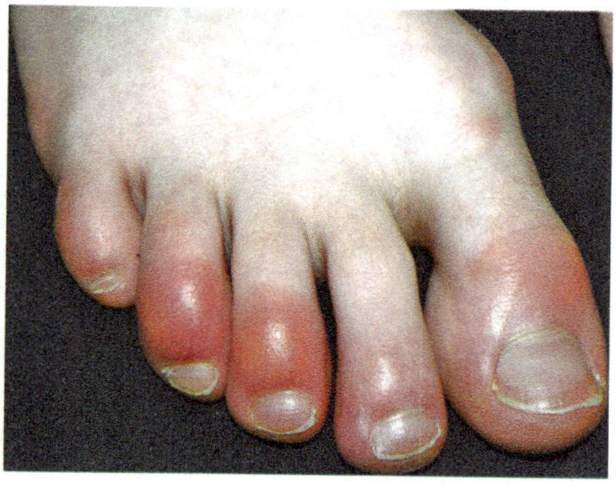

Fig. 2.42 Chilblains (Sapp 2007 from Wikimedia Commons 2011: Wintertenen.jpg)

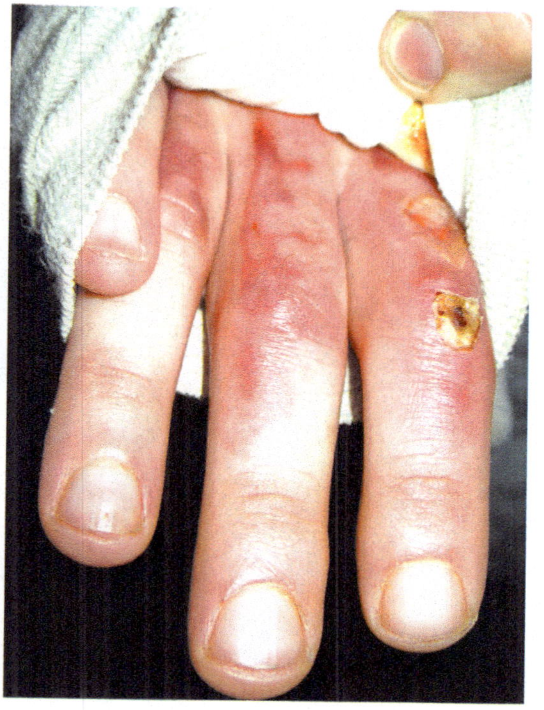

Fig. 2.43 Frostbite (Eli Duke 2010 from Wikimedia Commons 2011: Injuries at Antarctica – ouch!.jpg)

determinant in tissue damage than current. The pathway that the electrical current follows through the victim's body and the duration of the contact with the source of the current also play a role.

2.6.4 Other Nonmechanical Traumata

Radiation injuries are usually caused by the transfer of ionizing energy, for example, during the exposure to the ultraviolet (UV) spectrum in sunlight, resulting in sunburn. Sunlight, however, also may damage the skin by radiant heat (infrared). Radiation injuries may also occur from radiant energy from X-rays or radiation therapy for cancer treatment. Most victims with radiation injuries were seen in 1945 and the following years after the atomic bombs were dropped in Japan (Figs. 2.51 and 2.52).

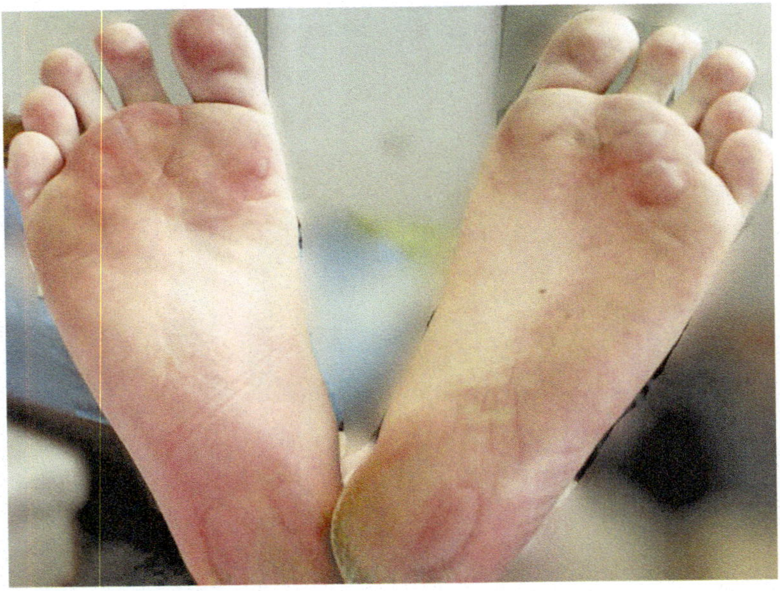

Fig. 2.44 Friction blisters (AndryFrench 2009: Friction Blisters On Human Foot.jpg)

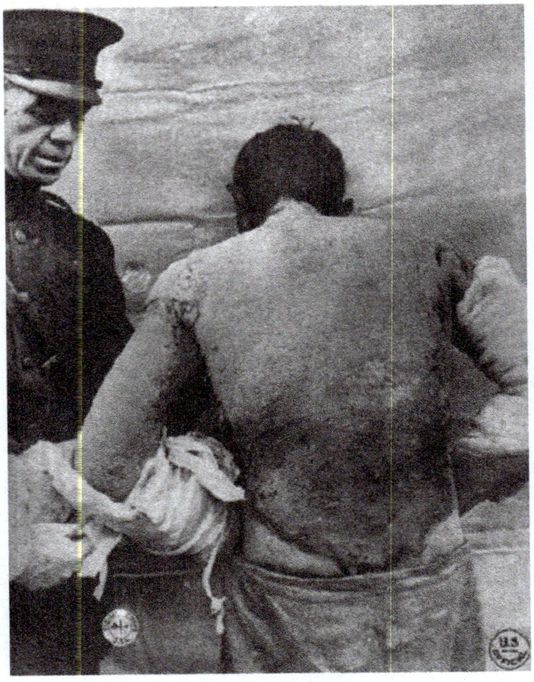

Fig. 2.45 Chemical burns caused by mustard gas (US photographer 1918 from Wikimedia Commons 2011: MustardGasChemicalBurns.jpg)

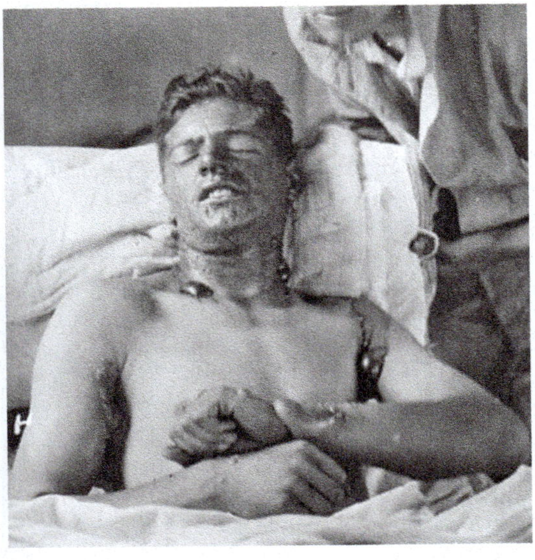

Fig. 2.46 Chemical burns caused by mustard gas (1916–1918 from Wikimedia Commons 2011: Mustard gas burns.jpg)

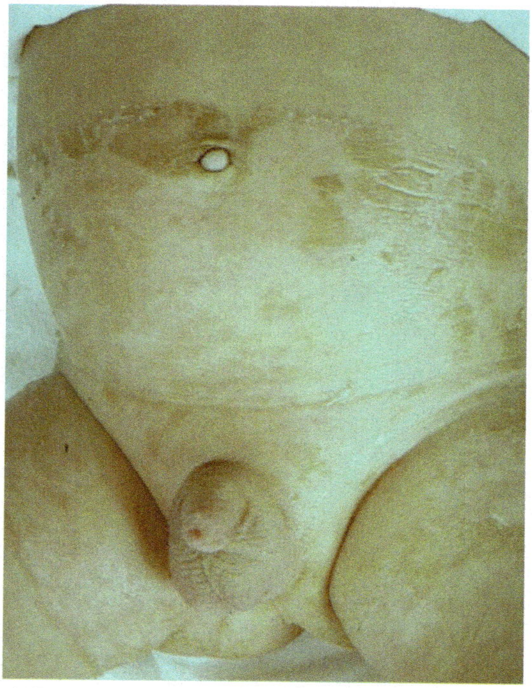

Fig. 2.47 Chemical trauma: bleaching agent

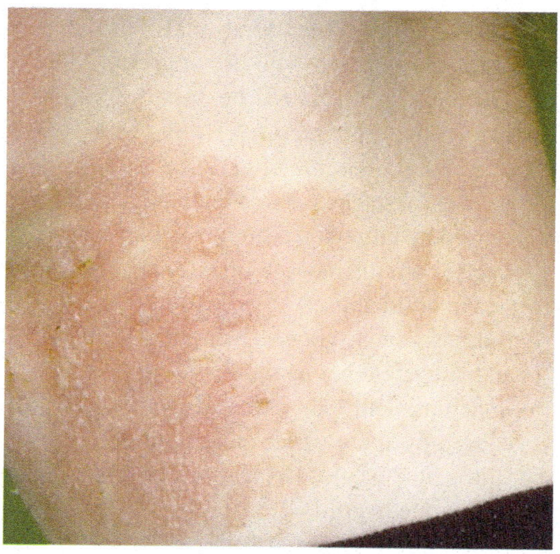

Fig. 2.48 Chemical trauma, due to self-mutilation – unknown substance

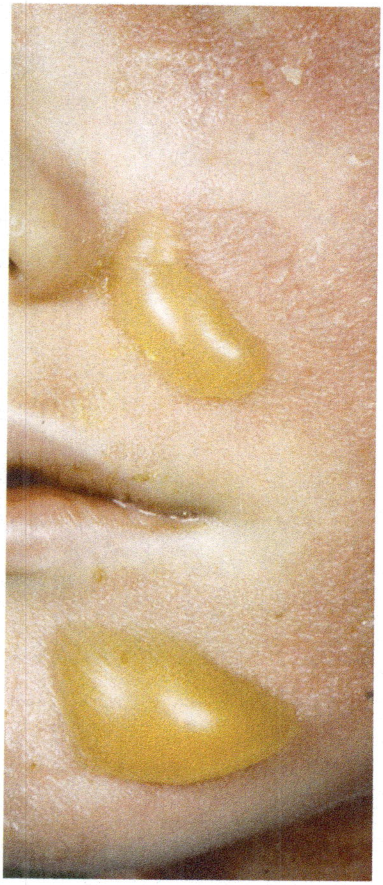

Fig. 2.49 Same patient as in Fig. 2.48: chemical trauma, due to self-mutilation – unknown substance

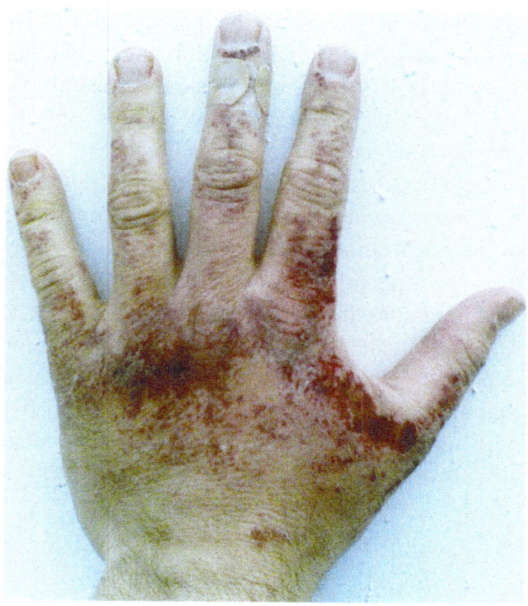

Fig. 2.50 Chemical burn, caused by exposure to a less than 10% sodium hydroxide solution (lye), 44 h after exposure (Blazius 2009 from Wikimedia Commons 2011: Sodium hydroxide solution burn.png)

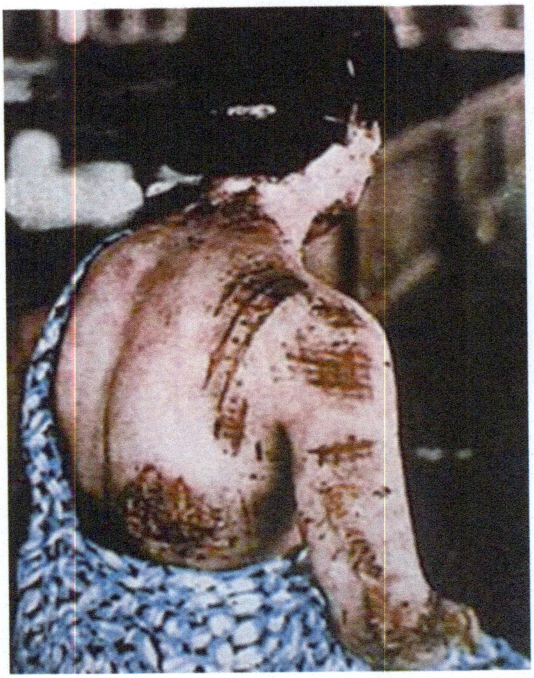

Fig. 2.51 Radiation burns: victim of atomic bomb, Hiroshima, 1945

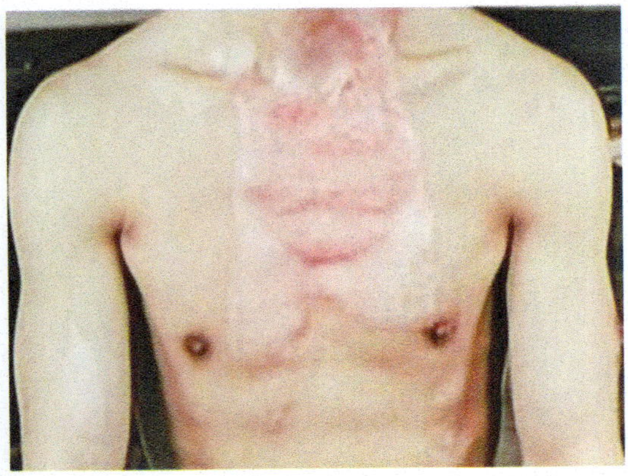

Fig. 2.52 Radiation injury: victim of atomic bomb, Hiroshima, 1945

2.7 Why and How: Physical Injuries in Child Abuse

2.7.1 Abusive Injuries

As stated in Chap. 1, the presence of injuries is not essential in establishing whether a child is a victim of physical abuse/physically aggressive behavior by parents or others. Trocmé et al. (2003) evaluated the data of 3,780 cases in which child maltreatment was substantiated and found that some type of physical injury was documented in 18%, mostly superficial injuries such as bruises, cuts, and abrasions. Trocmé concluded that the rates of physical injuries were lower than they expected. Nevertheless, other authors stated that at any given moment injuries can probably be found in up to 90% of victims of physical assault (Stephenson 1995; Nobuyasu 2001). Maguire et al. (2005) did a comprehensive review of the medical literature on bruising in childhood related to suspicions of child abuse and found prevalence figures for child abuse-related bruising in 28% of abused school age children up to 98% in infants with suspected abuse. Maguire concluded that "bruising is common in children who are abused." Most of the inflicted injuries will be superficial, externally visible, and include (Hobbs et al. 1999; Coulter 2000; Trocmé et al. 2003):

- Bruises, scratches, abrasions, and lacerations, caused by blunt-force trauma (Chaps. 3 and 7). Bruises are the most frequently observed injuries in child abuse.
- Baldness due to abusive hair pulling (Fig. 2.53) and subgaleal hematoma.
- Incisions and stab wounds, shot wounds, caused by sharp penetrating trauma.
- Burns and scalds from various causes and injury due to cold.

Other more severe inflicted injuries involve skeleton, central nervous system, and internal organs. These can be demonstrated by the use of supplementary investigations including:

- Imaging techniques (e.g., fractures, intracranial hemorrhages/injuries to the central nervous system, eye, intra-abdominal injuries)

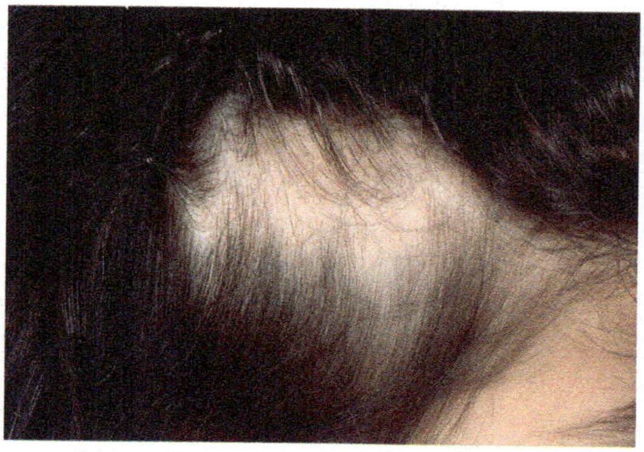

Fig. 2.53 Trichotillomania as differential diagnosis of (abusive hair pulling)

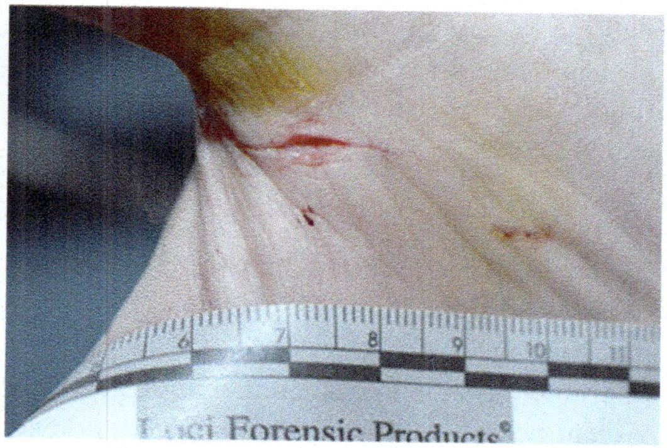

Fig. 2.54 Incised wound: self-defense injury on the palm between the thumb and index finger

- Laboratory investigation (e.g., intra-abdominal injuries)
- Fundoscopy (e.g., retinal hemorrhages, retinoschisis)
- Forensic light sources (e.g., old and new superficial and deeper subcutaneous injuries)

The severity of inflicted injuries varies from superficial injuries which cause pain and psychological harm to life threatening or fatal outcome. Trocmé et al. (2003) found that in only 4% of 3,780 substantiated cases of child abuse and neglect, the injuries were severe enough to require medical attention. McCurdy (1993) found that in 3.2% of children, the injuries were so serious that medical treatment or admission to hospital was required.

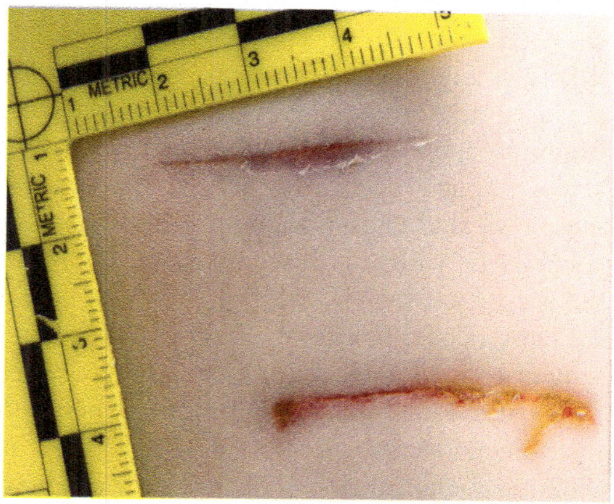

Fig. 2.55 Abrasion and superficial incised wound: self-defense injuries on the forearm

2.7.2 Self-Defense Injuries

Injuries and wounds resulting from self-defense against violence constitute a subcategory of non-accidental injuries (Figs. 2.54 and 2.55). This type of injuries is comparable in nature with those mentioned earlier but is sustained in a different manner. They are the result of an attempt by the child/person to defend himself/herself (often instinctively) in which he/she assumed a protective posture so as to sustain minimal damage during the assault or to reduce the risk for severe injury. Consequently, the injury may initially not show any recognizable form or pattern. In such cases, it may be useful to have the child show the posture he/she had possibly assumed during the assault. Generally, this concerns a protective posture, for example, a raised arm in front of the face or assuming a fetal position. The form or pattern will be clear when the child assumes this position once again. In principle, the injuries that may be sustained through self-defense can be all types of injury: bruises, abrasions, lacerations, incisions, stab and shot wounds, burns, and fractures.

2.7.3 Injuries Caused by Instrumental Violence

Instrumental violence is another subcategory of violent behavior against children. The violence is used as an "instrument" of behavior control and is goal directed. It occurs in the absence of emotional arousal and without provocation by the victim (Hodges 2007). It is premeditated and motive driven. The perpetrator has complete control over his/her actions and knows exactly why he or she is using violence. In child abuse, it is seen in situations in which power and pain are used to force the child to cooperate, for example, in child sexual abuse or in physically abusive education of children, comparable to the physically abusive training of military personnel. The violent behavior may cause injuries but is not motivated by the desire to cause physical harm per se. Injuries caused by instrumental violence are the same as injuries caused by other forms of physical abuse. The difference between instrumental violence and physical abuse is found in the motivation of the perpetrator: abuse of power in instrumental violence versus a variety of feelings, including powerlessness in physical abuse.

2.8 Assessment

2.8.1 "The Kipling Principle" in the Assessment of Child Abuse

> Like ballistic tests and fingerprints, medical evidence is only as good as the physician who assembles it. Findings taken by hurried, inexperienced or indifferent doctors in busy clinics or hospital emergency rooms often turn out to be worthless… (Crewdson 1988)

A careful and detailed history, a comprehensive physical examination, and, if indicated, additional laboratory and radiological investigations are essential to differentiate between inflicted and accidental injuries. Experience has taught that in numerous cases, explanations for injuries in children are too readily accepted without any questioning by medical personnel. Sometimes, this is due to the acute nature and the severity of the injury that requires immediate treatment.

Sometimes, the medical assessment is the first step in the process by which physical abuse is recognized. It is usually essential to have the child examined medically at some stage. The examination should be conducted in a quiet, private, and child-friendly room, which is appropriately equipped. The room must be well lit (preferably daylight or artificial light resembling daylight). The examination itself requires a calm, unhurried approach. This is why it should not be planned, if possible, during a normal outpatient clinic or in a busy hospital emergency department. It is essential that there is sufficient time for detailed and thorough recording of findings (Hobbs et al. 1999).

Attention should be paid to interactions between the child and parents, and of both with health-care personnel during history taking and examination. Attention should also be paid to the way the parents interact with one another.

Establishing whether an injury can be explained based on the provided history is a specific task for forensically trained physicians. Physicians and other professionals are primarily trained to diagnose and treat injuries/abnormalities; however, they are not trained to explain how a certain injury may occur, how it could not have occurred, or how the injury could be explained in a different way. One should not expect professionals who have not been trained in forensic medicine/forensic pediatrics to be competent at this.

2.8.2 History

Taking a history is primarily aimed at obtaining clarity in the context of physical complaints/abnormalities and the findings during the physical examination. This means that in the first phase of contact with the child and the parents (introduction, history, and physical examination), the physician, or other medical personnel, does not have to confront the parents with any inconsistencies in the history and hence with the suspected abuse. In case of ambiguity, questioning must continue in the interest of the child, the parents, and the treatment. Every plausible explanation must be considered to reconcile conflicting information.

At the start of the contact, the parents are usually given the benefit of any doubt, unless the situation is life threatening and involvement of the child protection service or the police may be indicated. Physicians and other medical personnel should treat the parents with respect, regardless of whether or not they are responsible for harming the child. However, acting in the best interest of the child is the paramount principle, and one cannot always act in the parent's best interest. If serious doubt remains, then the needs of the child should take precedence.

2.8.2.1 Special History

In fact, the history in suspected child abuse should be as comprehensive and detailed as the history for any other serious and complex pediatric condition (Thomas et al. 1991; AAP 2002; Hettler and Greenes 2003; Sibert 2004; Pierce et al. 2005; Kellogg 2007). There may be several starting points at the moment a child, either alone or together with his/her parents/care providers, presents to a physician. The reasons for which medical care is sought may have:

1. A direct relationship to (suspected) child abuse or lead to suspected child abuse, such as a child with subdural bleeding, retinal bleeding, encephalopathy, posterior rib fractures, and in whom an immediate suspicion of "inflicted traumatic brain injury" is justified.
2. No obvious relationship to child abuse. Concerns about child abuse arise while obtaining the history or examining the child. This could involve, for example, a child with an extensive hematoma, in whom a clotting disorder had been ruled out by laboratory investigation. It may also concern an unrelated finding, for example, a child with a dermatological disorder in whom scars of burns are found.

2.8.2.2 History of the Presenting Problem

As stipulated in the previous section, the reasons for seeking medical care should firstly be clarified. A careful and detailed description of the following aspects is essential if complaints or abnormalities that justify suspected child abuse are encountered:

- What abnormality (any finding at physical examination such as inherited or acquired abnormalities, accidental or non-accidental injury, or dermatological findings) is involved?
- What explanations are offered by the parents, guardians, or the child?
- When did the abnormality arise?
- Who was present when it happened?
- How did the child react?
- How did the parent(s) and other individuals present during the incident react?

It is important to repeat or to discuss the history with others for further clarification of the findings. The consequence of repeating may be that the history may either change completely or partially in some detail during discussion(s) with the parents (e.g., because their whole explanation, or details therein, was improbable or contradicted the explanations given by others), the child, and/or witnesses.

2.8.2.3 History Given by the Child

Children who have been abused are often unable to provide a reliable explanation for their injuries for various reasons. They may be too young, fearful for their lives or the consequences of telling the truth. They may be unable to accept that a trusted parent has harmed them in this way and may deny the abuse. Moreover, abused children frequently remain silent when they recover out of loyalty to or fear of the parents or perpetrator.

It is important to pay attention to the past history of the child and other members of the family. There may have been earlier injuries or "accidents," sometimes numerous, or admissions to hospital of the child or sibling. There may also be indications that violence had been directed toward other members of the family including a partner and other children.

A child that is raised in a violent home is at greater risk of experiencing severe forms of corporal punishment and intense verbal aggression from his or her parents than a child from a nonviolent home (Straus et al. 1980; Jouriles and LeCompte 1991; McCloskey et al. 1995). Studies show that children who are witnesses of intimate partner violence or live in homes where there is violence between adults are always emotionally abused and in addition are two to three times more likely to be physically abused than other children (McCloskey et al. 1995; Straus and Smith 2009). According to Appel and Holden (1998), the median co-occurrence rate between intimate partner violence and child physical abuse is about 40% (based on a large review). Other studies show a co-occurrence of intimate partner violence and child physical abuse or neglect in 30–60% of the cases (Edleson 1999; Herrenkohl et al. 2008; Casanueva et al. 2009). More than 90% of the mothers who were physically maltreated by their partners admitted that they used physical violence against their children, compared to 50% of the non-maltreated mothers (Moore and Pepler 1998).

Even if the child is not the direct target of the physical violence, the child will suffer as a witness of the aggression between his or her parents, which can be considered to be a severe form of psychological/emotional abuse or neglect (Henning et al. 1996; Osofsky 1998; Berry 2000; Levendosky and Graham-Bermann 2001). Witnessing domestic violence may have negative effects on the relationships between siblings and may even lead to violence between siblings after prolonged exposure to domestic violence (Moore et al. 1990). Furthermore, there may have been previous contacts with the child protection agency or the police due to domestic violence. Alcohol and/or drug abuse may also be a contributing factor to violence.

If the child immediately and spontaneously mentions how the injury occurred, there may be two explanations. Firstly, the child is telling the truth. Secondly, the child in rare situations may be coached and is telling a false history immediately and "spontaneously."

When taking the history, contradictory explanations may be given. There may also be a conspicuous discrepancy between the explanations of the child and the parents, between the parents themselves, and between the parents and a witness. Sometimes, no explanation is given because no witnesses were present. Explanations may constantly change. This may occur during further questioning regarding the explanation or when the history is taken on successive days. It may also be conspicuous when the child and the parents provide different explanations to different people.

The age and the developmental level of the child must be taken into account when evaluating the validity of the history. It may be that the explanation contradicts the developmental level of the child. The nature and/or the location of the injury may contradict the explanation given by the parents. It may well be that the explanation by the parents only partially explains the injuries. Finally, an explanation may be given whereby the child in question or one of the siblings is held responsible for the injuries.

2.8.2.4 History Given by the Parents

The contradiction between the severity of the injury and the degree of reaction by the parents may raise suspicions regarding maltreatment. A relatively minor injury may provoke an exaggerated reaction, or the reverse may occur, i.e., a totally inadequate (distant, indifferent) reaction is seen following serious injury. This may reflect on the parents' poor resistance to stress. An abusive parent may react aggressively to questioning. The parent may threaten or actually withdraw the child from medical care as soon as child abuse is mentioned. Non-abusive parents are more likely to act in the best interests of the child.

The reaction of the parents with regard to suspected child abuse will vary from conscious denial to complete ignorance. Conscious denial of knowing what happened is probably the most prevalent reaction. Feelings of guilt and shame may also been seen because the parent knows that his/her behavior has resulted in harm to the child. In rare cases, the parent may be ignorant or unaware that his/her behavior caused harm to the child.

A physician must be aware when talking to the parents regarding the cause of an injury that generally parents will quickly realize that the physician doubts their explanation and suspects child abuse. This applies not only to abusive but also to non-abusive parents. It may lead to the adoption of a defensive attitude by the parents at the start of or during the interview.

2.8.2.5 History Given by Others

Other persons (professionals or laypersons) involved in the case may give statements of what happened to the child or how the injury to the child occurred. If so, one should keep in mind that there are several possibilities about the reliability of the statement. The witness is telling the truth, or they may also have been coached by others involved in the case. However, with witnesses, there is also a third consideration, because the witness will react from his/her own norms and values. On the one hand, the witness may put his/her observations into perspective, whereas on the other hand, the observations may be exaggerated, because the witness wants to help the child or the parents. Finally, the witness may also act in his/her own interest by providing their own explanation for the injury.

2.8.2.6 Seeking Medical Care

One of the most conspicuous facts in the medical history of some cases is a delay or complete failure to seek medical care by the parents. Delay may vary from hours to days after the injury occurred. There are several explanations for this phenomenon, such as shame, incorrect evaluation of the situation, hope of spontaneous recovery, and hope that the injury is no longer recognizable as resulting from abuse.

Parents may consult other health-care providers in novel situations or as second or third opinion, when they think their pediatrician is suspecting child abuse (escape behavior), thus avoiding their usual general practitioner or pediatrician, without having to provide an acceptable explanation other than, for example, the urgency of the consultation. Care is often sought at an unusual hour, for example, in the evening, weekend, or outside normal working hours. This means that information on the child's medical care may be held by various physicians (e.g., general practitioners, pediatricians, surgeons, and others) and different departments (e.g., the departments of pediatrics and surgery, and the emergency rooms). Sometimes care for the child is sought by someone other than the parent(s), for example, the grandparents or a teacher.

2.8.2.7 Supplementary General History

The supplementary history is important in the evaluation of possible or probable medical causes of the actual complaints and physical findings. Moreover, it provides further insights into the manner in which the parents fulfill their parental tasks, the attitude of the parents toward the child and other children in the family, and the functioning of the family as a whole (Kellogg 2007):

- Pregnancy and birth – wanted/unwanted, planned/unplanned, prenatal care, peri- and postnatal complications, postpartum depression or other psychiatric disorder of mother or father, supervised or unsupervised delivery
- Growth and developmental disturbances influencing the personality and the temperament of the child
- Actual use of medication and drugs, prescribed and non-prescribed present and past
- Previous health-care contacts, both outpatient contacts and hospital admissions, trauma (accidental and non-accidental), congenital abnormalities, acute and chronic ailments, including allergies and metabolic disturbances
- Review of old notes and records
- Family history
- Clotting problems, bone abnormalities, and metabolic or genetic disorders
- Alcohol, drug, and medicine use in other family members
- Particulars of other siblings
- Earlier child abuse in other family members (children and adults)
- Parenting: care and control
- Mental health problems in parents including suicide and self-harm
- Social history

2.8.3 Physical Examination and Documentation of Findings

Considering the possible short- and long-term effects of child abuse, each case of suspected child abuse will demand a careful and thorough physical examination. Special attention should be paid to the age and the developmental level of the child, which may assist in differentiating between accidental and inflicted injuries. An example of the importance of establishing the developmental level of the child is that bruises are rarely seen in children of less than 9 months or immobile children: "those who don't cruise rarely bruise" (Chaps. 3 and 4) (Sugar et al. 1999).

Every inch of the body (from head to toe, including the anogenital area – Table 2.6) must be inspected, including locations where physical-abuse-related injuries would not be expected. Hobbs and Wynne (1990) showed that physical abuse may coexist with other abuse. Physically abused children are often also sexually abused and/or neglected (Hobbs and Wynne 1990). Their findings are confirmed by MacMillan et al. (1997) and Finkelhor et al. (2005). Body parts without injuries and/or skin abnormalities must be recorded.

Sometimes, the child has older or historical injuries for which the parents are unable or unwilling to provide an adequate explanation. Such injuries may be identified from history or found at physical examination or at supplementary investigations, for example, imaging techniques.

Furthermore, during the examination, attention should not only be paid to the physical examination and description and recording of the physical findings (Table 2.7) but also to the behavior of the child and his/her parents.

Table 2.6 Complete physical examination

General impression	Functioning and physical condition of the child Level of care, signs of neglect Symmetry in movements, loss of function of body parts Sensitivity and any pain reactions during the examination
Vital functions and temperature	
Growth parameters and nutritional state	Height, weight, head circumference Mid-upper arm circumference
Development	Developmental history and assessment, including language and social skills
Emotional state and demeanor	How does the child present? How would the child's emotional state be described?
Careful and structured inspection of all parts of the body – head to toe	
Skin	Erythema Bruises, petechiae, bitemarks (in case of bitemarks – DNA – see Chap. 8) Abrasions Lacerations Burns and scalds, cold-related injuries Incisions/stab wound, shot wound Pattern injuries Scars Tattoos Symptoms of skin disease (e.g., redness, scratch marks)
Head/neck	Scalp: e.g., swelling, bruising; traction alopecia Fontanel: level, fullness Face: e.g., bruising, petechiae, pattern injuries; symmetrical movements (smiling, crying) Nose: drainage of liquor or blood from the nostrils Neck: bruising, abrasions (nail imprints), ligature marks, or other signs of strangulation
Eyes	Periorbital bruising or petechiae Conjunctival (petechial) hemorrhage Retinal hemorrhage
Ears	Bruising of the pinna, retro-auricular bruising/mastoid bruising (Battle's sign) Fluid or blood drainage Ear canals and drums (laceration, hemotympanum)

(continued)

Table 2.6 (continued)

Oropharynx	Injuries inside the mouth: inner surface of the lips and cheeks, the gums, tear of lip, or tongue frenulum
Thorax	Deformities of the thorax Rachitic rosary (rickets may be related to neglectful care) Flail chest (caused by blunt trauma; paradoxical or reverse motion of a chest-wall segment while breathing spontaneously)
Abdomen	Distension on inspection Bruising of the abdominal wall Tenderness during palpation Bowel activity
Female genitalia and anus	Hymenal damage or scarring Bruises, abrasions, fissures, burns/scalds, scars Female genital mutilation
Male genitalia and anus	Bruises, abrasions, fissures, burns/scalds, scars
Back	Deformities Tenderness and bruises
Buttocks	Bruises, burns/scalds, scars Pattern injuries (e.g., tramline or vertical gluteal cleft injuries)
Extremities	Bruises on the inner sides of arms and legs Fractures (callus), luxations, deformities Symmetry in movements/loss of function
Neurological examination	

When child abuse is suspected, physical examination is usually supplemented with extensive laboratory investigations and imaging techniques. However, this is not always necessary, and children should not have to go through unnecessary medical investigations, when the cause of the injuries is obvious. For example, in case of extensive pattern bruises, one might consider a comprehensive coagulation screening for completeness sake or to avoid discussions about coagulation disorders, but this is in almost all cases unnecessary because the pattern tells the story of physical abuse (see also Chaps. 3 and 5).

Certain aspects are seen more frequently in inflicted than in accidental injuries and should arouse suspicion during the examination:

- Multiple injuries of different ages and in various stages of healing
- Injuries in different areas of the body (front – back, left – right)
- Injuries with a clearly recognizable pattern (pattern injuries), for example, handprint, iron burn, implement shape
- Self-defense injuries (Sect. 2.7.2)
- Injuries in protected sites (e.g., neck, pubis, perianal area) which are normally or only rarely injured in an accident

In Table 2.7 an overview of the aspects that must be recorded in the description (and the evaluation) of the injuries/skin abnormalities is given. Every injury and all other findings, including skin abnormalities, should be recorded and described correctly (Table 2.7).

2.8.4 Supplementary Investigations

The reader is referred to the relevant chapters for details of the various supplementary investigations in various types of injuries. Here, only supplementary radiodiagnostics are dealt with. A complete skeletal survey according to the guidelines of either the "American College of Radiology" or the "Royal College of Radiologists and the Royal College of Paediatrics and Child Health" must be compiled for every child <2 years old in whom child physical abuse is suspected, and in case of other serious external or internal

Table 2.7 Description of physical findings

1.	Nature	Traumatic: Mechanical (static or dynamic loading) (Sect. 2.5) (Near) contact with physical agents (Sect. 2.6) Artificial (e.g., scars or tattoos) Dermatological disease
2.	Shape	Flat lesions: Pattern injuries Recognizable pattern for a dermatological disorder Non-flat lesions: Particularly important in sexually transmitted diseases
3.	Number	
4.	Size	Always in centimeters – never in symbols Measurement: vertical, horizontal/vertical x horizontal
5.	Site	Anatomically correct Left/right From fixed anatomical orientation points, preferably in relation to the skeleton Distribution of the injuries over the body Use body plans
6.	Border	Well demarcated Less well demarcated Varyingly demarcated
7.	Color	Generally only indicative because the description of the color of an abnormality is subjective Always use a standard color scale for photographs

Table 2.8 The standard child protection skeletal survey for suspected non-accidental injury

Skull	AP, lateral, and Towne's views (the latter if clinically indicated) Skull radiographs should be taken with the skeletal survey even if a CT scan has been or will be performed
Chest	AP including the clavicles Oblique views of both sides of the chest to show the ribs ("left and right oblique")
Abdomen	AP including the pelvis and the hips
Spine	Lateral (this may require separate views of the cervical, thoracic, and thoracolumbar regions) If the whole spine is not clearly visible on the AP view of the chest and abdominal radiographs, then additional views will be required AP views of the cervical spine are rarely diagnostic at this age and should only be made at the discretion of the radiologist
Limbs	AP of both upper arms AP of both forearms AP of both femurs AP of both lower legs PA of hands AP of feet

RCR and RCPCH (2008)
AP anteroposterior, *PA* posteroanterior

injuries in children >2 years old (American College of Radiology 2006; Royal College of Radiologists, Royal College of Paediatrics and Child Health 2008). The complete guidelines are available for downloading without cost. The guidelines of the "Royal College of Radiologists and the Royal College of Paediatrics and Child Health" are given in Table 2.8.

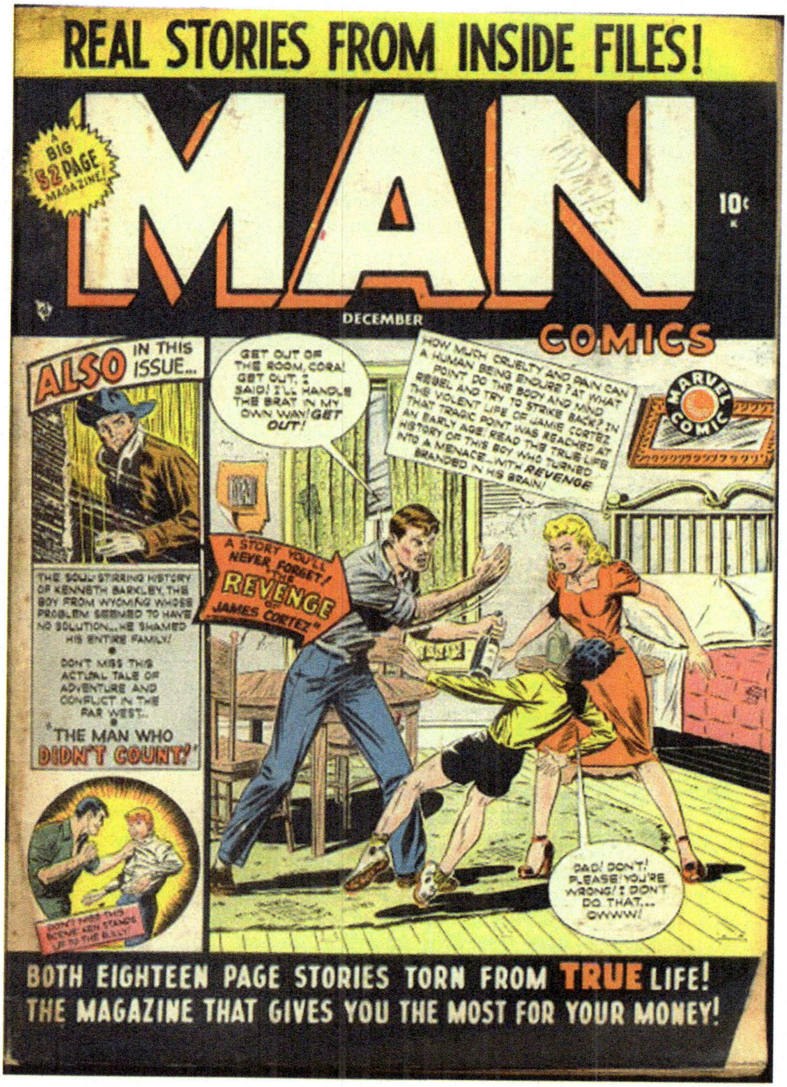
REAL STORIES FROM INSIDE FILES!
A BIG 52 PAGE MAGAZINE!
MAN
10¢
DECEMBER
COMICS
ALSO IN THIS ISSUE...
THE SOUL-STIRRING HISTORY OF KENNETH BARKLEY, THE BOY FROM WYOMING WHOSE PROBLEM SEEMED TO HAVE NO SOLUTION...HE SHAMED HIS ENTIRE FAMILY!
DON'T MISS THIS ACTUAL TALE OF ADVENTURE AND CONFLICT IN THE FAR WEST...
"THE MAN WHO DIDN'T COUNT!"
GET OUT OF THE ROOM, CORA! GET OUT, I SAID! I'LL HANDLE THE BRAT IN MY OWN WAY! GET OUT!
HOW MUCH CRUELTY AND PAIN CAN A HUMAN BEING ENDURE? AT WHAT POINT DO THE BODY AND MIND REBEL AND TRY TO STRIKE BACK? IN THE VIOLENT LIFE OF JAMIE CORTEZ THAT TRAGIC POINT WAS REACHED AT AN EARLY AGE! READ THE TRUE LIFE HISTORY OF THIS BOY WHO TURNED INTO A MENACE...WITH REVENGE BRANDED IN HIS BRAIN!
MARVEL COMIC
A STORY YOU'LL NEVER FORGET! "THE REVENGE OF JAMES CORTEZ"
DAD! DON'T! PLEASE! YOU'RE WRONG! I DON'T DO THAT... OWWW!
BOTH EIGHTEEN PAGE STORIES TORN FROM TRUE LIFE!
THE MAGAZINE THAT GIVES YOU THE MOST FOR YOUR MONEY!

Fig. 2.56 Who did it: dynamic impact loading!

2.9 Who Did It?

The question of who was responsible for the occurrence of the injury can rarely be answered based solely on the injuries found in a child. It is not the task of the examining forensic doctor to prove who did it. Finding and proving who did it is the task of behavioral analysts, the police, and the court (Fig. 2.56).

References

AAP American Academy of Pediatrics Committee on Child Abuse & Neglect (2002) When inflicted skin injuries constitute child abuse. Pediatrics 110(3):644–645

American College of Radiology (2006) ACR practice guideline for skeletal surveys in children. http://www.acr.org/. Accessed on 2008

Appel AE, Holden GW (1998) The co-occurrence of spouse and physical child abuse: a review and appraisal. J Fam Psychol 12(4):578–599

Arieff AI, Kronlund BA (1999) Fatal child abuse by forced water intoxication. Pediatrics 103(6 Pt1):1292–1295

Barnes PM, Norton CM, Frank D, Dunstan FD et al (2005) Abdominal injury due to child abuse. Lancet 366(9481):234–235

Berry D (2000) The domestic violence sourcebook, 3rd edn. McGraw-Hill, New York

Bowkett B, Kolbe A (1998) Traumatic duodenal perforations in children: child abuse a frequent cause. Aust N Z J Surg 68(5):380–382

Brannon H (2007) Skin anatomy. About.com dermatology. http://dermatology.about.com/cs/skinanatomy/a/anatomy.htm. Accessed on 2009

Burton D (2007) Static v. dynamic loading: why the WTC towers fell so fast. http://www.burtonsys.com/staticvdyn/. Accessed on 2009

Casanueva C, Martin SL, Runyan DK (2009) Repeated reports for child maltreatment among intimate partner violence victims: findings from the National Survey of Child and Adolescent Well-Being. Child Abuse Negl 33(2):84–93

CDC (Center for Disease Control and Prevention) Injury Center (2007). http://www.cdc.gov/ncipc/wisqars/nonfatal/definitions.htm. Accessed on 2011

Coleman R (2001) The skin. Technion University. http://www.technion.ac.il/~mdcourse/274203/lect12.html. Accessed on 2007

Coulter K (2000) Bruising and skin trauma. Pediatr Rev 21(1):34–35

Crewdson J (1988) By silence betrayed – sexual abuse of children in America. Little Brown and Company, Boston

Edleson JL (1999) The overlap between child maltreatment and woman battering. Violence Against Women 5(2):134–154

el Awad ME (1994) Overheating in neonates in Saudi Arabia. East Afr Med J 71(12):805–806

Finkelhor D, Ormrod R, Turner H et al (2005) The victimization of children and youth: a comprehensive, national survey. Child Maltreat 10(1):5–25

Fridman I (2001) Surface area of human skin. In: Elert G (ed) The physics factbook. http://hypertextbook.com/facts/2001/IgorFridman.shtml. Accessed on 2009

Gaines BA, Shultz BS, Morrison K et al (2004) Duodenal injuries in children: beware of child abuse. J Pediatr Surg 39(4):600–602

Goldsmith LA (1990) My organ is bigger than your organ. Arch Dermatol 126(3):301–302

Health Canada (2003) Injury surveillance in Canada: current realities, challenges. Health Canada. http://www.hc-sc.gc.ca/hl-vs/securit/index-eng.php. Accessed on 2010

Henning K, Leitenberg H, Coffey P et al (1996) Long term psychological and social impact of witnessing physical conflict between parents. J Interpers Violence 11(1):35–49

Herr S, Fallat ME (2006) Abusive abdominal and thoracic trauma. Clin Pediatr Emerg Med 7(3):149–152

Herrenkohl TI, Sousa C, Tajima EA et al (2008) Intersection of child abuse and children's exposure to domestic violence. Trauma Violence Abuse 9(2):84–99

Hettiaratchy S, Dziewulski P (2004) ABC of burns – pathophysiology and types of burns. Br Med J 328(7453):1427–1429

Hettler J, Greenes DS (2003) Can the initial history predict whether a child with a head injury has been abused? Pediatrics 111(3):602–607

Hobbs CJ, Wynne JM (1990) The sexually abused battered child. Arch Dis Child 65(4):423–427

Hobbs CJ, Hanks HGI, Wynne JM (1999) Chapter 4. Physical abuse. In: Hobbs CJ, Hanks HGI, Wynne JM (eds) Child abuse and neglect – a clinician's handbook, 2nd edn. Churchill Livingstone, London, pp 63–104

Hodges HJ (2007) Psychopathy as a predictor of instrumental violence among civil psychiatric patients. A thesis. Drexel University

Johnson CF (1990) Inflicted injury versus accidental injury. Pediatr Clin North Am 37(4):791–814

Jouriles EN, LeCompte SH (1991) Husband's aggression toward wives and mothers' and fathers' aggression toward children: moderating effects of child gender. J Consult Clin Psychol 59(1):190–192

Kaczor K, Pierce MC, Makoroff K, Corey TS (2006) Bruising and physical child abuse. Clin Pediatr Emerg Med 7(3):153–160

Kellogg ND (2007) Evaluation of suspected child physical abuse. Pediatrics 199(6):1232–1241

Kernerman English Multilingual Dictionary (2006–2010)

Kipling R (1902) The elephant's child. In: Just So Stories. Macmillan & Co, New York

Koumbourlis AC (2002) Electrical injuries. Crit Care Med 30(11 Suppl):S424–S430

Langlois NEI, Gresham GA (1991) The ageing of bruises: a review and study of the colour changes with time. Forensic Sci Int 50(2):227–238

Ledbetter DJ, Hatch EI, Feldman KW et al (1988) Diagnostic and surgical implications of child abuse. Arch Surg 123(9):1101–1105

Levendosky AA, Graham-Bermann SA (2001) Parenting in battered women: the effects of intimate partner violence on women and their children. J Fam Violence 16(2):171–192

MacMillan HL, Fleming JE, Trocmé N et al (1997) Prevalence of child physical and sexual abuse in the community. Results from the Ontario Health Supplement. JAMA 278(2):131–135

Maguire S, Mann MK, Sibert J, Kemp A (2005) Are there patterns of bruising in childhood which are diagnostic or suggestive of abuse? A systematic review. Arch Dis Child 90(2):182–186

Martos Sánchez I, Ros Pérez P, Otheo-de-Tejada E et al (2000) Fatal hypernatremia due to accidental administration of table salt. An Esp Pediatr 53(5):495–498 [in Spanish]

Mathew MO, Ramamohan N, Bennet GC (1998) Importance of bruising associated with paediatric fractures: prospective observational study. Br Med J 317(7166):1117–1118

McCloskey LA, Figueredo AJ, Koss MP (1995) The effects of systemic family violence on children's mental health. Child Dev 66(5):1239–1261

McCurdy (1993) cited from Nobuyasu S. Cost and benefit simulation analysis of catastrophic maltreatment. In: Franey K, Geffner R, Falconer R (eds) The cost of child maltreatment: who pays? We all do. Family Violence & Sexual Assault Institute, San Diego 2001

Meyer-Heim A, Landau K, Boltshauser E (2002) Treatment of acne with consequences – pseudotumor cerebri due to hypervitaminosis A. Praxis (Bern 1994) 91(1–2):23–26 [in German]

Moore TE, Pepler DJ (1998) Wounding words: maternal verbal aggression and children's adjustment. J Fam Violence 21(1):89–93

Moore T, Pepler D, Weinberg B et al (1990) Research on children from violent families. Can Ment Health 38(2–3):19–23

NCECI (2007) NOMESCO classification of external causes of injuries, 4th rev edn. Nordic Medico-Statistical Committee, Copenhagen

Nobuyasu S (2001) Cost and benefit simulation analysis of catastrophic maltreatment. In: Franey K, Geffner R, Falconer R (eds) The cost of child maltreatment: who pays? We all do. Family Violence & Sexual Assault Institute, San Diego

NYU (2003) The MathMol hypermedia textbook. New York University. http://www.nyu.edu/pages/mathmol/txtbk2/. Accessed on 2011

Osofsky JD (1998) Children as invisible victims of domestic and community violence, Chapter 4. In: Holden GW, Geffner R, Jouriles EN (eds) Children exposed to marital violence: theory, research, and applied issues. American Psychological Association, Washington, DC

Panke TW, McLeod CG (1985) Pathology of thermal injury – a practical approach. Grune & Stratton, Orlando, pp 298–302

Paterson CR (1987) Child abuse or copper deficiency? Br Med J 295(6591):213

Patient.co.uk (2007) Body surface area calculator (Mosteller). http://www.patient.co.uk/doctor/Body-Surface-Area-Calculator-%28Mosteller%29.htm. Accessed on 2009

Pierce MC, Bertocci GE, Janosky JE et al (2005) Femur fractures in resulting from stair falls among children: an injury plausibility model. Pediatrics 115(6):1712–1722

Pounder DJ (2000) Burns and scalds. In: Siegel J, Knupfer G, Saukko P (eds) Encyclopedia of forensic sciences, 1st edn. Elsevier Academic Press, London, pp 326–330

Quereshi UA, Bhat JI, Ali SW et al (2010) Acute salt poisoning due to different oral rehydration solution (ORS) packet sizes. Indian J Pediatr 77(6):679–680

Richardson AC (1994) Cutaneous manifestations of abuse. In: Reece RM (ed) Child abuse. Lea & Febiger, Philadelphia, pp 167–184

Royal College of Radiologists, Royal College of Paediatrics and Child Health (2008) Standards for the radiological investigations of suspected non-accidental injury. RCP and RCPCH, London. www.rcpch.ac.uk/doc.aspx?id_Resource=3521. Accessed on 2009

Sibert J (2004) Bruising, coagulation disorder, and physical child abuse. Blood Coagul Fibrinolysis 15(Suppl 1):S33–S39

Starling SP, Sirotnak AP, Heisler KW et al (2007) Inflicted skeletal trauma: the relationship of perpetrators to their victims. Child Abuse Negl 31(9):993–999

Stephenson T (1995) Bruising in children. Curr Paediatr 5(4):225–229

Straus M, Smith C (2009) Family patterns and child abuse. In: Straus M, Gelles R (eds) Physical violence in American families: risk factors and adaptations to violence in 8,145 families. 4th printing, Transaction Publishers, 245–62

Straus M, Gelles R, Steinmetz S (1980) Behind closed doors: violence in the American family. Doubleday, Garden City, New Jersey

Sugar N, Taylor J, Feldman K (1999) Bruises in infants and toddlers: those who don't cruise rarely bruise. Arch Pediatr Adolesc Med 153(4):399–403

Taitz LS (1991a) Child abuse and metabolic bone disease: are they often confused? Br Med J 302(6787):1244

Taitz LS (1991b) Child abuse: some myths and shibboleths. Hosp Update 17:400–408

Thomas SA, Rosenfield NS, Leventhal JM et al (1991) Long-bone fractures in young children: distinguishing accidental injuries from child abuse. Pediatrics 88(3):471–476

Trocmé N, MacMillan H, Fallon B et al (2003) Nature and severity of physical harm caused by child abuse and neglect: results from the Canadian Incidence Study. CMAJ 169(9):911–915

Wheeler DS, Shope TR (1997) Depressed skull fracture in a 7-month-old who fell from bed. Pediatrics 100(6):1033–1034

WHO (World Health Organisation) (2006). Regional office for Europe. Unintentional child injuries in the WHO European Region, Geneva

Wikipedia (2011) Mass versus weight. http://en.wikipedia.org/wiki/Mass_versus_weight. Accessed on 2011

Williams J (2003) Bruises. In: Strachan-Peterson M, Durfee M, Coulter K (eds) Child abuse and neglect. Guidelines for identification, assessment, and case management. Volcano Press, Volcano, pp 23–33

Wilson EF (1977) Estimation of the age of cutaneous contusions in child abuse. Pediatrics 60(5):750–752

Zhu BL, Ishida K, Fujita MQ, Maeda H (1998) Infant death presumably due to exertional self-overheating in bed: an autopsy case of suspected child abuse. Nihon Hoigaku Zasshi 52(2):153–156

3 Blunt-Force Trauma: Bruises

3.1 Introduction

In humans, the skin is the most visible organ, and it is also the most frequently damaged organ when children sustain injuries. The injuries most commonly seen are bruises and abrasions. These injuries are usually the result of everyday activities at home, including play, sports, or during participating in traffic. In most cases, a skin injury is the only abnormality. However, sometimes an external injury is an indication for more serious internal damage (the "tip of the iceberg" phenomenon).

In physical abuse, the skin often is the "primary target" organ. Bruises and other skin injuries may be an indication of physical abuse in children. Bruises are the most commonly seen injuries that result from blunt-force trauma in physical violence against children (Hobbs et al. 1999a; Maguire et al. 2005a, b; Hammond 2009).

3.2 Bruises

3.2.1 Defining Bruise, Hematoma, and Petechia

The definition and nomenclature of bleeding and blood accumulation in the skin and subcutaneous tissues vary greatly in the medical literature. Some of the terms used are bruise, bruising, contusion, hematoma, intra-/subcutaneous bleeding/hemorrhage, purpura, ecchymosis, and petechia. In this chapter, only three terms for localized collections of blood in the skin or subcutaneous tissue will be used: bruise, hematoma, and petechia.

A bruise is defined as a localized collection of blood in the skin and or subcutaneous tissue occurring as a result of damage to the capillaries or larger blood vessels allowing blood to leak into the tissues leading to skin discoloration (RCPCH 2008b). A bruise is almost always caused by blunt-force trauma (Robinson 2000; DiMaio and DiMaio 2001b; Brenner 2004). Only rarely bruises are manifestations of a medical condition, for example, a coagulation disorder, leukemia, or vasculitis (Chaps. 5 and 6). Bruises can also be mimicked in many different ways (Chap. 6).

A hematoma is defined a collection of blood forming a fluctuant mass under the skin (RCPCH 2008b). Petechiae are defined as small, distinct bruises (<2 mm) that occur when arterioles or venules rupture (RCPCH 2008b) (Sect. 3.3). It is advised not to use other terms like contusion, purpura, or ecchymosis in a forensic context to prevent confusion.

3.2.2 Clinical Features

Generally, bruises will be located superficially in the skin and subcutaneous tissues. Superficial bruises will almost always show externally visible surface discoloration (immediately or after a delay of hours to days, which will change over time), more or less prominent local swelling, and

R.A.C. Bilo et al., *Cutaneous Manifestations of Child Abuse and Their Differential Diagnosis*,
DOI 10.1007/978-3-642-29287-3_3, © Springer-Verlag Berlin Heidelberg 2013

pain without the skin being abraded or lacerated necessarily by blunt-force trauma. A bruise at a certain site does not necessarily indicate the point of impact of the blunt force.

Bruises can also be located internally: each organ can be damaged through blunt-force trauma, for example, muscle tissue, brain, heart, lungs, and kidneys (DiMaio and DiMaio 2001b; Brenner 2004).

3.2.2.1 The Visibility of Bruises

As stated previously, bruises are the most frequent posttraumatic findings in accidents and in child abuse. Unfortunately, they are not always visible. The external visibility of a bruise depends on the depth of the location (externally visible bruises are most commonly located in the dermis), the amount of extravasated blood, the presence of underlying solid structures, and the structure of the perivascular area and the looseness of the surrounding tissues.

Superficial bruises may become visible immediately or within minutes after the incident, whereas deeper bruises may not be visible until several hours or even days later. This depends on the persistence of the bleeding, the diffusion of blood from the deeper to the more superficial structures, the displacement of pooled blood (e.g., under the influence of the gravity in combination with anatomical characteristics), and on the hemolysis. Deep bruises are sometimes not visible externally and are only found after incising the skin and subcutaneous tissues (DiMaio and DiMaio 2001b).

As stated before, following injury to the skin, it may take minutes to days for a bruise to become visible. Hammond (2009) illustrates this with the example of a bruise from a fractured femur that may become visible around the knee after a couple of days. It is also seen in blunt-force trauma to the upper abdomen, in which the bruise becomes visible in the skin of the lower abdomen days after the trauma. According to Hammond (2009), this phenomenon is caused by the tracking of blood through tissue planes following blunt-force trauma. Delayed “coming out” is also described in subgaleal bleeding, which may lead to externally visible bruises around the eyes, behind the ears, and in the neck. These bruises may become visible 1–8 days after blunt-force trauma in infants and young children (Kuban et al. 1983), but it may take up to 14 days until enough blood is collected in the subgaleal space to be visible or palpable for a caretaker or during a physical examination (Vu et al. 2004) (Figs. 3.1 and 3.2).

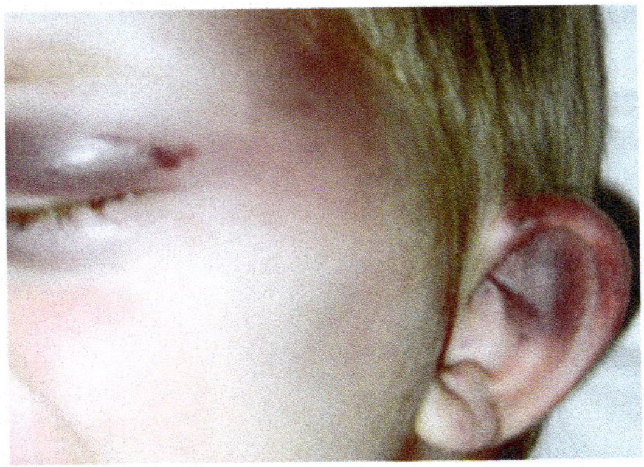

Fig. 3.1 Typical distribution of a subgaleal bleeding: the bleeding became visible almost 24 h after an observed accidental fall on the head

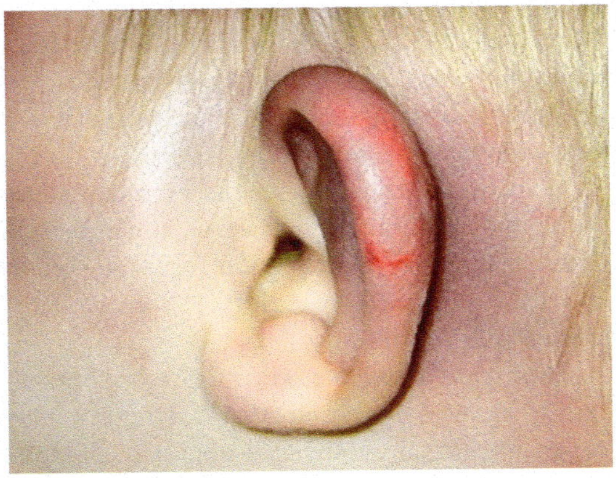

Fig. 3.2 Same child as in Fig. 3.1: typical auricular and retro-auricular distribution of bruising in a subgaleal bleeding

Bruises often appear to be either invisible or hardly visible when located on the trunk (because the thickness of the skin) or in people with a dark-colored skin (Robinson 2000). Bruises were even statistically more obvious in white children

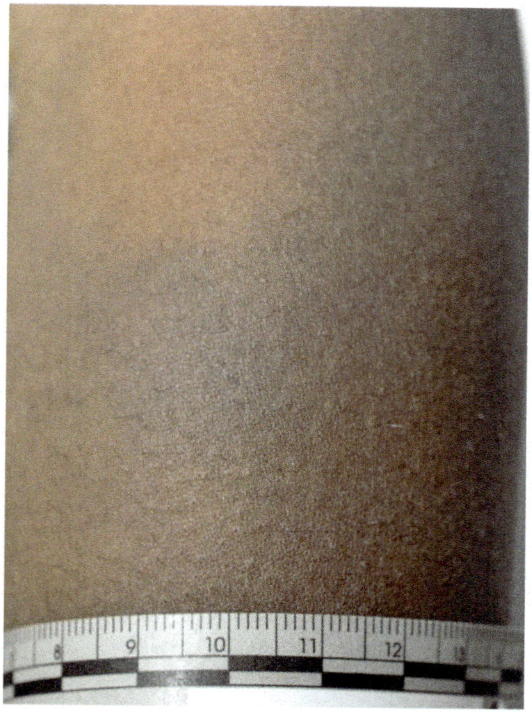

Fig. 3.3 Bruising in a child with *dark-colored* skin

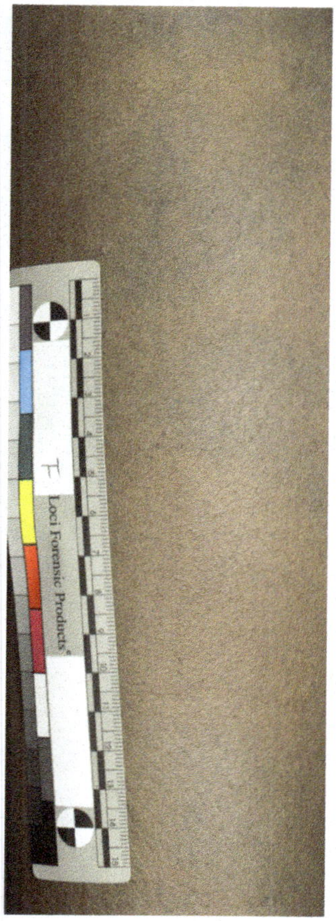

Fig. 3.4 Bruising in a child with *dark-colored* skin

than in African-American children due to skin tone ($P<.007$) (Sugar et al. 1999). Sugar found this difference not surprising. Although she stated that it could be possible that dark-colored children do have fewer bruises, she found it more likely that bruises are recognized more easily in children with lighter pigmentation (Figs. 3.3, 3.4, 3.5, 3.6, 3.7, 3.8, and 3.9).

Wood's lamp illumination (ultraviolet light at a wavelength of approximately 365 nm) has been reported to be useful in identifying bruises that are faint or not visible to the naked eye (Vogeley et al. 2002). Forensic light sources (containing the light components ultraviolet, visible, and infrared) can also be used during physical examinations to investigate (body) fluids such as blood, saliva, semen, urine, vaginal secretions, and sweat but may also reveal old and new bruises, bitemarks, healed burns, and patterned wound details that are invisible when illuminated by normal white light (Figs. 3.10 and 3.11) (Crimescope 2003) (see Sect. 9.7).

3.2.2.2 Size of Bruising and Applied Force

To a certain extent, the size of the bruise will indicate the level of force exerted on the body (= the amount of energy that has been transferred during the impact between the object and the body). Generally, it can be maintained that the size of the bruise is proportional to the force used. However, size does depend not only on the amount of force used but also on the structure and the supply of vessels to the affected tissue. In other words, in children, it is difficult to "read" the level of force that was used from the size of the bruise. In children, bruises develop relatively easier and generally somewhat faster than in adults, although the

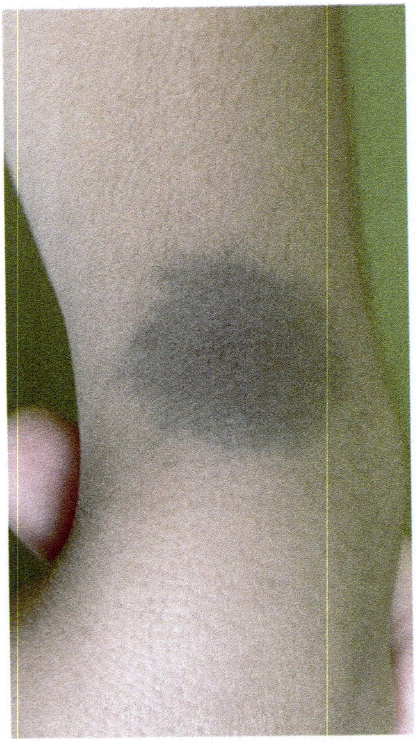

Fig. 3.5 Mongolian spot on the wrist of a child with a *dark-colored* skin (less typical location) (see also Chap. 6)

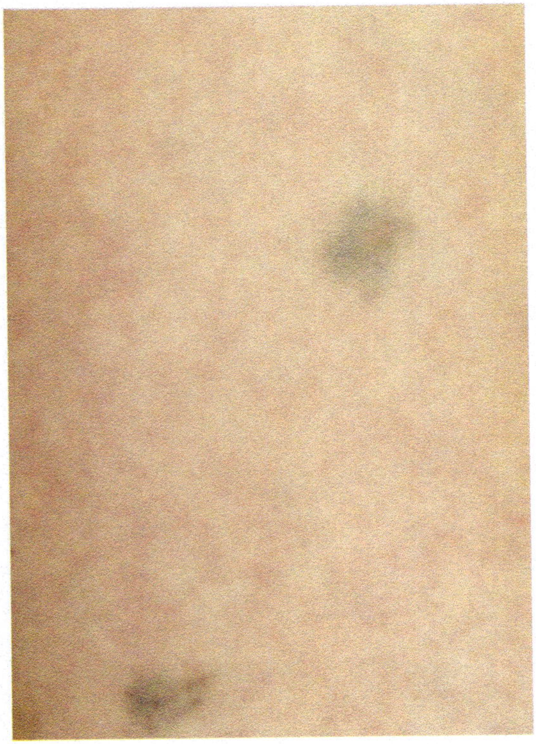

Fig. 3.6 Bruises in a "white" child

Fig. 3.7 Fading bruise in a "white" child

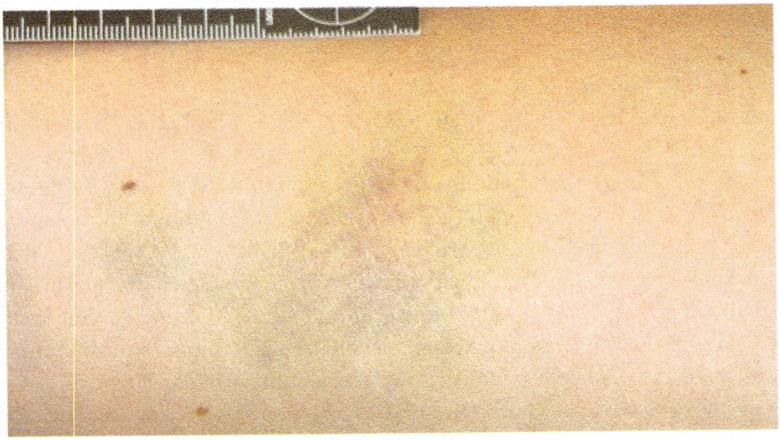

exact amount of force that is required to cause bruises remains unknown. Other factors that play a role are the location of the injury, the type of tissue that is damaged additionally to the skin (e.g., bone, muscle, or subcutaneous fat) and the tension of the skin during the development of the injury (Watson 1990; DiMaio and DiMaio 2001b).

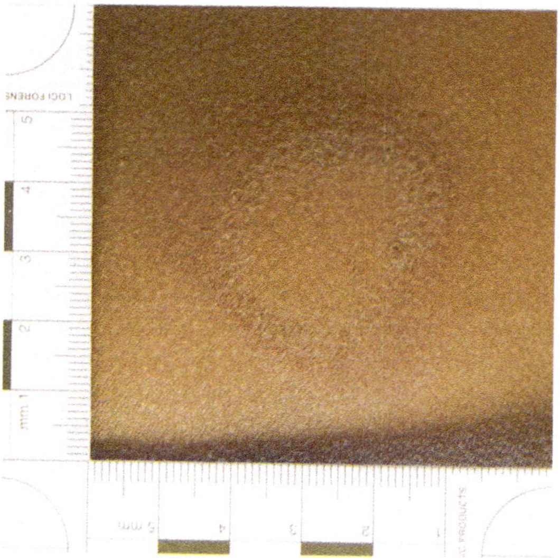

Fig. 3.8 Bitemark in a child with *dark-colored* skin (see also Chap. 8)

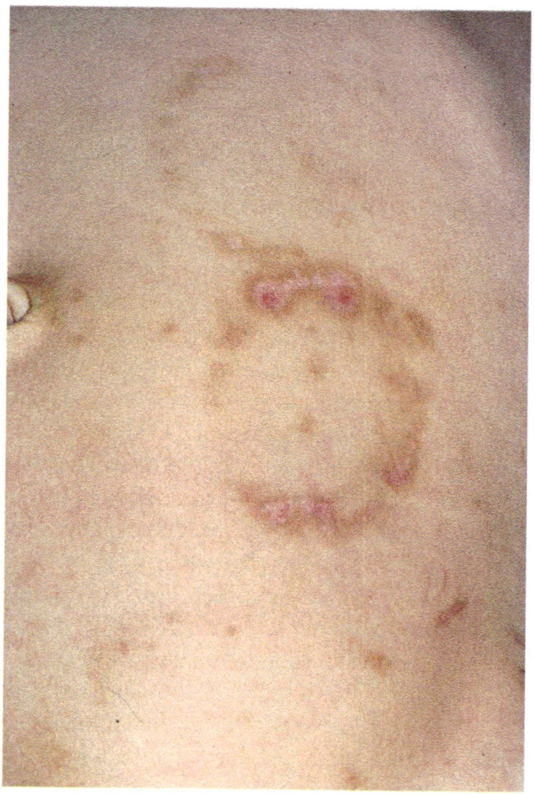

Fig. 3.9 Bitemark on the abdomen in a "white" child (= Fig. 8.13)

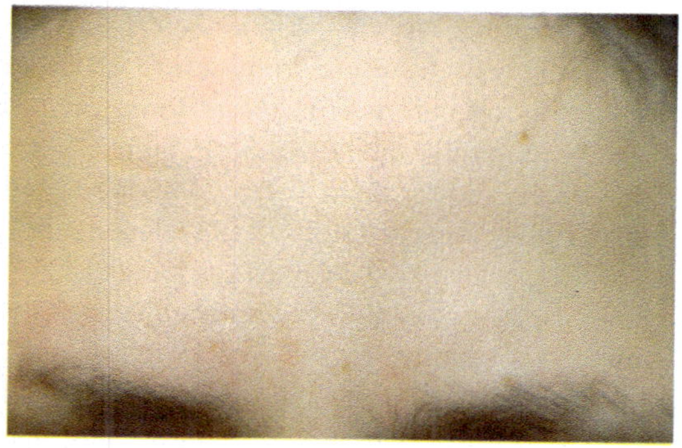

Fig. 3.10 Hardly visible bruising on the forehead (= Fig. 9.23)

Fig. 3.11 Using forensic light: rectangular pattern (= Fig. 9.24)

3.2.2.3 Complications of Bruising in Children

In general, it can be maintained that skin bruises are not life-threatening, and most bruises will not lead to complications. Complications, however, cannot completely be excluded. In assaulted adults, multiple and extensive bruises may lead to hypovolemia, shock, and ultimately death through massive loss of blood in the bruised areas (Robinson 2000; DiMaio and DiMaio 2001b). It is not known whether this also happens in children, but theoretically, this may happen. Also, as a result of accidental or non-accidental bleeding, clotting disturbances may occur on the basis of consumption coagulopathy. This has been described in children with intracranial bleeding but may also be expected in children with extensive bleeding in other locations (Hymel et al. 1997; Becker et al. 1999).

Furthermore, several articles on traumatic rhabdomyolysis resulting from severe abuse in the form of repeated assaults (blunt-force trauma) have been published (Rosenberg et al. 1983; Schwengel and Ludwig 1985; Mukherji and Siegel 1987; Leung and Robson 1987; Knottenbelt 1994; Roy et al. 1999). Peebles and Losek (2007) reported that 14 children with traumatic rhabdomyolysis have been described in the medical literature. All children appeared to have had extensive "soft-tissue muscle injuries" on the buttocks and/or the legs. Nine children developed acute kidney failure.

3.2.2.4 Postmortem Development of Bruises and Livor Mortis

Although it can generally be stated that the development of bruises must be regarded as an intravital reaction (happening during life), it is known that under certain conditions, postmortem bruises may develop. DiMaio cites Robertson (1957) that postmortem bruises may develop in case of a substantial blow within several hours after death. Capillaries and venules are damaged by the blow, and the blood migrates into the connective tissue. Such bruises may look the same as those developed prior to death, although swelling is likely to be absent (Robinson 2000). Postmortem bruises occur very infrequently and are found on sites where the skin is close to the bone.

Histological investigation to distinguish postmortem bruises from those that had developed prior to death is not meaningful because generally most of the bruises develop just prior to death, and thus, the time for a tissue reaction is insufficient. However, the proof for the development of bruises when alive is provided by an inflammatory reaction at histological investigation.

Postmortem and perimortem bruising should be differentiated from livor mortis (lividity, hypostasis), which is, like rigor mortis (stiffening of the muscles) and algor mortis (decrease of body temperature), a normal postmortem phenomenon. Livor is the reddish purple discoloration of the skin (and organs) that develops as soon as the circulation stops and is the result of gravitational settling or pooling of blood in dilatating capillaries/venules (Gilbert-Barnes et al. 2005). In adults, livor may start to develop within 30–60 min after death and is usually fixed after 8–12 h. In infants, lividity may develop more quickly than in older children or adults because of their thinner skin (Griest 2010). The time course in older children is not exactly known but may be comparable to that in adults. Sometimes, however, in very young children, one will hardly find any development of livor. Livor is sometimes misinterpreted as antemortem bruising. Livor tends to be more diffuse with indistinct borders, while bruising mostly will show distinct borders and is rarely diffuse. Before the livor is fixed, it will blanch under pressure with an object or under diascopy, while bruises do not blanch. In doubt, livor mortis and bruising can be differentiated by incising the skin. In bruises, the bleeding is present in the subcutaneous tissues. In livor, the blood will stay confined to the vascular system (Griest 2010).

Sometimes, one may see findings in livor which may resemble patterned injuries (Figs. 3.12, 3.13, 3.14, 3.15, 3.16, 3.17, and 3.18).

3.2.3 Dating of Bruises

3.2.3.1 Supposed Principles of Dating

In the past, the attempts to globally date bruises were based on the color changes that occurred while the bruise was healing. However, the initial color of a bruise depends on the natural color of the skin (in humans, this varies from very pale to deeply pigmented), the depth below the surface, and the viscosity of the accumulated blood. A superficial and fresh bruise tends to appear as red (Fig. 3.19), a deep bruise as blue or even almost black, and a less deep bruise as purple (Robinson 2000).

The color changes are the result of hemoglobin degradation during the hours and days after the bruise was sustained. During the initial period after a bruise has developed, hemoglobin pigment is released by hemolysis. The pigment is subsequently taken up by the phagocytes where

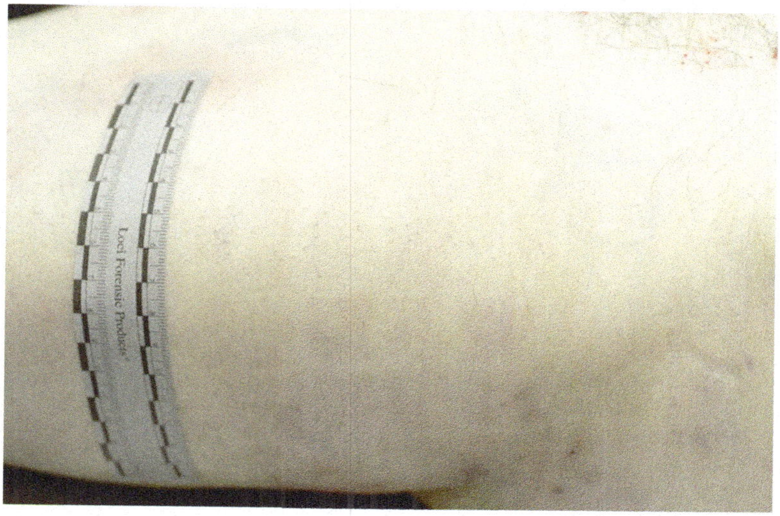

Fig. 3.12 Findings in livor mortis resembling pattern injuries

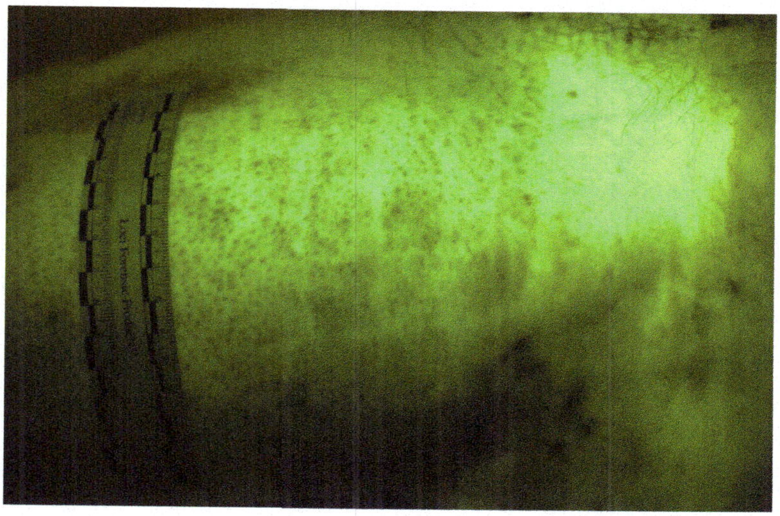

Fig. 3.13 Findings in livor mortis resembling pattern injuries (forensic light)

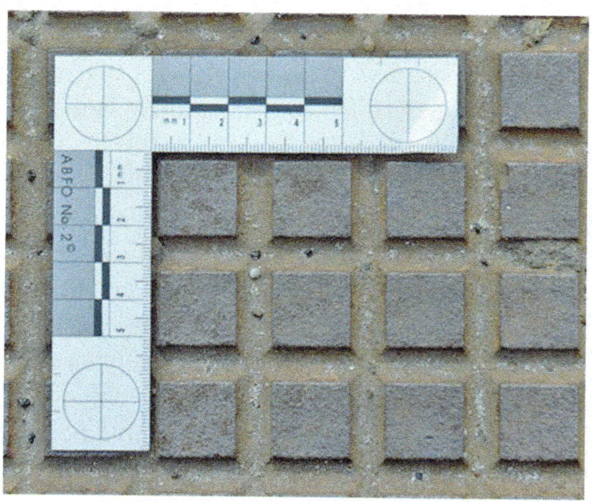

Fig. 3.14 Findings in livor mortis resembling pattern injuries: pattern caused by a manhole cover

Fig. 3.15 Findings in livor mortis resembling pattern injuries

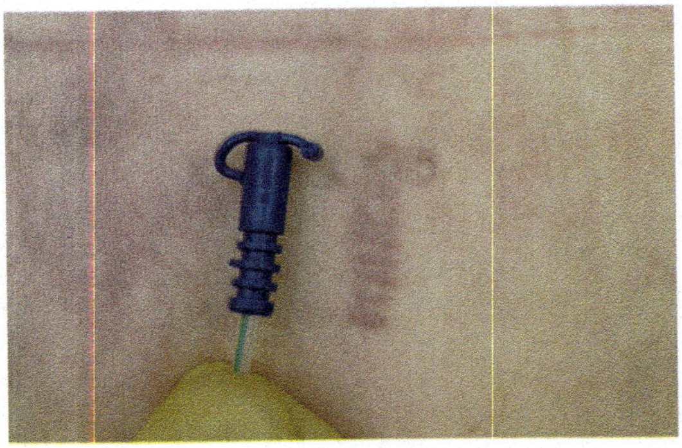

Fig. 3.16 Findings in livor mortis resembling pattern injuries

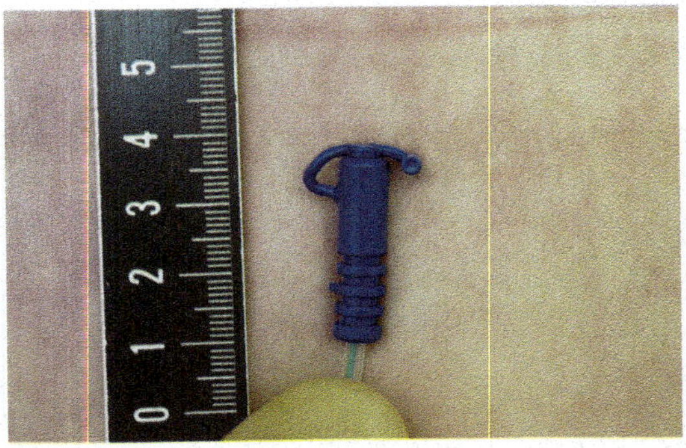

Fig. 3.17 Findings in livor mortis resembling pattern injuries: pattern caused by a medical device

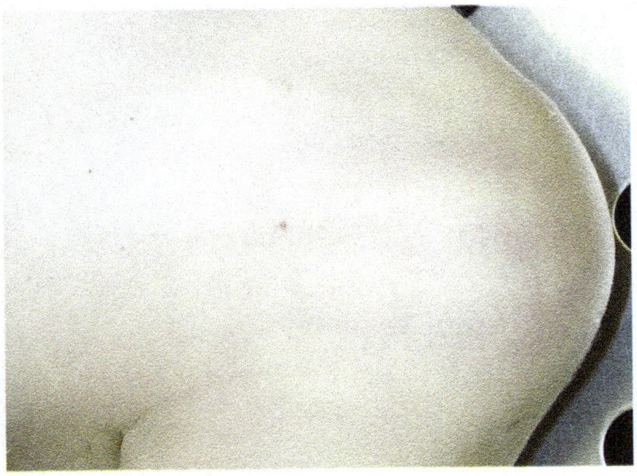

Fig. 3.18 Findings in livor mortis resembling pattern injuries: handprint

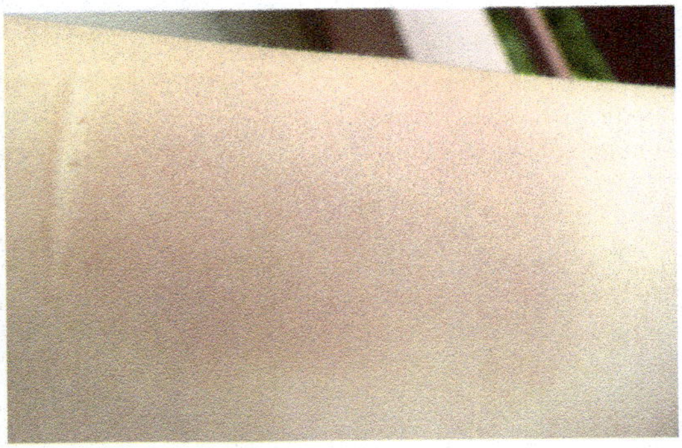

Fig. 3.19 Superficial bruise: uniform *red* color – fresh, less than a couple of hours (Rama 2005 from Wikimedia Commons 2007: Hematome-p1000482.jpg)

degradation to iron pigment takes place. Finally, the degradation products are converted into hemosiderin, which remains present for months or years (Busuttil 2004; Saukko and Knight 2004a; Harris and Flaherty 2011).

The change is first and most prominently seen at places where the blood deposit is thinnest, mostly around the margins of the bruise, whereas in the thickest areas, the bruise retains its initial color longest (Robinson 2000). Consequently, a bruise can show multiple colors at the same time, for example, red to purple in the center to yellow at the edges of the bruise (Figs. 3.20 and 3.21).

Not all colors (described in Table 3.1) will appear during the healing process of a bruise. Bruises of different shades of color on different locations may have developed simultaneously as well in children as adults. The speed with which the color changes take place depends on the age and health of the individual concerned, the lymphatic and the venous drainage of the damaged skin, and the phagocytic activity at the site of the bruise. In children, bruises heal rapidly, unless the bruises are substantial, and may reabsorb over a number of days. An overview of the color changes seen during the degradation of hemoglobin is provided in Table 3.1.

Many schemes have been used in the past, for example, the empirical schemes of Wilson (1977) and Reece and Grodin (1985). Speight even proposed a time scale in hours for superficial bruises (Speight 1997). When these schemes are compared, they show that dating based solely on color changes is not reliable.

In bruises, color changes (the visible healing process) are influenced by numerous factors (David 2005). Due to intra- and interindividual

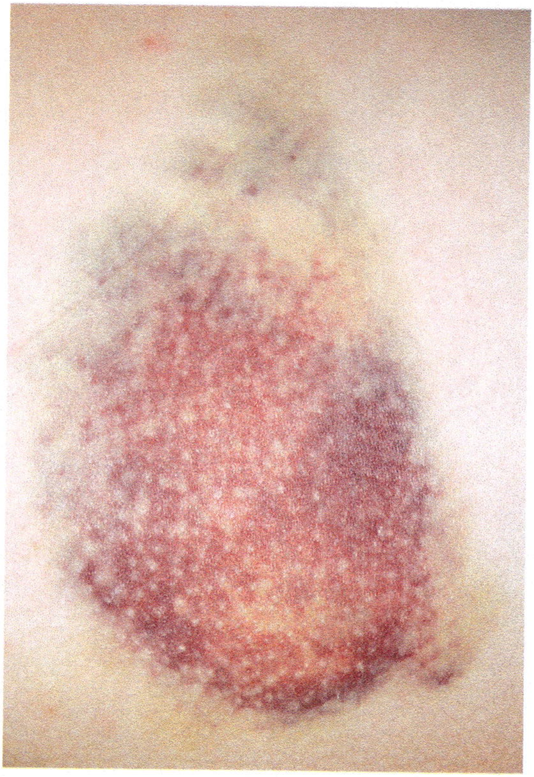

Fig. 3.20 Healing bruise: *red*, *green*, and *yellow* discoloration – at least 18-h-old (Kos and Shwayder 2006 from Wikimedia Commons 2011: Hématome.jpg)

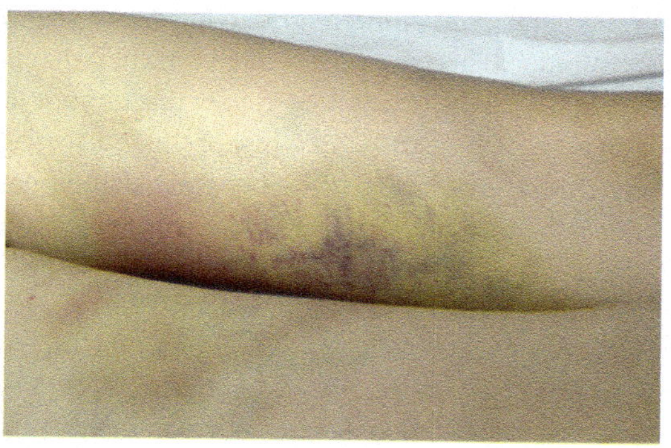

Fig. 3.21 Healing bruise: *red*, *green*, and *yellow* discoloration – at least 18-h-old

differences in healing, it is difficult to date bruises in children. Moreover, the depth of the bruise also plays a role: in superficial bruises, the yellow discoloration is visible earlier than in deeper bruises. The location of the bruise is also important: bruises on the face (eyelids, lips, cheeks) and on the genitalia (vulva, scrotum) (in "loose" tissues) and bruises on the back of the hand, the wrists, the elbows, the eye sockets, the eyebrows, and on the hip shaft will become visible earlier than those at other sites. After an assault, a bruise may develop almost immediately on the eyelids, whereas deeper bruises may not be visible even after a number of days (body-site variations).

Table 3.1 Color changes during the degradation of hemoglobin (Busuttil 2004; Saukko and Knight 2004a; Harris and Flaherty 2011) (Figs. 3.19, 3.20, 3.21, 3.22, 3.23, 3.24, and 3.25)

Color	Hemoglobin and degradation products
Red	Hemoglobin pigment + local inflammatory reaction
Blue	Deoxygenated, unsaturated Hb
Purple	
Brown	
Greenish	Biliverdin – hematoidin
Yellow	Bilirubin
Straw color	
Disappearance	Hemosiderin

3.2.3.2 Subjective and Objective Interpretation of the Color

Stephenson and Bialas (1996) conducted a prospective study into the color and the changes in color of bruises for which they used the photographs of 50 accidental bruises in 23 children. The individual who was assigned to evaluate the photograph was unaware of the moment of accident. It appeared that it was not possible to establish the dating accurately. The participants in the study were able to establish correct dating in 55% of the photographs. It also appeared that the individual who had conducted the physical examination was generally more accurate in dating the injury than those who did this on the basis of the photographs. In this study, red coloring was observed in 15 of the 37 bruises within a week after developing. In 10 of the 42 bruises, discoloration was already present after 1 day.

The findings of Stephenson were confirmed in a study by Munang et al. (2002). Three clinicians were asked to date 58 bruises in 44 children. The bruises were then photographed, and the same

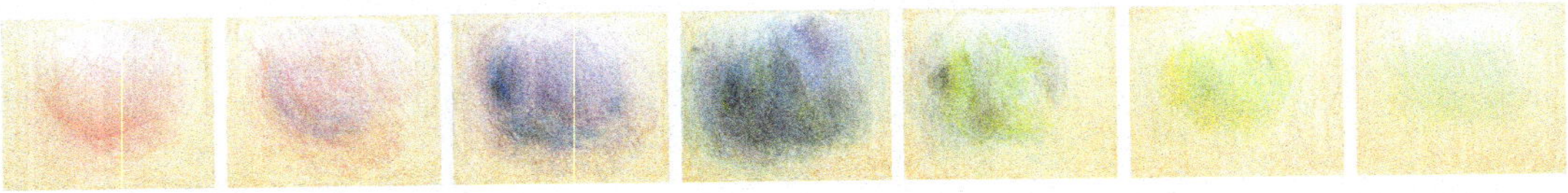

Fig. 3.22 Most common changes in color of a bruise in time (from immediately after the trauma up to weeks)

Fig. 3.23 Healing bruise: *greenish* discoloration

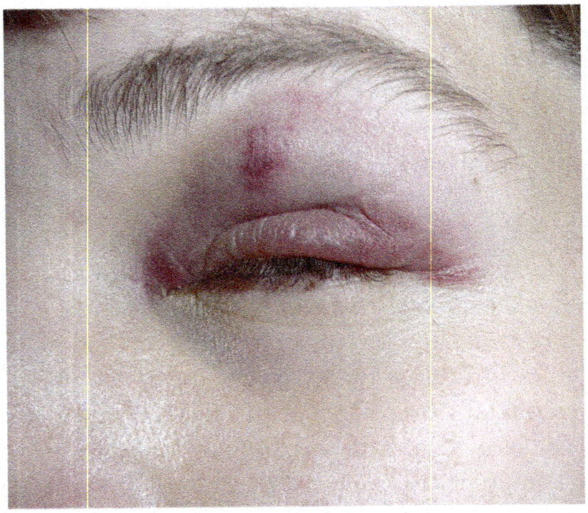

Fig. 3.24 Black eye, 2nd day (Pavel Ševela 2010 from Wikimedia Commons: Black eye (2).jpg)

observers described the bruises at a later date. In only 27% of cases, the observers reached consensus when evaluating the bruise during physical examination. When the observers were asked to evaluate the same bruises on photographs, consensus was reached in only 24%. In 31% of cases, the descriptions of the observers completely concurred with the later description of a photograph of the same bruise.

Langlois and Gresham (1991) conducted a prospective study using 369 photographs of

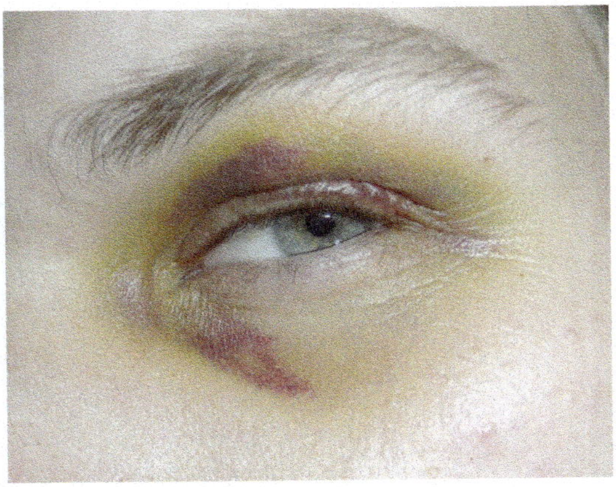

Fig. 3.25 Black eye, 3rd day (Pavel Ševela 2010 from Wikimedia Commons: Black eye (3).jpg)

bruises of known cause and time of development (varying from less than 6 h to 21 days) in 89 Caucasians aged 10–100 years. They concluded that after a trauma, yellow discoloration developed after a minimum of 18 h and that this discoloration appeared more rapidly in individuals who were older than 65 years. Moreover, they determined that in the absence of yellow discoloration, it could not be established whether the bruise was less than 18-h-old. Other colors are less reliable, even when taking the fact into account that no consensus could be reached between the various investigators on which color was visible. A red, blue, purple, and black discoloration of the bruise may either be visible or become visible at any time, ranging from 1 h after development to its disappearance (up to 21 days). Redness may be present at all stages, from development to healing. They also noted that bruises of the same age and cause presented with different colors and showed different color changes per individual. Based on the above study, the only conclusion that can be reached is that the yellow discoloration shows that the bruise is at least 18-h-old (Langlois and Gresham 1991).

Vanezis (1997), (quoted from Robinson 2000) used and so on color photometry to date bruises and concluded that yellow discoloration is visible after about 24 h. Vanezis also concluded that using color photometry did not improve the accuracy of the dating.

Bariciak et al. (2003) showed that there was no significant relation between the colors red/blue and purple and recent bruises and between the colors yellow/brown and green and older bruises. Bariciak also reported that all colors can be found at all stages (fresh, average old, and old). Similar findings were also reported by Stephenson and Bialas (1996).

The results concerning the yellow discoloration were confusing in the studies by Stephenson and Bialas (1996), Carpenter (1999), and Bariciak et al. (2003), although they did not contradict the initial findings reported by Langlois and Gresham (1991). Stephenson found a yellow discoloration in ten bruises only after 24 h, Carpenter found a yellow discoloration after 48 h, and Bariciak always found a yellow/green/brown discoloration within 48 h.

The review by Maguire et al. (2005a, b) showed that the accuracy of physicians to date bruises within 24 h after occurrence was less than 40%. The accuracy with which the physicians were able to determine whether it was a fresh, an average old, and an old bruise varied from 55–63%. Intra- and interobserver reliability was poor.

3.2.3.3 The Role of Histology/Histopathology in Dating

According to DiMaio, histological investigation is still only indicative for dating bruises (DiMaio and DiMaio 2001b). David's (2004) view differs from DiMaio's. According to David, color change schemes are unreliable, but sometimes, histopathological investigation is useful in deceased children. The pathologist can distinguish between very fresh bruises (no visible cellular reaction), recent bruises (visible neutrophil infiltration), and (by estimation) those older than 2–3 days (incontinence of hemosiderin present – iron deposition) (Fig. 3.26).

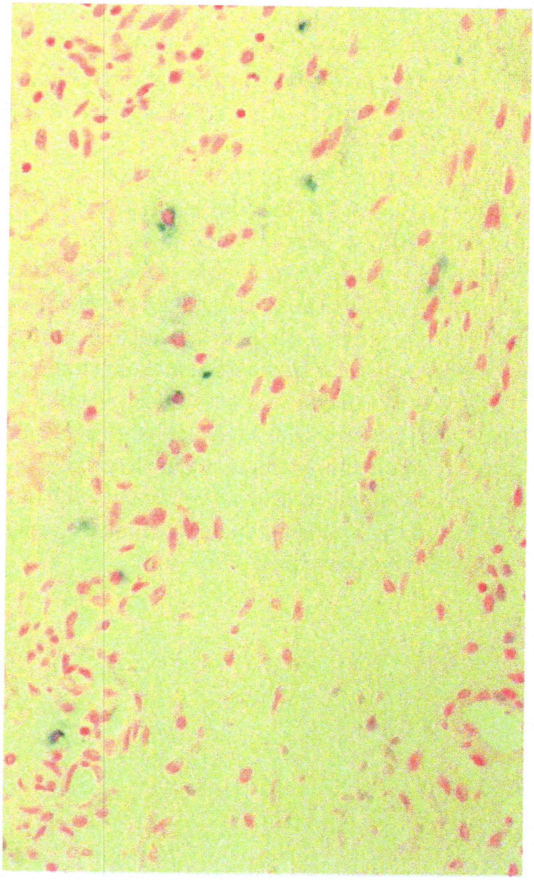

Fig. 3.26 Iron deposition visible (*blue color*): most probably at least 2- to 3-days-old

3.2.3.4 Conclusion on Dating Bruises

It can be concluded that at present, there is no scientific basis for an accurate dating of bruises based on color changes (Schwartz and Ricci 1996; Stephenson and Bialas 1996; Carpenter 1999; Munang et al. 2002; Bariciak et al. 2003; David 2004, 2005; Maguire et al. 2005a, b). Only yellow discoloration indicates that a bruise is at least 18-h-old (Langlois and Gresham 1991). If absent, however, it cannot be concluded that the bruise is less than 18-h-old. Yellow discoloration does not give an indication of the maximum age of the bruise (Fig. 3.27).

There are no reliable data known at what age bruises are no longer visible. Disappearance of the visibility of a bruise depends on many factors, including the type of loading (static or dynamic), the depth of the injury, the type of injured tissue, diffusion of the blood through the damaged tissue, and may take days to many weeks (Wilson 1977; Reece and Grodin 1985; Schwartz and Ricci 1996; Payne-James 2003).

According to Maguire et al. (2005a, b), dating should not be used within the scope of child protection. Based on color changes, no definite statement can be made regarding the age of a bruise. The dating of bruises can and should only be used in order to estimate whether the explanation provided by the parents or the child at which time the injury was sustained is correct. In fact, in order to distinguish between accidental and non-accidental cause, it is more important to establish whether the appearance of the bruise is consistent with the mentioned cause rather than establishing the probable time it was sustained (Table 3.2).

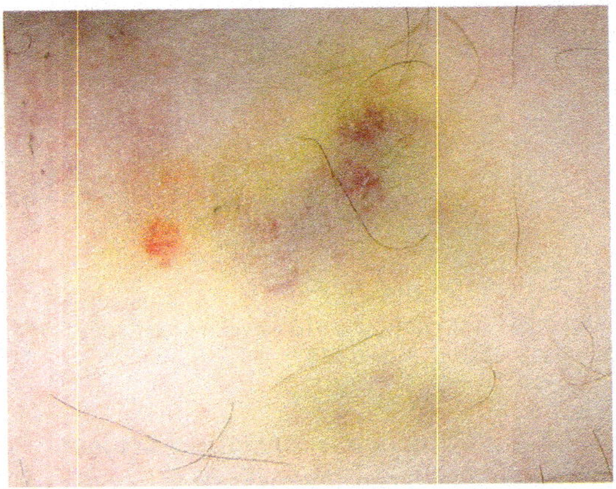

Fig. 3.27 Bruise, 9 days after taking a blood sample (MykReeve 2005 from Wikimedia Commons 2011: Myk-haematoma.jpg)

3.2.3.5 Dating of Subconjunctival Hemorrhage and Bleeding Under Mucous Membranes

It is impossible to date subconjunctival bleeding based on color changes since the bleeding changes color rarely or not at all. It is suggested that the hemoglobin continues to be oxygenated by the surrounding air via the epithelial membrane of the conjunctiva and therefore would not undergo the same degradation as in the skin (Busuttil 2004). A subconjunctival bleeding will almost always disappear completely and spontaneously within 1–2 weeks (Merck Manual 2007), although it may take longer (Figs. 3.28, 3.29, 3.30, and 3.31). Discoloration may subside from red (fresh bleeding) via a little greenish to yellow in a few days (Merck Manual 2007).

According to Lee (2008), bleeding under the mucous membranes does not undergo color changes and for that reason can never, not even indicatively, be dated.

3.2.4 Types of Bruising

When the force applied is sufficient to deform the skin and subcutaneous tissues and to rupture blood vessels (subcutaneous venules and capillaries), it will lead to bruising. Damage to the vessels leads to loss of blood from the intravascular space into the skin and subcutaneous tissues. Because of this extravasation of blood, bruises do not blanch under pressure and show a characteristic color, which usually changes in time (Hobbs et al. 1999a, b). However, in the first stage, the bright red color of the bruises is not just determined by

Table 3.2 Indicative dating of bruises (Simpson 1979; Busuttil 2004; Saukko and Knight 2004a)

Dating	Histopathology	Color
Very fresh (<several hours)	No visible cellular reaction	Red (red color may be present at any stage of healing)
Recent	Neutrophilic infiltration	
>18 h		Yellow/green
<24 h		Even discoloration
>24 h	Hemosiderin present in minority of cases	
<48 h		No observable color change
>2–3 days	Hemosiderin present in most cases	
>1 week	Hematoidin	Yellow-brown

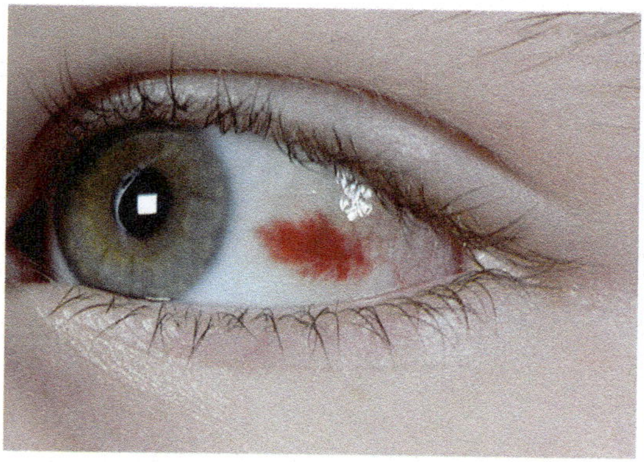

Fig. 3.28 Subconjunctival bleeding: unknown date

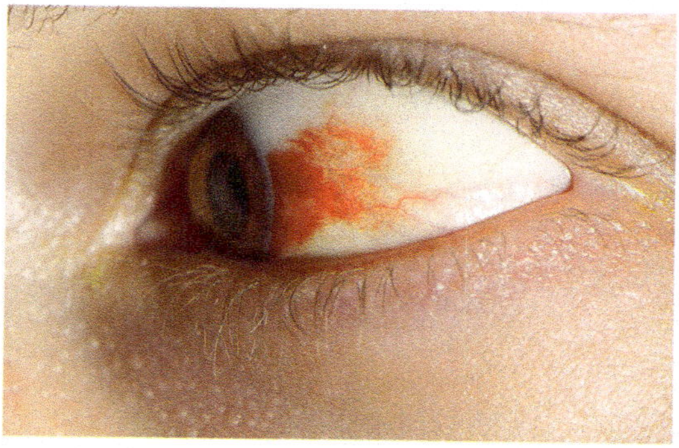

Fig. 3.29 Subconjunctival bleeding: 48-h-old (Daniel Flather 2011 from Wikimedia Commons 2011: Subconjunctival hemorrhage eye.jpg)

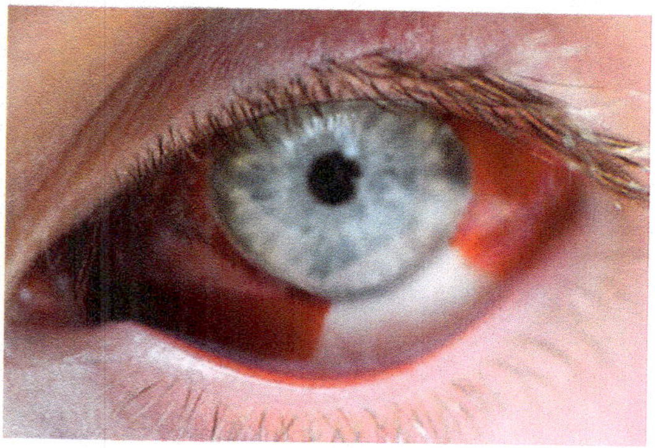

Fig. 3.30 Subconjunctival bleeding: 1-week-old (Therealbs2002 2010 from Wikimedia Commons 2011: Subconjunctival hemorrhage before after.jpg)

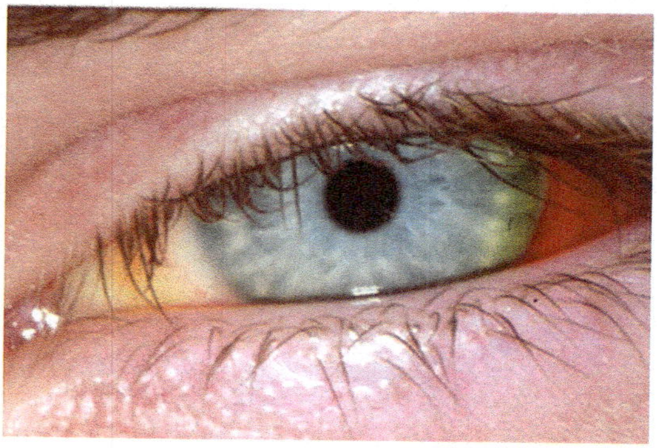

Fig. 3.31 Subconjunctival bleeding: 4-weeks-old (Therealbs2002 2010 from Wikimedia Commons 2011: Subconjunctival hemorrhage before after.jpg)

the extravasation of blood into the dermis and the loose subcutaneous connective tissues but also by local capillary dilatation and an inflammatory reaction (red, tender, and swollen) of the impact site and the surrounding area, which is due to the release of histamines (Jenny and Reece 2009). The major part of the swelling that develops in a bruise is due to the inflammatory response to the trauma and only partially the result of the extravasation of blood.

Deformation of the skin, ultimately leading to extravasation of blood, is caused by either static (compression) or dynamic (collision) loading of the skin (Chap. 2). Bruises (but also other injuries like burns) may show a recognizable grouping or a specific shape, which will reflect how the injury was caused. These injuries are termed tell-tale injuries, pattern injuries, shaped injuries, or mirror injuries (Sect. 2.5.3) (Fig. 3.32).

3.2.5 Bruises and Child Abuse

3.2.5.1 Introduction

Bruises are the most frequently observed injuries in child abuse and are present in up to 90% of physically abused children (Hobbs et al. 1999a, b; Maguire et al. 2005a, b; Hammond 2009). Johnson and Showers (1985) mention that in a children's hospital, bruising was the reason for reporting suspected child physical abuse in 52% of cases.

The nature, size, and location of non-accidental bruises vary and depend largely on the "object" used, the actions of the perpetrator during the assault, and the type of loading (Sect. 2.5) (Table 3.3). Static or dynamic loading combined with a specific object and a specific action may

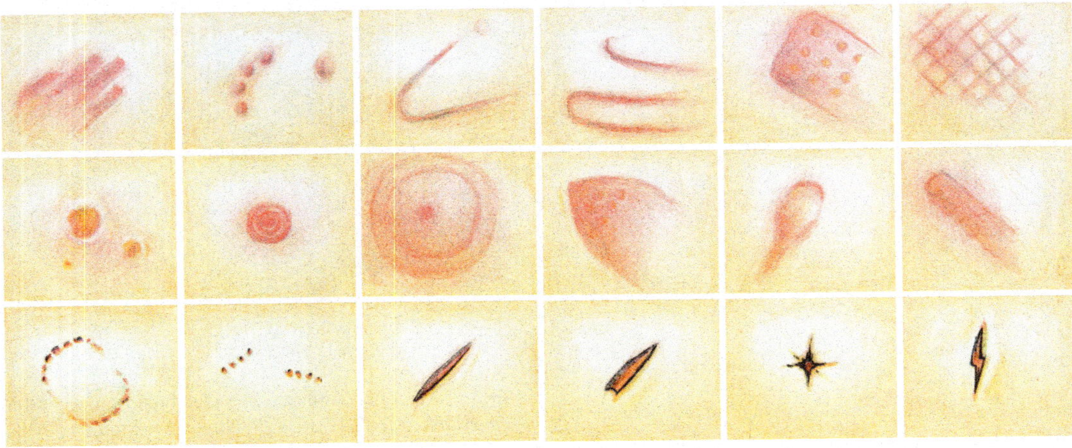

Fig. 3.32 Tell-tale injuries (Johnson 1996)

Table 3.3 Bruising in child abuse

Objects	Actions
Dynamic (rapid) impact loading	
Body parts	
Hands, fingers, fist	Hitting, slapping
Elbow	Punching
Feet (with or without wearing shoes)	Prodding, poking
Knee	Kicking
Head (forehead)	Butting
Implements	
Flexible (cable, rope, belt)	Beating
Rigid (stick, baseball bat, buckle, shoe, slipper, hairbrush, clothes hanger, kitchen utensils, bottle)	Poking, prodding
Static loading	
Body parts	
Hand/fingers	Pinching Grabbing, gripping Compressing: choking, strangulating
Teeth (Chap. 8)	Biting
Implements	
Flexible (cable, rope, belt)	Tying Gagging Choking, strangulating
Rigid (clothes peg, bench vice)	Compressing

lead to injuries that biomechanically fit the type of loading, object, and action, so-called pattern injuries, tell-tale injuries, shaped injuries, or mirror injuries (Sect. 2.5.3). One of the "tell-tales" of some injuries will be that the pattern or shape and location mirror the infliction and cannot be explained through play or normal interactions with other children or adults.

According to Johnson and Showers (1985), the diversity of abnormalities seen in child abuse indicates that in most cases, an angry perpetrator grabs the object that is directly at hand during a

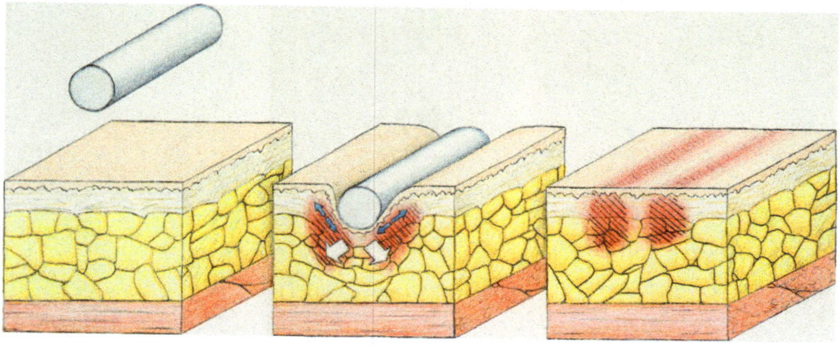

Fig. 3.33 Tramline bruising caused by hitting with a round subject

crisis and uses it to hit the child. This also indicates that in most of the physical assaults, there is no preconceived plan to inflict damage to the child.

In principle, the range of objects that may be used during the assault is unlimited. The only limitation is determined by the objects at hand during the crisis that provokes the assault. Consequently, the objects involved may be potentially life-threatening, for example, a knife or a fork, which may cause deep penetrating injuries.

In case of "planned" abuse, the "fantasy" of the perpetrator for "disciplining" the child is the only limitation for the object used. The perpetrator may use any object, which he or she is accustomed to use for "disciplining" the child.

The nature, size, and location of the bruises are not only determined by the object, actions, and type of loading but also by the posture of the child during the assault. The type of clothing worn by the child during the assault may also play a role. The pattern of the weave of the clothing may lead to a more or less superimposed imprint in the injury caused by the actions of the perpetrator.

Bruises in child abuse do not only occur as a result of an object hitting the child but also because the child is dropped, thrown, swung (dynamic loading), or pushed (static loading) against a solid object, for example, the floor or a wall.

3.2.5.2 Dynamic Impact Loading: Tramline Bruising

Dynamic impact loading may lead to a typical phenomenon known as "tramline" bruising. "Tramline bruising" or "railway bruising" results from a "high-velocity" impact on the skin with a round or rectangular object. Tramline bruising is characterized by two parallel lines of bruising with an undamaged zone in between the lines (Saukko and Knight 2004a) (Figs. 3.33, 3.34, and 3.35). This type of bruising often shows a curved closed end, which implies the use of a cylindrical implement, for example, a baton, baseball bat, or stick (Robinson 2000). It can also be seen

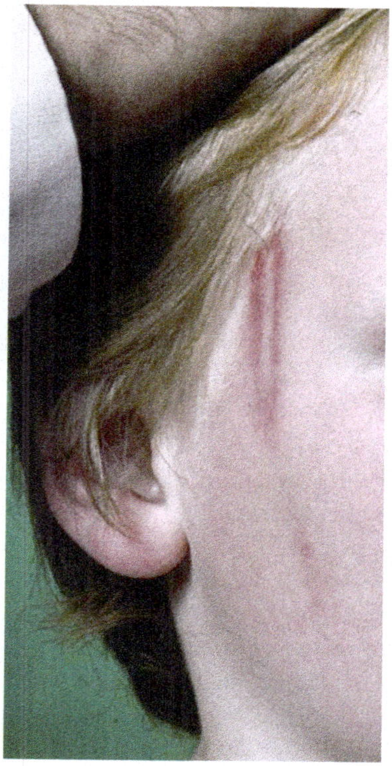

Fig. 3.34 Tramline bruising caused by hitting with a stick

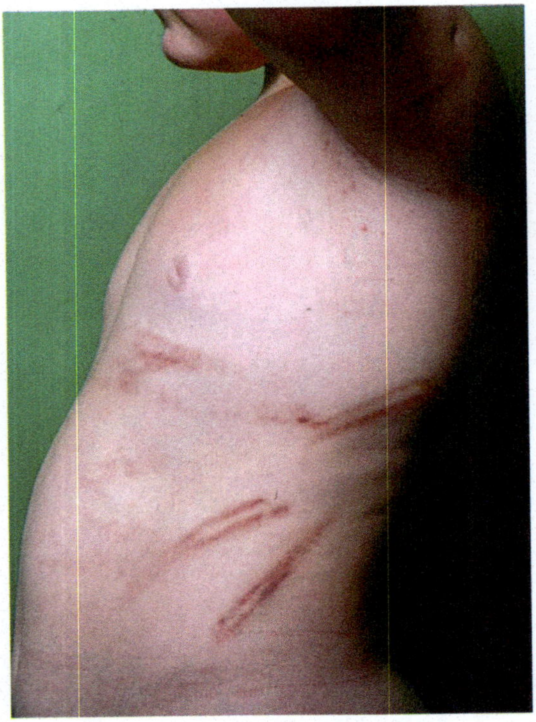

Fig. 3.35 Same patient as in Fig. 3.34

when a child is slapped in the face with an open hand (outline bruising).

In case of using a rigid implement like a baton, the bruising will not or only partially follow the body contours. Tramline bruising may follow the body contours, which implies the use of a flexible implement. In that case, the bruising may show a somewhat broadening curved closed end (Nathanson 2000). According to Robinson (2000), tramline bruising can also be seen if a person has been beaten with a flat strip like a ruler.

The two parallel lines of a tramline bruise are caused by the subjection of the skin to maximal distortion of the capillaries and venules at the "stretching" margins during the impact. This will lead to the rupture of vessels and extravasation of blood. During the impact, the vessels at the site of compression are not or only slightly damaged.

Oval bruising with a pallid center is a variant of tramline bruising and is indicative for injuries which were inflicted with an object with a rounded surface, such as a baseball or squash ball, which impacts the skin. It can also be caused

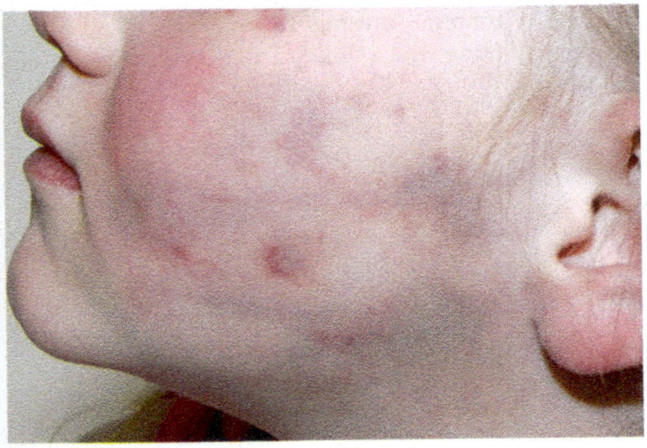

Fig. 3.36 Slapping in the face

by, for example, fast poking with a truncheon or beating with a wooden spoon (Robinson 2000).

3.2.5.3 Dynamic Impact Loading: Using of Hands and Feet

Hand Marks

The perpetrator almost always uses his or her dominant hand in a physical assault against a child. This creates a possibility to differentiate between right- and left-handed perpetrators. If one suspects hand marks, it is convenient to see if the suspicious bruise matches one's own hand. This makes it easier to identify a hand imprint and to distinguish between bruises resulting from an adult hand and those from a child's hand.

Slapping

Parallel lines, consisting of grouped petechiae and corresponding to the interphalangeal spaces (Glasgow and Graham 1997), often finger-sized and demarcating two or three fingers, may be found during physical examination (outline bruising – hand mark). Especially in the acute phase, a hand imprint or linear finger marks may be visible when a child has been slapped with an open hand. These marks, caused by imprint of the fingers, resemble tramline bruising but are often less well demarcated than the typical tramline bruising caused by objects. The most prevalent location is the left cheek (most perpetrators are right-handed and will slap the child with their dominant hand while facing the child) or the buttocks (Figs. 3.36 and 3.37). Occasionally, the bruise merges at the site where the finger and the

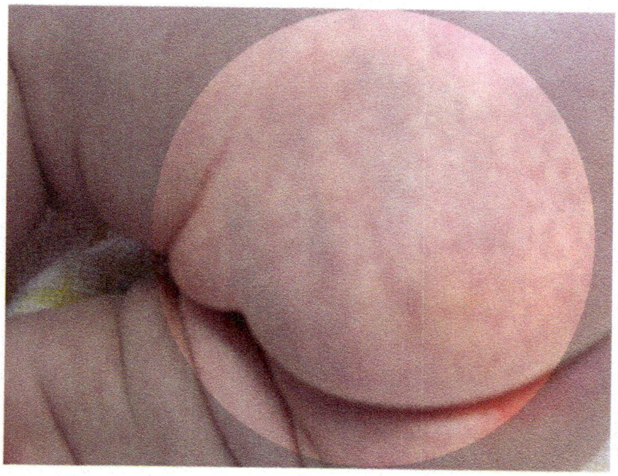

Fig. 3.37 Slapping on the buttocks

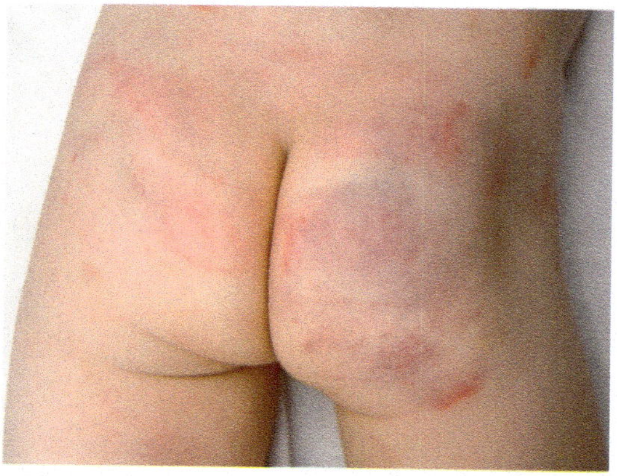

Fig. 3.38 Extensive bruising of the buttocks with vertical gluteal cleft injuries: always non-accidental – caused by severe beating with hand, implement, or both

palm come together, sometimes resulting in a more diffuse and extensive bruising on the cheek or the buttocks (Fig. 3.38). Sometimes, a conspicuous bruise is seen at the site of a ring (e.g., on the face and on the buttocks) if the perpetrator is wearing a ring on the hand used for slapping – a typical tell-tale mark (Robinson 2000). Also, superficial abrasions caused by the fingernails can sometimes be found near slapping injuries (Glasgow and Graham 1997). A combination of two or three parallel linear "outline" bruises of fingerbreadth may be encountered in a more diffuse bruise on the cheek (Schmitt 1987). If a slapmark is found on the cheeks, one should always look for retro-auricular bruising and for a laceration of the tympanum (Herrmann et al. 2008).

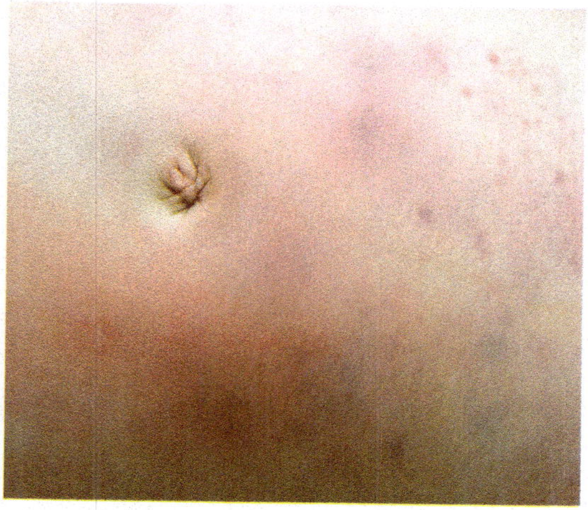

Fig. 3.39 At least four larger and several smaller bruises on the lower abdomen

Bruises resulting from slapping with an open hand may fade rapidly (Kornberg 1992).

When a child is slapped with the open hand or when the perpetrator is wearing a ring, a laceration may develop at the site where the skin is most taut.

Sometimes, bruising does not "follow" the shape of the inflicting object, to "create" a pattern injury, for example, the hand, but follows the contours of the anatomic structures. This is the case in the so-called vertical gluteal cleft injuries (Feldman 1992), sometimes also referred to as crimping bruising of the buttocks (Hammond 2009). The child squeezes the buttocks and the gluteal cleft together when slapped there. Bruising is not found in the gluteal cleft, but linear bruises are found on the edges that run parallel to the gluteal cleft.

Punching

The injury that results from punching with a fist depends on the body site involved. The most targeted body part in punching is the face. Sometimes, imprints of the "knuckles" (also known as a "monocle bruising") as a series of round bruises are visible, and sometimes, there is diffuse, often severe bruising of the face (penetrating recesses such as the eye socket) (Hobbs et al. 1999a, b). One should always look for injuries of the eyes, intraoral damage (e.g., of the oral mucosa, especially on the inside of the

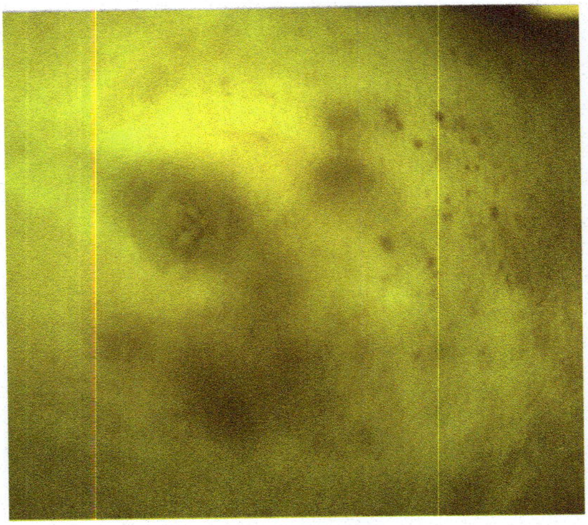

Fig. 3.40 Same patient as in Fig. 3.39: using forensic light – at least four dark lesions in a partially semicircular configuration suggestive for repetitive punching or kicking

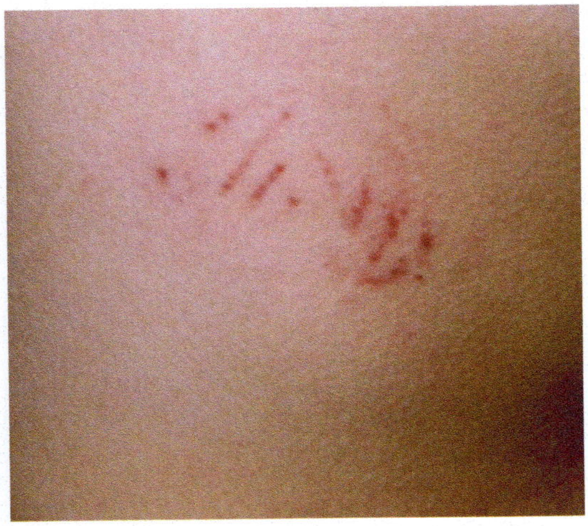

Fig. 3.41 Shoe print

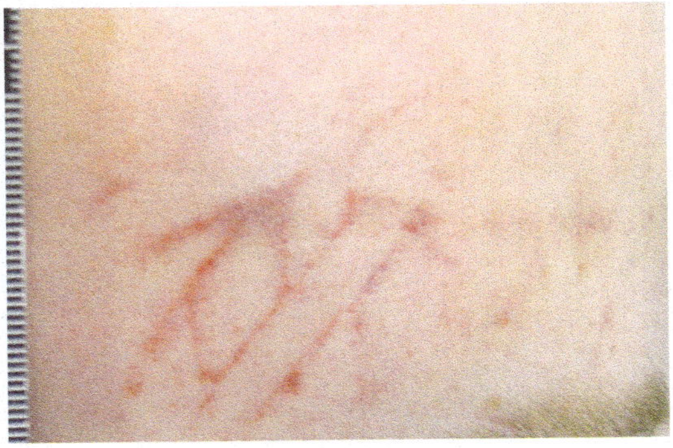

Fig. 3.42 Shoe print on forehead

lips), and dental fractures (Herrmann et al. 2008). The second most targeted body part is the abdomen, which can lead to contusions and lacerations of the intra-abdominal organs, often without externally visible bruising and sometimes with significant bruising (Figs. 3.38, 3.39, and 3.40).

Poking

After heavy-handed poking, clusters of 3–4 round or oval bruises of about 1 cm in diameter may be found, which are predominantly seen on the anterior upper chest (Wynne 2003). Poking with one finger may also result in one bruise of about 1 cm in diameter. Rough poking may leave fingernail cuts on the skin (Hobbs et al. 1999a, b). If the child falls during prodding, bruising may also be found on the opposite side of the body (Schmitt 1987).

Foot Marks: Kicking and Stamping

The severity of the injuries in kicking depends on the speed of the kick, the position of the child (standing or lying down), the site of impact, whether the perpetrator is wearing shoes or not, and the part of the foot (toes, sole, or heel) used to kick.

Kicking with the toes or the toecap results in large, irregularly shaped bruises. These are usually seen on the lower half of the body (Hobbs et al. 1999a, b), although all parts of the body, for example, the head or the thorax, can be affected. Sometimes, the bruise reflects the shape of the shoe (Figs. 3.41, 3.42, 3.43, and 3.44). Bruises are usually located at the site where the child has been kicked. However, sometimes, especially when the child has been kicked in the belly, bruising will only become visible after several days, whereby the bruise is eventually found at a site other than the trauma site, for example, in the groin. If one suspects that the child has been kicked in the belly, liver functions should be determined.

If the child is already lying down on the floor, the perpetrator may stop kicking with the toes or the toecap and stamp down (bringing the foot

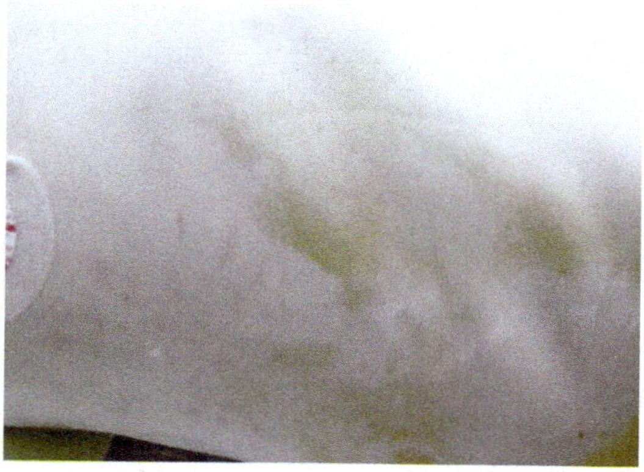

Fig. 3.43 Hardly visible shoe print on the left side of the thorax

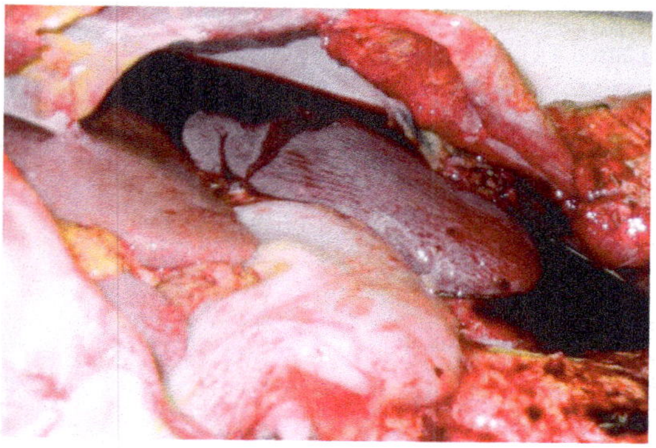

Fig. 3.44 Same patient as in Fig. 3.43: fatal rupture of the spleen, probably caused by the kicking which left the shoe print on the left side of the thorax

vertically down) on the body with a bare foot or the sole/heel of the shoe. If the perpetrator is wearing a shoe, this may lead to a recognizable pattern injury.

Kicking or stamping will lead to more serious complications than hitting or slapping with the hand. On the one hand, this is due to the severity of the bruising and the amount of extravasated blood in the skin and/or internal organs and, on the other hand, to the increased risk for underlying damage (fractures, contusion of or damage to internal organs). In case of intra-abdominal injuries, externally visible injuries may be absent.

3.2.5.4 Dynamic Impact Loading: Using of Implements

According to Newson and Newson (1986), at the age of 7 years ($n=700$ children), 26% of boys and 18% of girls had been hit by some kind of implement, in order of preference: strap or belt, cane or stick, slipper, and miscellaneous objects. However, in physical assault against children, implements are used less often than, the hands. The reasons for this are:

- Using implements is less accepted than using hands for disciplining children.
- Generally, it concerns an immediate action in a crisis, without any preconceived plan, whereby the child is beaten with whatever is at hand, usually the hand itself. If at that moment, there is an object, for example, a hairbrush, a comb, or a shoe at hand, then the perpetrator may use that object. However, sometimes the parent consciously chooses a particular object for disciplining children, for example, a belt or a stick.

When implements are used, characteristic pattern injuries may develop. Generally, it can be maintained that bruises and other cutaneous injuries with a markedly unusual appearance and a sharp border are the result of physical assault.

In order to establish whether a flexible or a rigid object was used in the assault, it is important to investigate whether the injury follows the natural contours of the child's body. If this is the case, then it is highly likely that the child was assaulted with a flexible object. If not, then the child was probably assaulted with a rigid object.

The violence used in striking on the back may be so severe that the underlying anatomical structures such as the ribs or the kidneys may be damaged (Raimer et al. 1981).

If one suspects that an implement is used, for example, because of a recognizable pattern injury, one should always try to obtain the object, so the object can be compared to the injury. The object should also be appropriately been measured and photographed.

Flexible Objects: Cable, Rope, and Belt

When a child is beaten with a flexible object, it may lead to various injuries (Figs. 3.45, 3.46, 3.47, 3.48, 3.49, 3.50, 3.51, 3.52, 3.53, 3.54, 3.55, and 3.56):

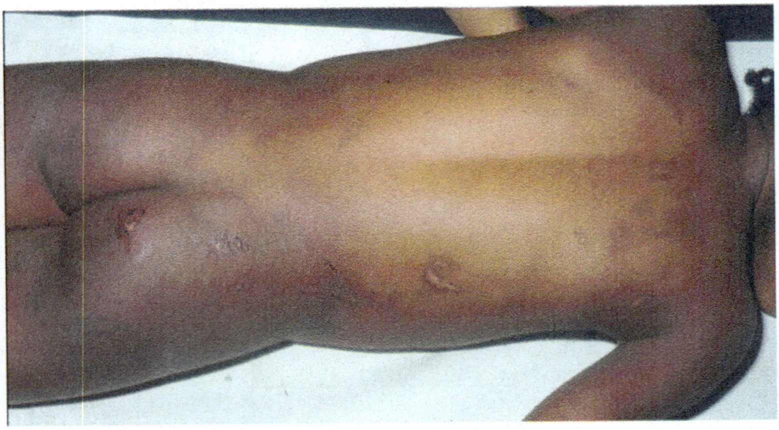

Fig. 3.45 Multiple injuries caused by hitting with an object. Some of the injuries are suggestive for beating with a flexible object, for example, on the back and on the front of the thighs (loop marks), other injuries are more suggestive for a more rigid object, for example, on the right leg (tramline bruising)

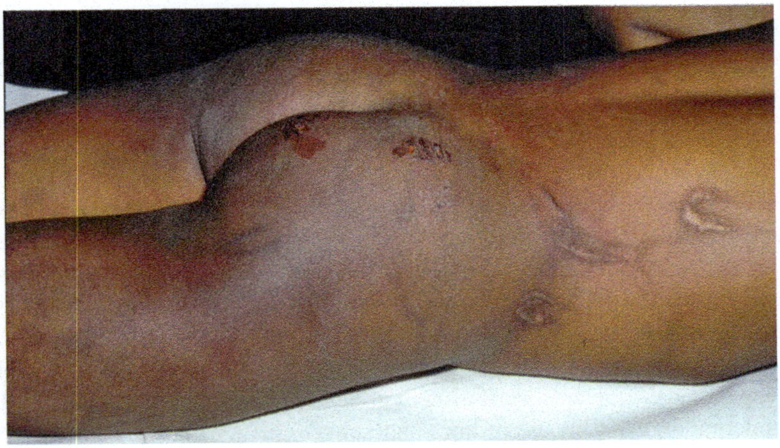

Fig. 3.46 Same child: scarring and loop marks

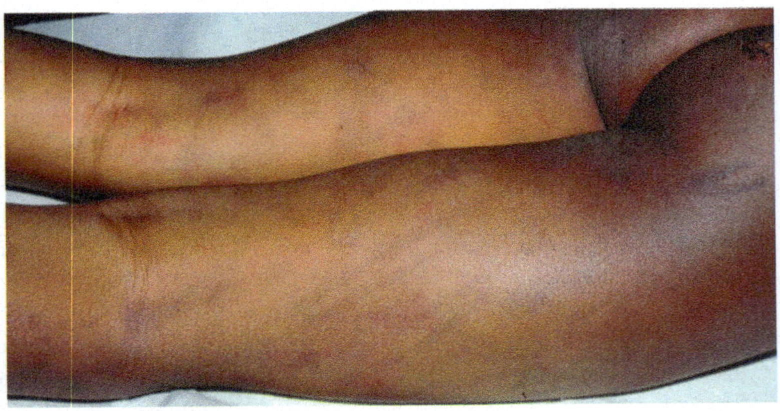

Fig. 3.47 Same child: tramline bruising

- Multiple loop-shaped bruises may develop when the cable/electrical cord or the rope was folded. Sometimes, this results in multiple looped-shaped lacerations and residual loop-shaped scars after healing (particularly on the extremities and on the back or buttocks): the distal part of the object impacts the skin with maximal force (Sussman 1968).
- Multiple linear bruises, sometimes with a characteristic shape and often sharp demarcation

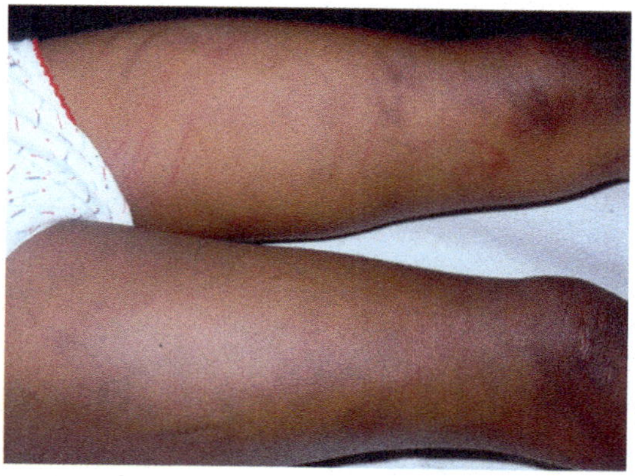

Fig. 3.48 Same child

(belt) or multiple linear lacerations (mainly on the extremities and on the back), may be seen when the cable or the rope was not folded. Similar small straight bruises or scratches will develop when the child is beaten with a twig or a branch.

Sometimes, similar injuries of the same age may be found on different parts of the child's body. This may indicate that the child has tried to protect itself as much as possible by changing position.

If sharply bordered rectangular bruises of varying length are encountered on the curved

Fig. 3.49 Same child: bruising of the right arm

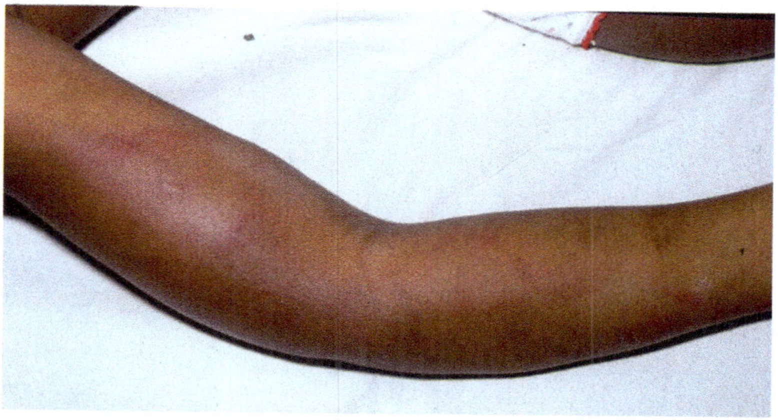

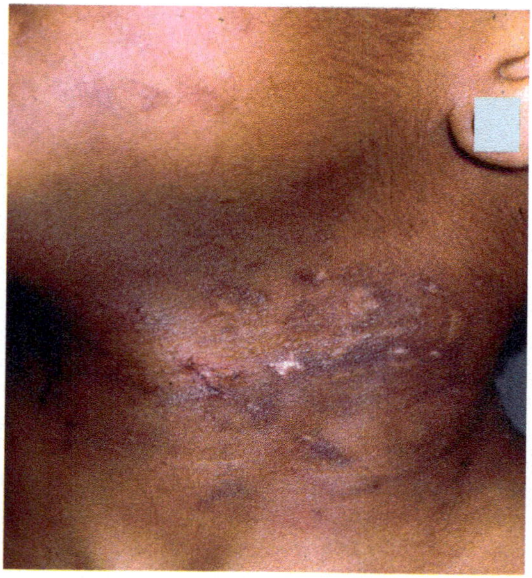

Fig. 3.50 Same child: scarring in the neck, suggestive for scratch marks and/or static fingernail imprints (see Chap. 7)

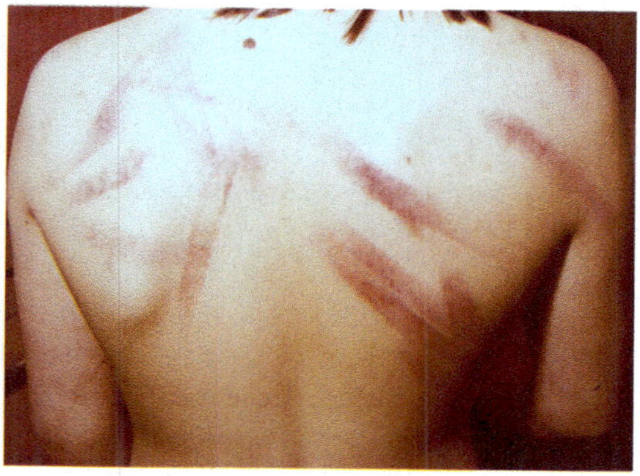

Fig. 3.51 Multiple belt marks

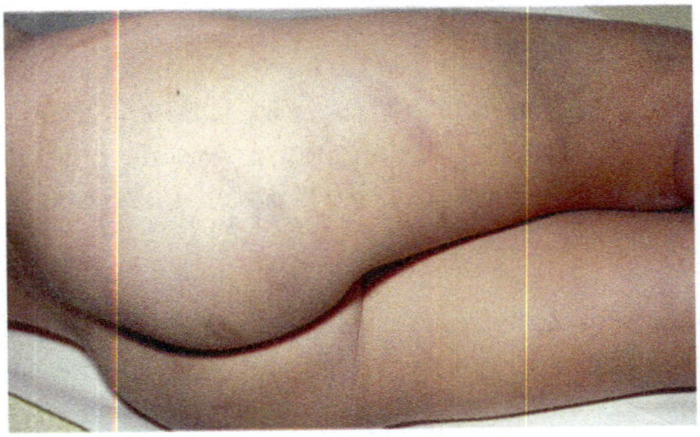

Fig. 3.52 Multiple bruises, probably belt marks

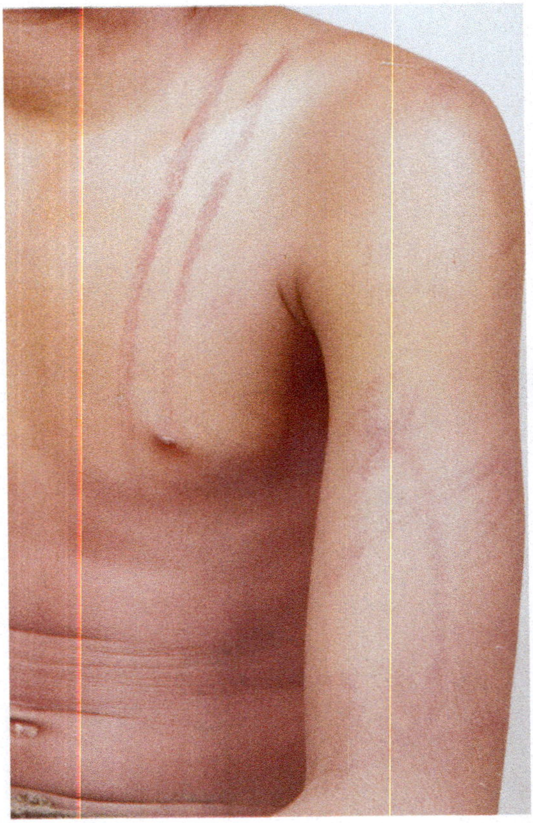

Fig. 3.53 Multiple loop-shaped bruises, caused by beating with a flexible object

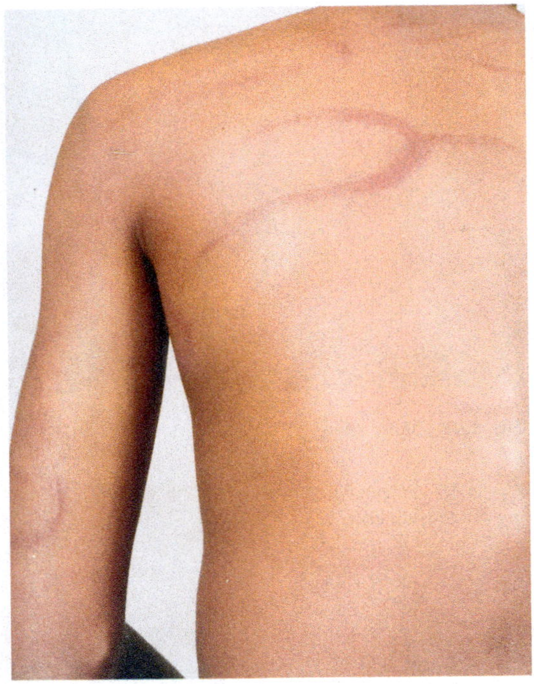

Fig. 3.54 Same child as in Fig. 3.53

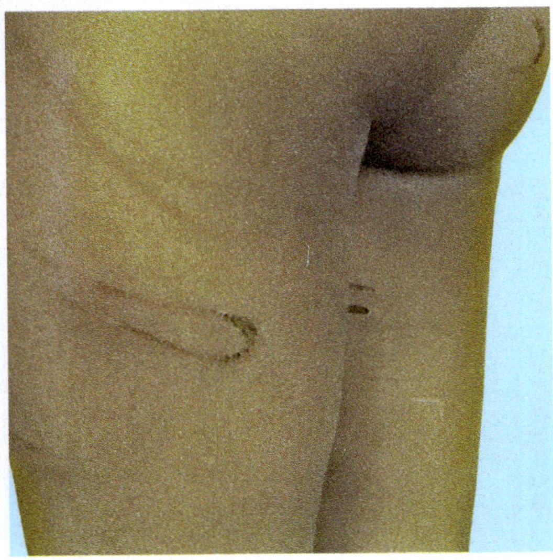

Fig. 3.55 Same child as in Fig. 3.53

surfaces of the body, such as the buttocks or the cheeks, then these are nearly always caused by an assault with a belt. Sometimes, imprints of the holes of the tongue of the belt or the shape of the buckle can still be seen (Sussman 1968).

If the perpetrator decides to use the rigid part (the buckle) instead of the flexible part of the belt, the resulting, usually deep, injury will have a characteristic shape. There may be damage to the skin in the form of a laceration and damage to the underlying structures.

An assault with the buckle instead of the flexible part of the belt may indicate more serious

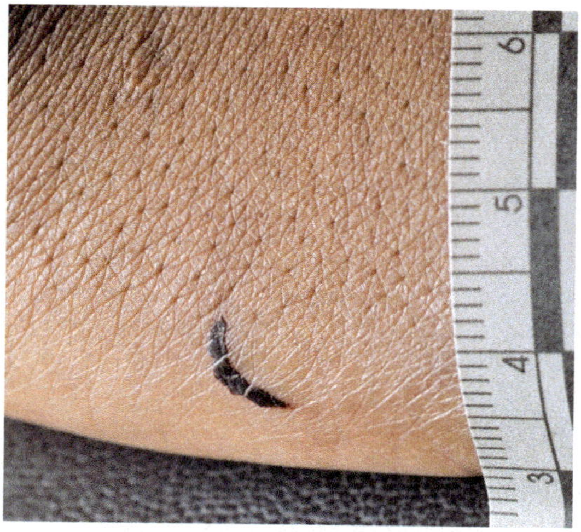

Fig. 3.56 Healing loopmark abrasion (electrical cord)

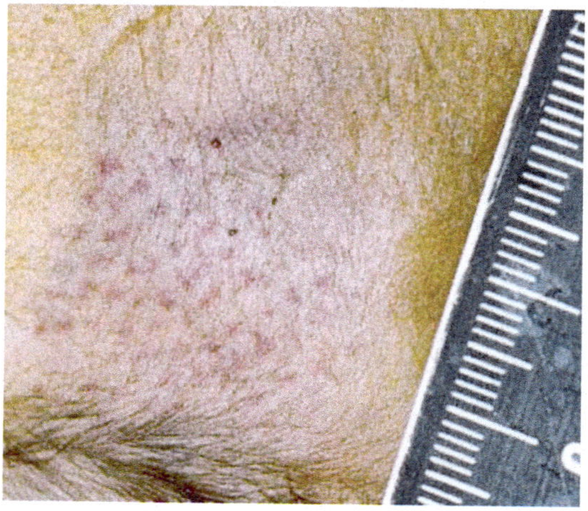

Fig. 3.57 Finding during forensic autopsy: (see Figs. 3.58, 3.59, 3.60, and 3.61)

problems in the perpetrator. The perpetrator must know that an assault with a buckle would result in a more severe injury. In a crisis, the perpetrator holds the buckle and folds the belt or winds it around the hand after removing the belt from the trousers. The same applies when the belt is hanging from the buckle on a nail in the wall. Therefore, in both situations, the perpetrator must carry out an extra maneuver, namely, to turn the belt around and hold it by the other end in order to assault the child with the buckle. Thus, the perpetrator consciously chooses to use the buckle to inflict injury to the child.

The slipper is a flexible object, and it is unlikely that it will leave a recognizable pattern. The resulting injury may be redness resembling first-degree burns during the first hours after the assault. Initially, the redness may be misinterpreted until the more characteristic bruising develops (Raimer et al. 1981). The individual bruises may merge to form one large bruise.

Rigid Objects: Cane, Stick, Shoes, Hairbrush, Clothes Hangers, Kitchen Utensils, Buckle, and Ring

Assaults in which a stick is used cause linear "tram-line" bruises or if severe even linear lacerations, which may be found particularly on the extremities and on the back during examination.

When a blunt object, such as a shoe or a hair-brush handle (non-bristled part), is used, bruises with a typical and often recognizable shape will develop. When the bristled part of the hairbrush is used, multiple pinpoint skin hemorrhages will develop (Figs. 3.57, 3.58, 3.59, 3.60, and 3.61).

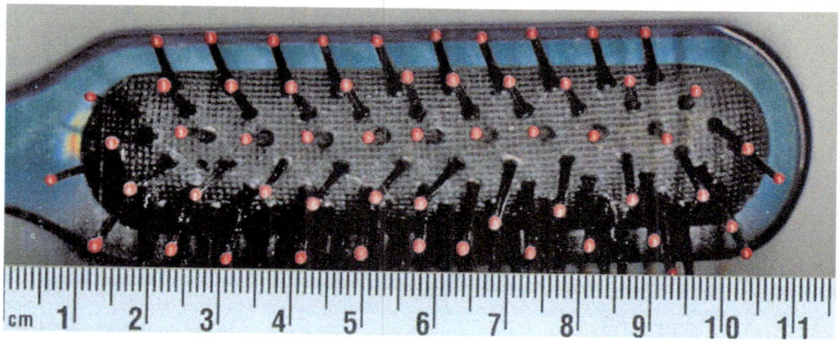

Fig. 3.58 Hairbrush, found on the scene of death (bristled part)

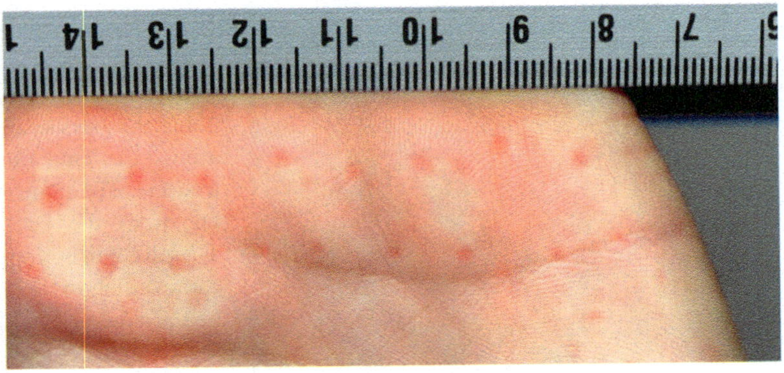

Fig. 3.59 Configuration of the imprint of the bristled part does not fit the finding during autopsy

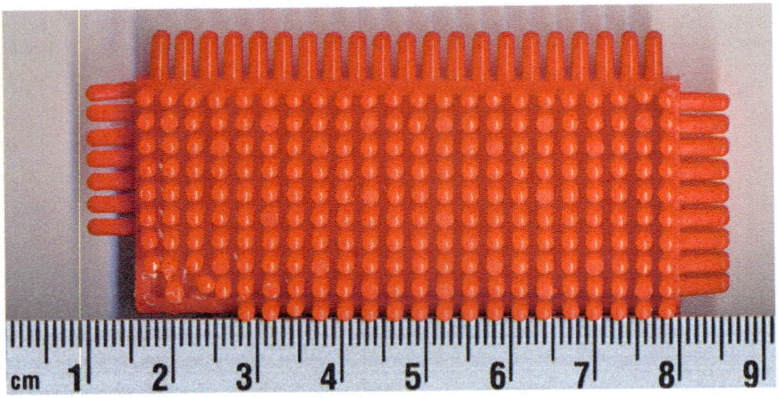

Fig. 3.60 Stickle brick, found on the scene of death

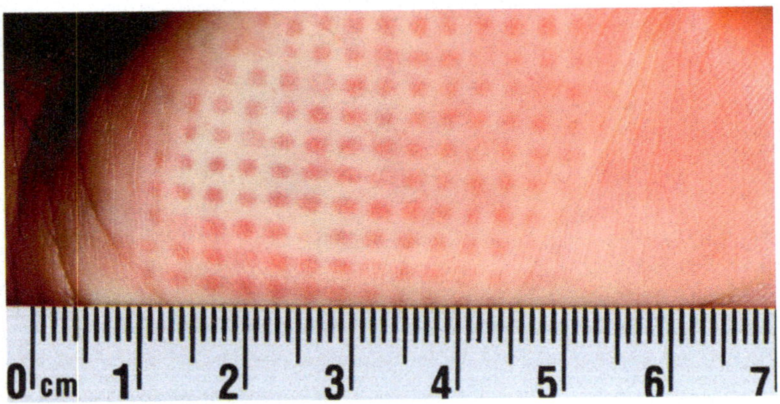

Fig. 3.61 The configuration of the imprint of the stickle brick does resemble the finding during autopsy

Scratching with a comb or a fork results in the development of linear bruising or abrasions. Stabbing causes grouped pointed wounds, depending on the number of prongs of the fork the child is pricked with. Slapping with a ring or a buckle will lead to specific pattern injuries (Figs. 3.62 and 3.63).

3.2.5.5 Static Loading: Using of Hands

Pinching

If a child has been pinched, the resulting bruising is often not characteristic (Herrmann et al. 2008). After pinching with the fingertips, one may see two circular or oval bruises side by side (particularly on the extremities, the cheeks, or the

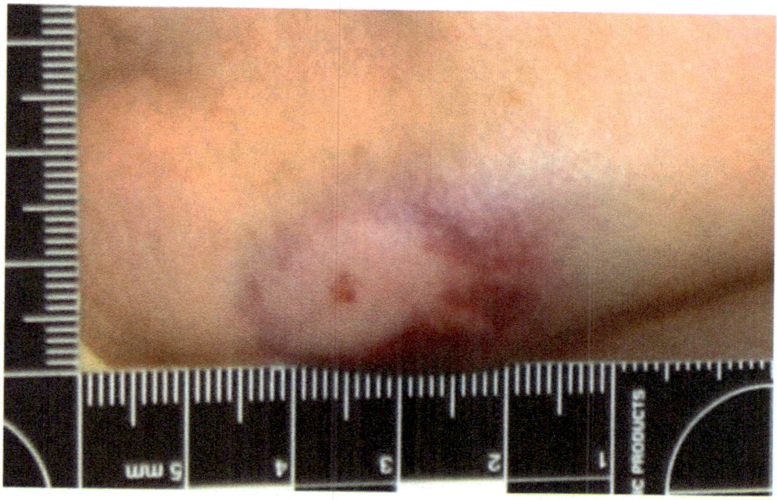

Fig. 3.62 Bruising caused by hitting with a rigid object (a ring, as stated by the victim)

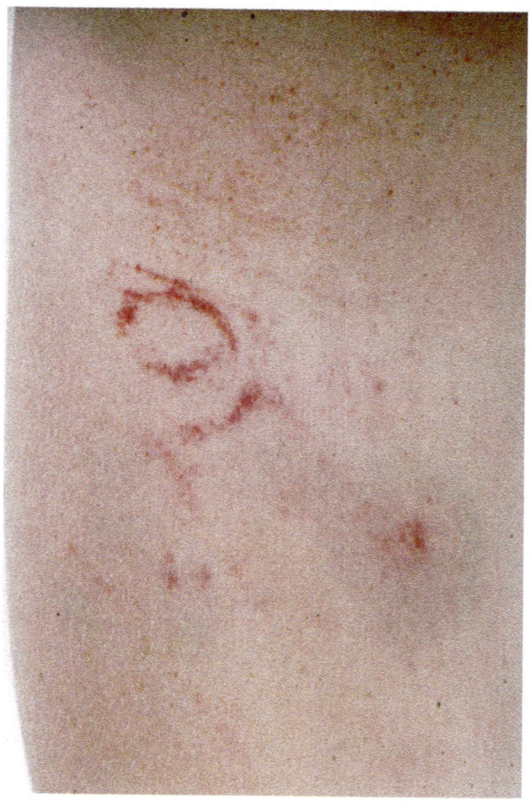

Fig. 3.63 Buckle print

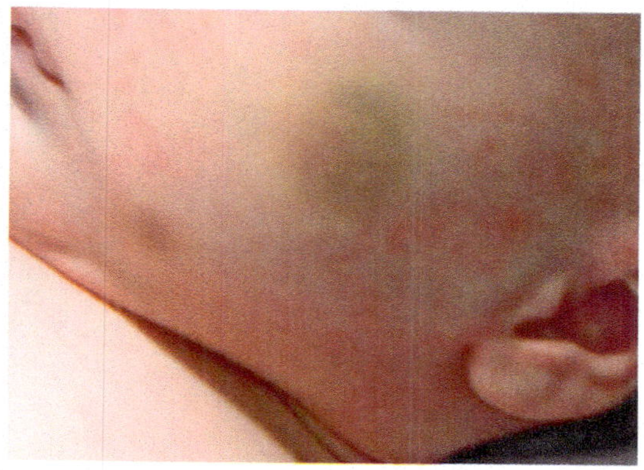

Fig. 3.64 Pinching: cheek

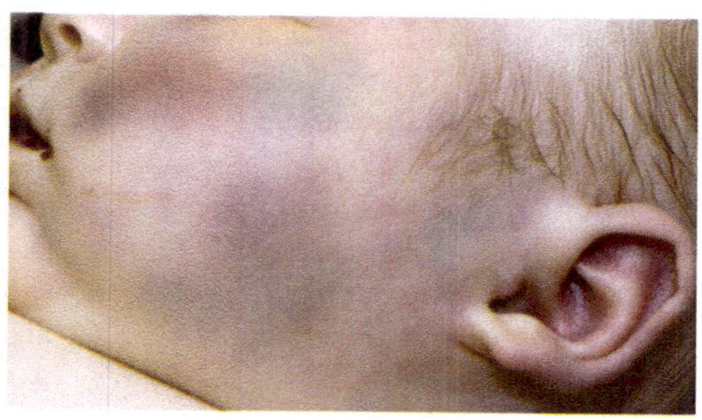

Fig. 3.65 Pinch marks in a fatally abused child. The bruising on the cheek was first noted 5 days before the incident, in which the child was killed. The initial bruising was less striking and smaller (pinching was admitted)

buttocks) with an unbruised area between the bruises (Figs. 3.64 and 3.65). Also, one may find a pair of bruises that face one another (circular, oval, or crescent-shaped), whereby the shape is mainly determined by the imprint of the fingernails (Schmitt 1987; Hobbs et al. 1999a, b) (see also Sect. 7.3.3). In self-infliction, one may find pinch marks on the arms (Hobbs et al. 1999a, b).

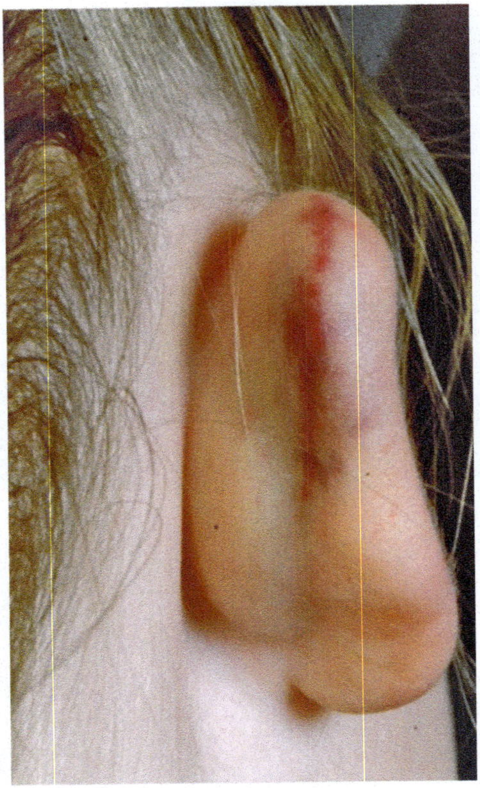

Fig. 3.66 Pinch mark on the ear

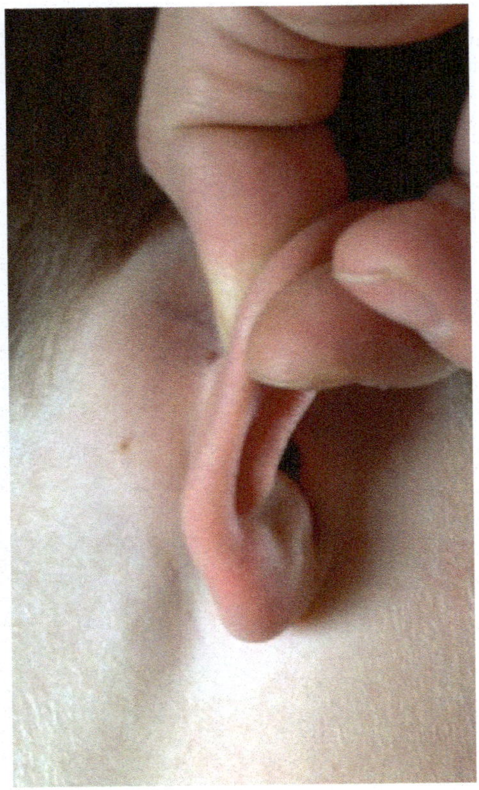

Fig. 3.67 Probable mechanism

Feldman (1992) described injuries in which the pattern appears to be determined by the anatomy/contours of the injured body part: vertical gluteal cleft injuries (Sect. 3.2.5.3) and a rim of petechial bruising along the helix, without bruising of the rest of the pinna. The exact mechanism of this typical pattern is not known, although Feldman thought it may be caused by crimping of the rim. Another explanation could be that during pinching of the helix, blood extravasates at the site with the least resistance to leakage (Figs. 3.66 and 3.67).

Grabbing/Gripping

Grabbing/gripping a child may result in fingertip bruising or grip marks: arc-shaped clusters of circular, oval, or crescent-shaped bruises, about 0.5–2.5 cm in diameter (Figs. 3.68, 3.69, 3.70, 3.71, 3.72, 3.73, and 3.74). Sometimes, these grip marks are accompanied by imprints or excoriations caused by fingernails. Grip marks tend to fade rapidly and may disappear within a few days (Glasgow and Graham 1997).

A grip mark is a typical tell-tale injury: the configuration and location of the grip marks provide a strong indication of what could have happened (see Table 3.4). A grip mark sometimes indicates the dominant hand of the perpetrator, especially when found in the face.

Tell-Tale Signs in Grip Marks: "Shaking"

The mode of "shaking" or "swinging" in an infant with a subdural hematoma can be "visualized" by the distribution of grip marks on the body (if present). If a child is shaken or swung, the perpetrator can hold the child in several ways:

- In face-to-face position
- In face-to-back position

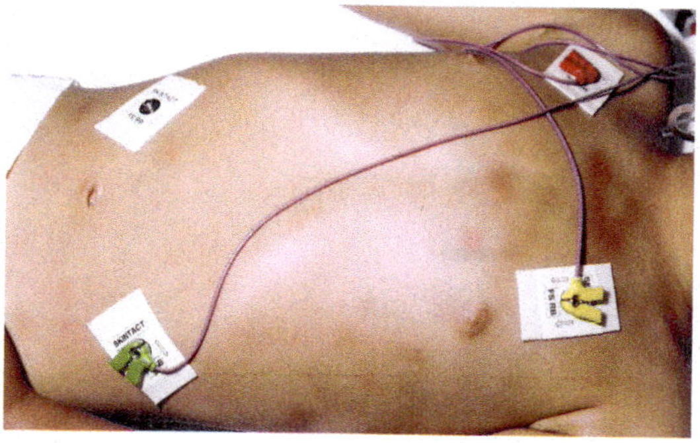

Fig. 3.68 Extensive bruising on the trunk of an abused child (suggestive for gripping, punching, and prodding): front

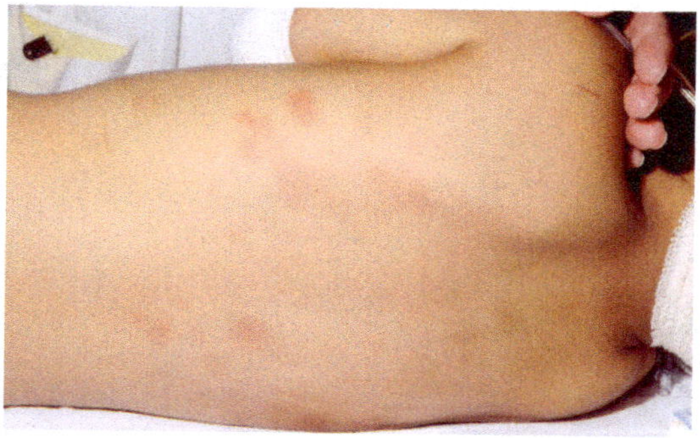

Fig. 3.69 Extensive bruising on the trunk of an abused child: back (= Fig. 2.23)

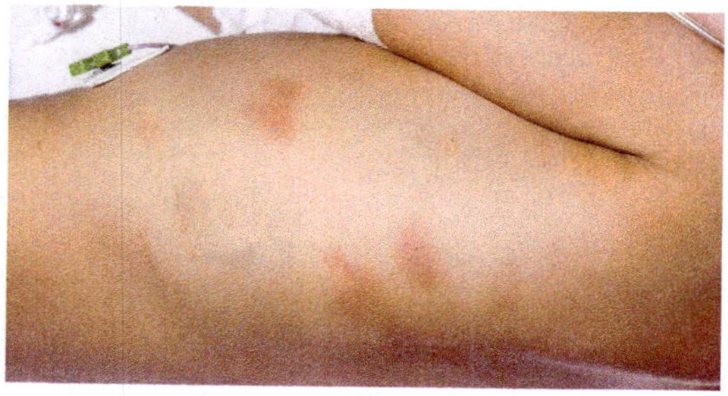

Fig. 3.70 Extensive bruising on the trunk of an abused child: left *side*

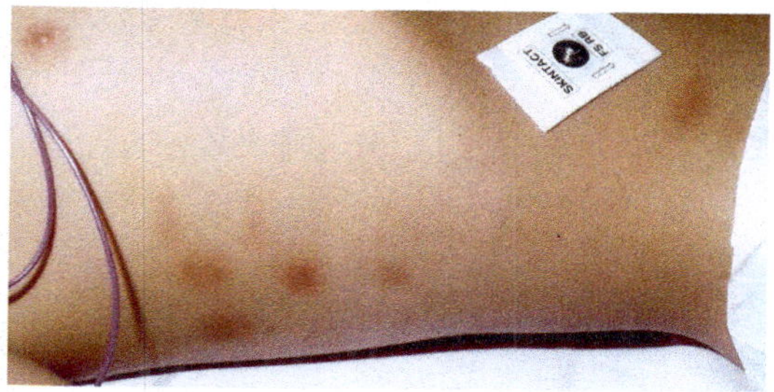

Fig. 3.71 Extensive bruising on the trunk of an abused child: right side

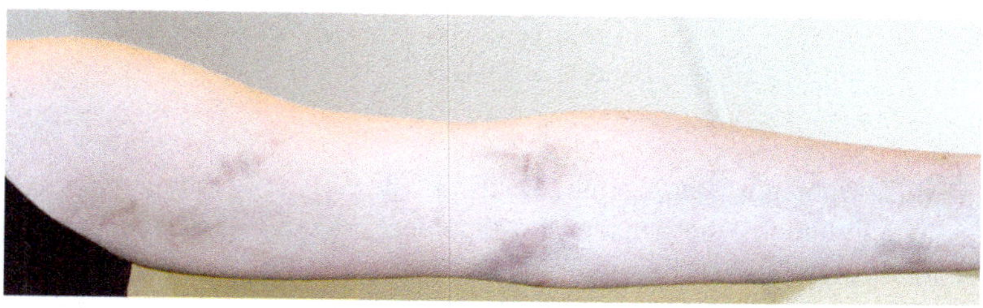

Fig. 3.72 Extensive bruising on the inside of the left arm of a victim of an assault (grabbing and kicking)

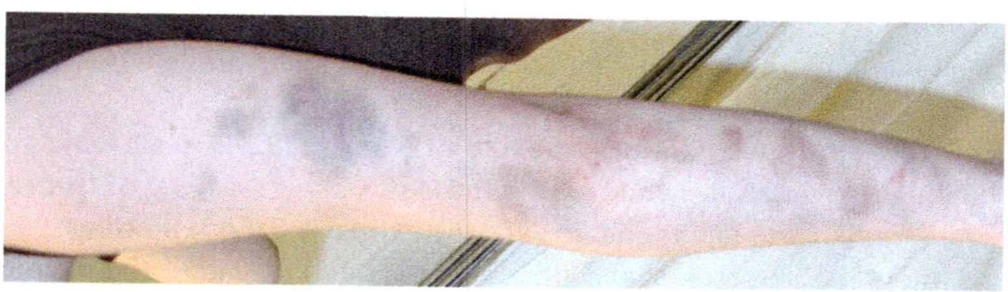

Fig. 3.73 Same person as in Fig. 3.72: extensive bruising on the outside of the left arm (grabbing and kicking)

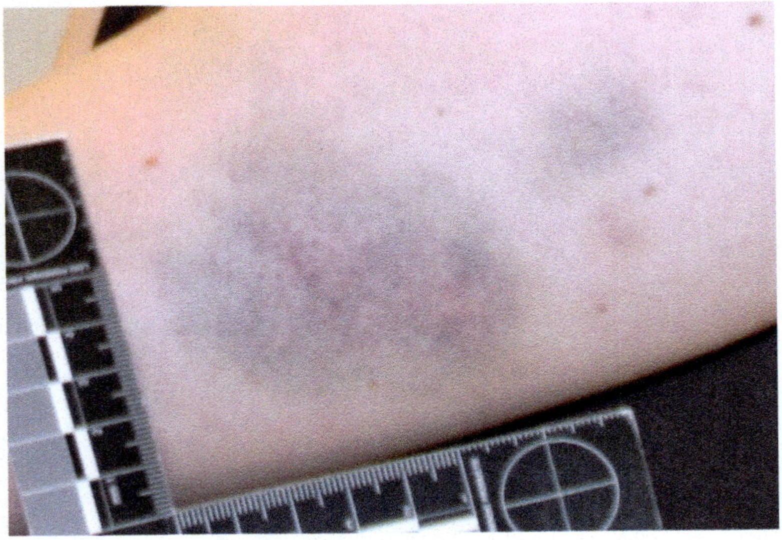

Fig. 3.74 Same person as in Fig. 3.72: detail of the large bruise on the outside of the left upper arm (grabbing and kicking)

Table 3.4 Tell-tale grip marks

Action	Anatomical location	Age of the child
"Shaking"	Often symmetrical Trunk Forearm, upper arm, shoulders Legs, for example, around ankles	Mainly <1 year
Forced feeding	Cheeks	Mainly <3 years
Choking	Cheeks Around the mouth and nose	Mainly <3 years
Grabbing/gripping	Arms Cheeks/chin	All ages
Strangulation	Neck	All ages
Sexual abuse	Often symmetrical Forearm, upper arm, shoulders, and sometimes around wrists Buttocks and thighs	All ages

- In upright position around the trunk (thorax and abdomen), the arms, or the shoulders
- In upside down position around the legs

If the child is held around the chest in a face-to-face position and there is bruising, these bruises can be found in clusters of up to eight fingerprints (two times four imprints) on the back and two (thumb) prints on the front.

Tell-Tale Signs in Grip Marks: Sexual Abuse

Finding grip marks in a child may indicate sexual abusive acts. Grip marks can indicate the various positions the perpetrator and the child were in (face-to-face, face-to-back, and so on):

- On the buttocks and the thighs, for example, in a face-to-face position: two sets of fingerprints on the back and two sets of thumbprints on the front
- Around the knees
- On the forearms or on the inner sides of the upper arms and the shoulders, sometimes around the wrists

3.2.5.6 Static Loading: Using of Implements

Tying: Binding

Ligature-like circumferential bruises and/or abrasions around the wrists and/or the ankles

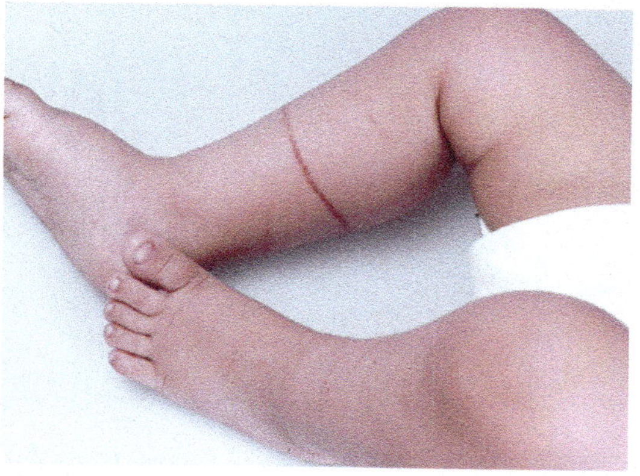

Fig. 3.75 Tying marks on the inside of the leg

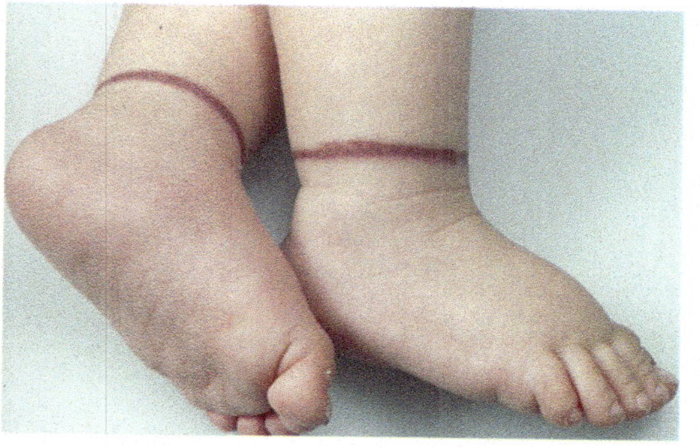

Fig. 3.77 Marks, due to being tied with a rope to the bed (= Fig. 7.39)

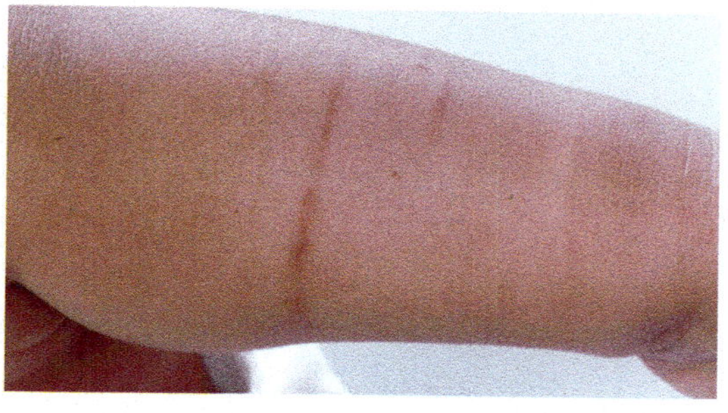

Fig. 3.76 Same child: outside of the leg

may imply binding injuries (Figs. 3.75, 3.76, and 3.77). This type of injury can also result in distal petechiae and edema (Kos and Shwayder 2006). If the binding is "too" tight, it may cause "cuts" and cut-off blood circulation in the tied extremities. After recovery, circular hyperpigmentations may be seen around the extremities. This type of injury is highly suggestive for child abuse. A circular friction burn may develop around the extremity if a child is bound with a belt or a piece of bed sheet (Raimer et al. 1981; Schmitt 1987).

Tying a child down in bed may have various reasons:

- The child continuously climbs out of the bed. The parents are afraid that the child may incur damage by falling out of the bed.
- The child is tied down in the bed as punishment.
- The child is tied down to prevent any resistance during sexual abuse.

If the child is lying down tied to an object such as the leg of a chair or a bedpost, the lesions will not be circular. The part of the extremity positioned against, for example, the bedpost will either show no abnormalities or an imprint of the object against which the child had been positioned.

Similar injuries as in tying (bruises and abrasions) can be found at the oral commissure and on the cheeks in gagging (Figs. 3.78, 3.79, 3.80, 3.81, and 3.82). Gagging in child abuse is an act in which the perpetrator tries to prevent or end crying, shouting, or speaking by securing an obstruction across or within the mouth (Purdue 2000). The mouth will be partially or completely blocked with fabric, for example, a handkerchief, towel, or adhesive tape. The direction of the lesions is determined by the direction of the gagging. Because of their location and shape, these marks are highly characteristic of abuse (Kos and Shwayder 2006). "Gagging" injuries can be accompanied by marks such as nail abrasions caused by the victim in trying to remove the gag. If a child has been gagged repeatedly, scarring may be found at the oral commissure. Gagging may lead to suffocation by mechanical asphyxiation, especially if the child is not able to breathe freely through the nose, for example, because of blockage with mucus or edema (Saukko and Knight 2004b).

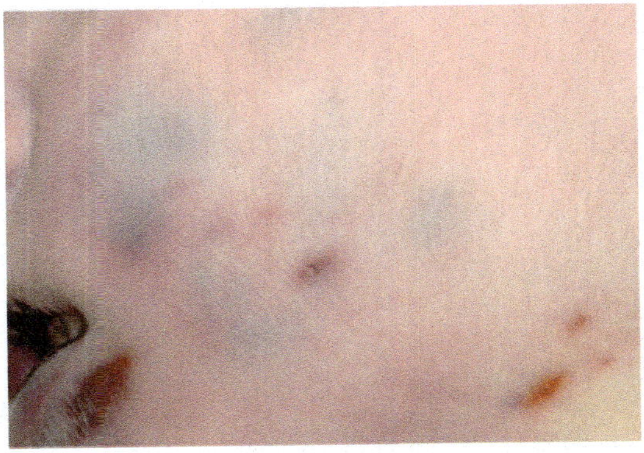

Fig. 3.78 Bruising on the left cheek suspicious for gagging

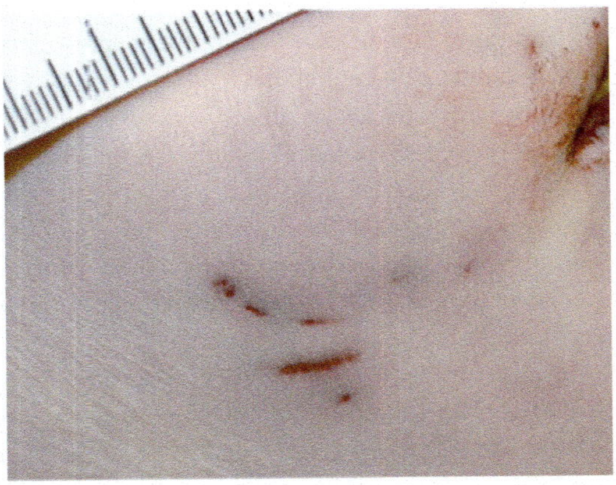

Fig. 3.79 Hardly visible bruising on the right cheek, suspicious for gagging. Scratching most probably caused by the child while trying to remove the gag

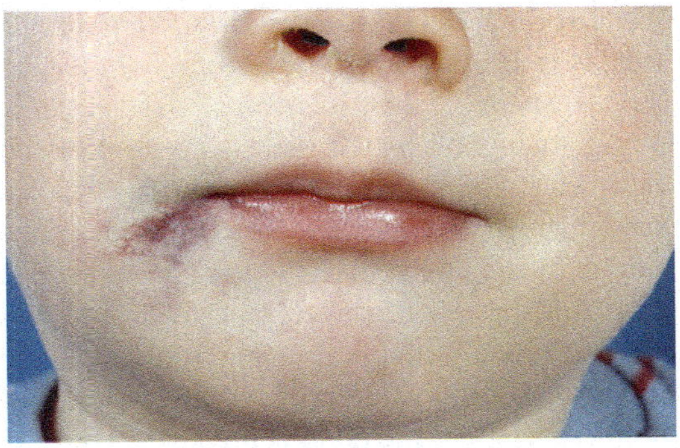

Fig. 3.80 Differential diagnosis of findings in gagging: vascular malformation (= Fig. 6.57)

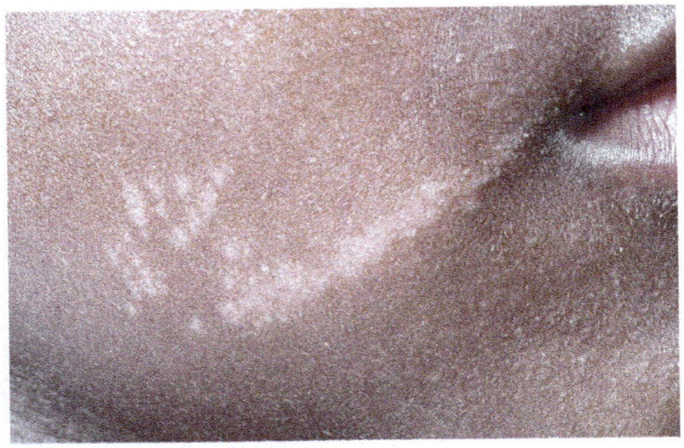

Fig. 3.81 Differential diagnosis of findings in gagging: lichen striatus

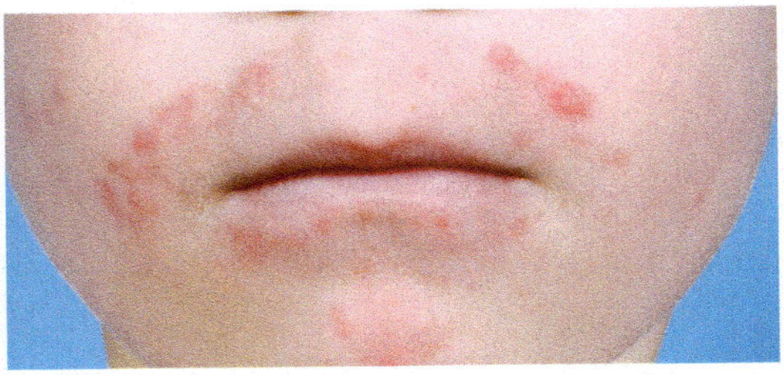

Fig. 3.82 Differential diagnosis of findings in gagging: liplick dermatitis

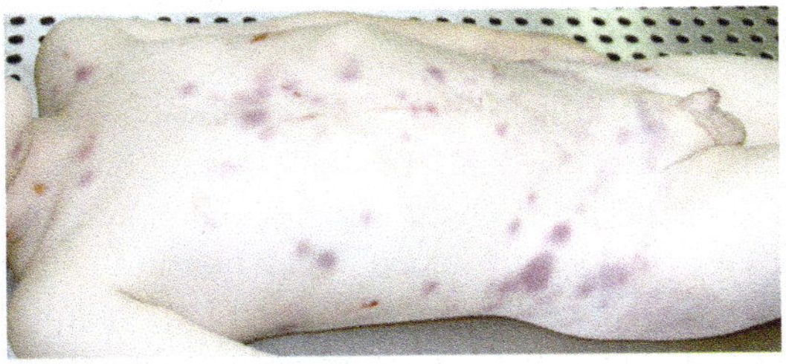

Fig. 3.83 Extensive bruising on the trunk of a fatally abused child

3.2.5.7 Particular Locations of Bruises in Child Abuse

Trunk

Accidental bruising of the trunk is rare, compared to accidental bruising of the forehead and limbs (Glasgow and Graham 1997) (Fig. 3.83). Accidental bruising will be found on bony prominences, such as the ribs and pelvic bone.

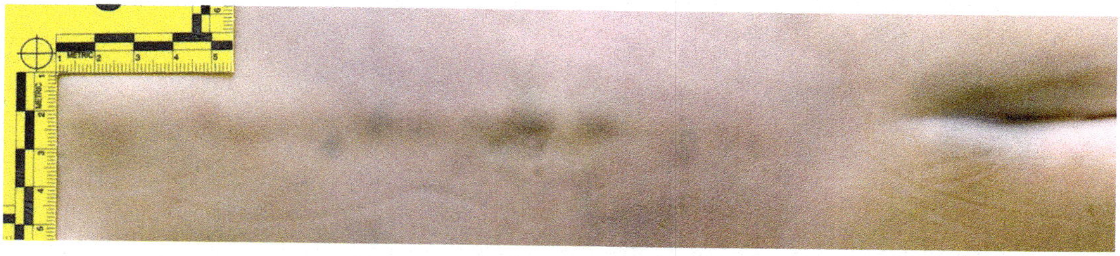

Fig. 3.84 Non-accidental bruising on the vertebral spinous processes plus a Mongolian spot in the gluteal cleft

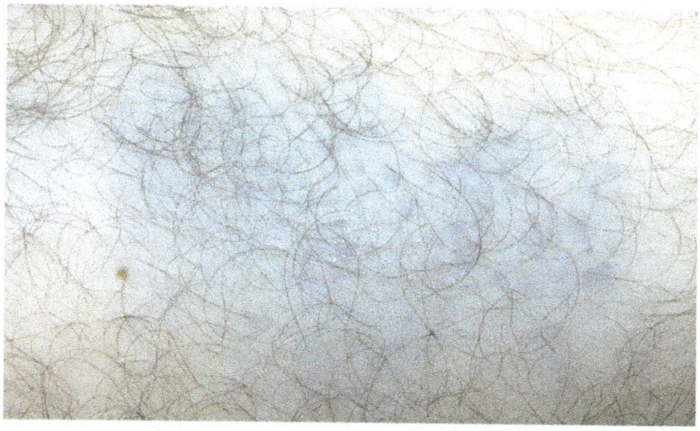

Fig. 3.85 Differentiating between a bruise and a Mongolian spot: bruise

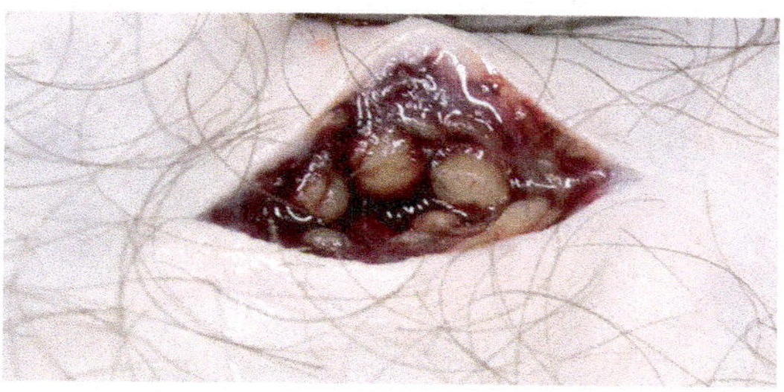

Fig. 3.86 Differentiating between a bruise and a Mongolian spot: incision with visible blood (= Fig. 2.11)

Fig. 3.87 Differentiating between a bruise and a Mongolian spot: Mongolian spot

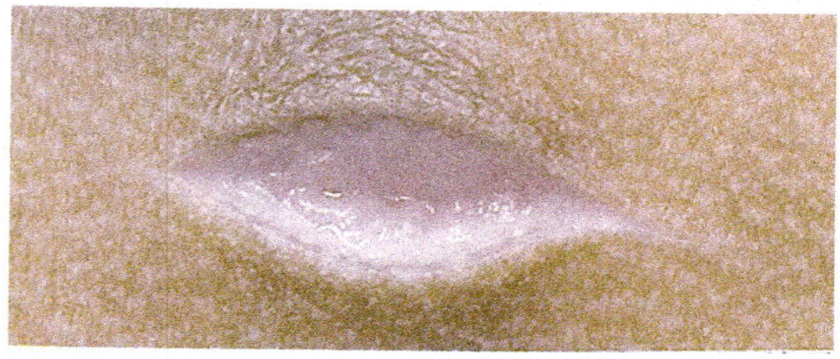

Fig. 3.88 Differentiating between a bruise and a Mongolian spot: incision, no visible blood (= Fig. 2.12)

On the back, one will find bruising on the vertebral spinous processes, sacrum, or pelvic bone, if a child tumbles backward (Glasgow and Graham 1997). However, in case of bruising on a large part of the processes, one should consider child abuse (Figs. 3.84, 3.85, 3.86, 3.87, and 3.88).

Non-accidental bruising of the thorax and abdomen is usually the result of beatings or grabbing (often leading to recognizable pattern injuries). Abdominal bruising rarely occurs due to the flexibility and padding of the abdominal wall, but when present, it usually indicates forceful grabbing or very forceful blunt impact. If abdominal bruising is found at physical examination, the physician must also look for associated internal injuries (Davis and Carrasco 2002).

Lower abdominal bruising may be associated with sexual abuse (Hobbs et al. 1999a, b).

Extremities

Gavin et al. (1997) described subungual bruising which developed because the perpetrator repeatedly bit on the fingertips of the victim, leading to hemorrhages under the fingernails (Gavin et al. 1997). Extreme short cutting of nails may be

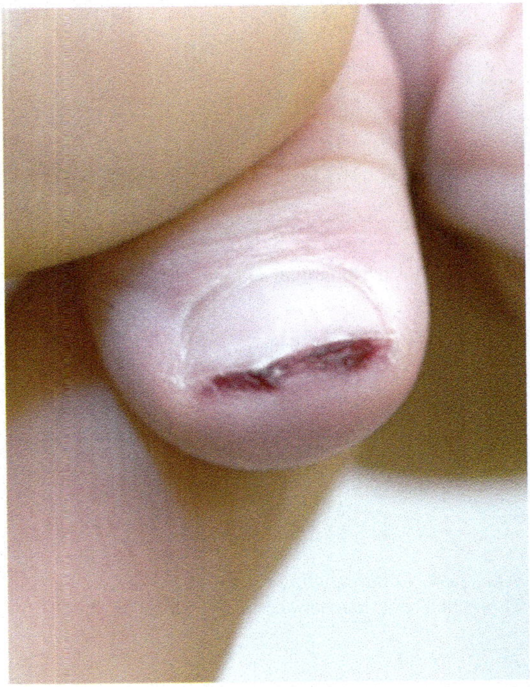

Fig. 3.89 Extremely short cutting of nails with bleeding

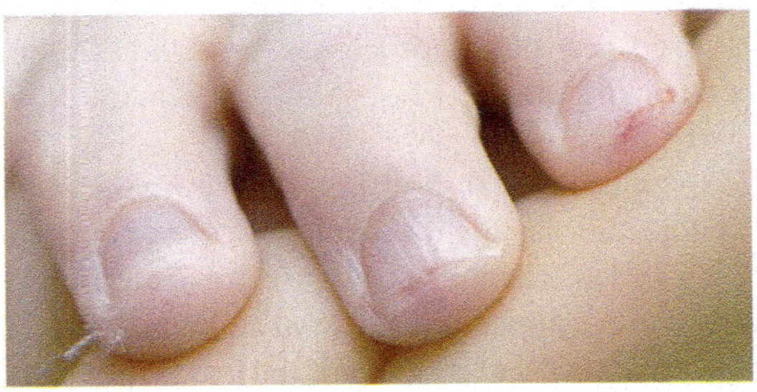

Fig. 3.90 Extremely short cutting of nails

connected to child abuse (Figs. 3.89 and 3.90) This should be differentiated from nail-biting (Fig. 3.91). Bruising of the palm of the hand in a nonmobile child should raise a suspicion of child abuse (Fig. 3.92).

Anogenital Region

Bruising in the anogenital region is highly suspect for abuse (including sexual abuse) since accidental injury of these areas is rare (Pascoe et al. 1979; Raimer et al. 1981; Hobbs et al. 1999a, b; RCPCH 2008a, b).

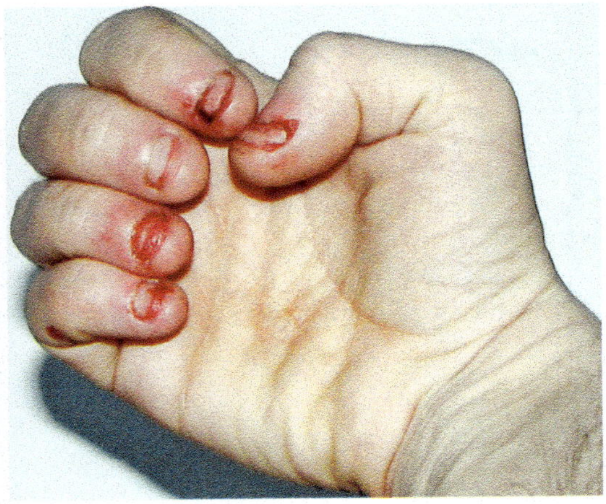

Fig. 3.91 Dermatophagia and nail-biting (6th Happiness 2009 from Wikimedia Commons 2011: Dermatophagia.jpg)

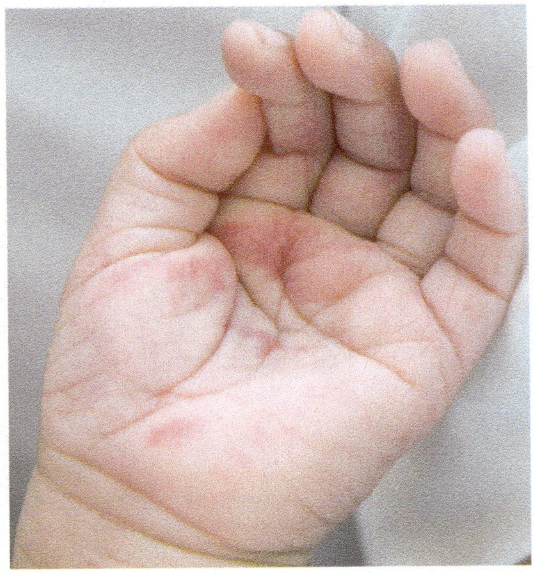

Fig. 3.92 Bruising on the palm of the hand, caused by violently compressing the hand

3.2.5.8 Differential Diagnosis of Non-accidental Bruising

> A bruise must never be interpreted in isolation and must always be assessed in the context of medical and social history, developmental stage, explanation given, full clinical examination and relevant investigations. Maguire et al. (2005a, b)

In 1986, Kaplan stated the following: "When a patient's problem is judged to be the result of child abuse and it is not, considerable harm may be done to the child, his parents, and the doctor-parent relationship" (Kaplan 1986). In the same article, he also mentioned the dilemma of many physicians, fearing to over- or underdiagnose child abuse: "Overdiagnosing the battered child syndrome can be as harmful as failing to consider it."

It emerges from the article of Kaplan and, for example, from the study by Wheeler and Hobbs (1988) that overdiagnosing of physical signs happens and that many of the findings in the differential diagnosis of bruising in child abuse are not even rare. It even appears that the manifestation of the finding is not always atypical. However, the differential diagnosis is sometimes made considerably more difficult either because of an atypical clinical course followed by the finding or because of its atypical location.

Additional investigations and a clinical evaluation are always indicated if bruises are found in a child under the age of 1 year. Bruising in these children may indicate child abuse but may also indicate a serious disorder, like a bruising or bleeding disorder.

Suspicions of non-accidental bruising in children may arise in accidentally bruised children (Chap. 4), in children with a bleeding disorder (Chap. 5), and in children with a dermatological disorder or in children which harm themselves (self-inflicted injuries) and in children with fictitious disorders (Chap. 6).

Although a thorough evaluation is important, one should also try to prevent that children have to undergo unnecessary medical investigations, when the cause of the injuries is obvious. For example, in case of extensive pattern bruises, one might consider a comprehensive coagulation screening for completeness sake or to avoid discussions about coagulation disorders, but this is in almost all case unnecessary because the pattern tells the story of physical abuse (Lee 2008).

3.3 Petechiae

3.3.1 Defining Petechiae

Petechiae are small red, purple, or brown spots caused by minor hemorrhages (0.1–2 mm – pinpoint to pinhead) in the skin (intradermal bleeding) and/or the mucous membranes and/or the serosal surfaces. Petechiae do not blanch under diascopy. There have been discussions whether petechiae are the result of damage to venules or capillaries (Purdue 2000; Saukko and Knight 2004 a, b; Kumar et al. 2007). Most probably, they are caused by damage to/leakage of the postcapillary venules. Bleeding from capillary damage will only be visible microscopically and not by visual inspection during a physical examination (Purdue 2000; Saukko and Knight 2004a, b; Busuttil 2009).

According to Saukko and Knight (2004a, b) and Purdue (2000), petechiae in trauma are caused by an acute rise in venous pressure (back pressure caused by mechanical obstruction of venous return to the heart) that leads to overdistension and rupture of the thin-walled peripheral venules, which again leads to rapid extravasation of blood, especially in lax tissues, such as the eyelid, or in unsupported serous membranes, such as the pleura and the epicardium. The role of focal hypoxia of the wall of the venules is controversial.

3.3.2 Clinical Features

Typical locations for petechiae in children are (among others Purdue 2000) (Figs. 3.93, 3.94, 3.95, 3.96, 3.97, 3.98, 3.99, 3.100, and 3.101):

- The loose skin around the eyes, on the cheeks, and on the face (often in a "butterfly" or "mask-like" distribution)
- The skin behind the ears and in the neck
- The mucous membranes of the eye sclera, the connective tissue of the eyelids, the lips, the gums, the epiglottis, and the genitalia
- The serous membranes of the heart (epicardium), the lung (pleura), the abdominal peritoneum, and the serosa of the bowel (rarely)
- The surfaces of the internal organs: thymus and brain

Petechiae and purpura must be evaluated according to the overall context of the patient, the severity and extent of the lesions, and the history and age of the patient (Pediatric Care Online 2009). Petechiae (and purpura) are not pathognomonic for asphyxiation or any other cause, whether trauma- or disease-related (Ely 2000; Busuttil 2009). There are many conditions in

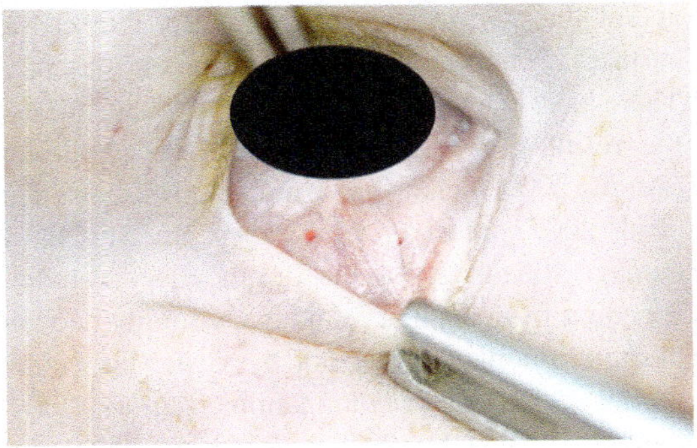

Fig. 3.93 Petechiae in a smothered child: petechiae in the conjunctiva and "fresh" (*red*) petechiae and old (*brown*) petechiae (or freckles) in the periorbital skin (the perpetrator confessed to two smothering incidents on 2 days, 4 days apart)

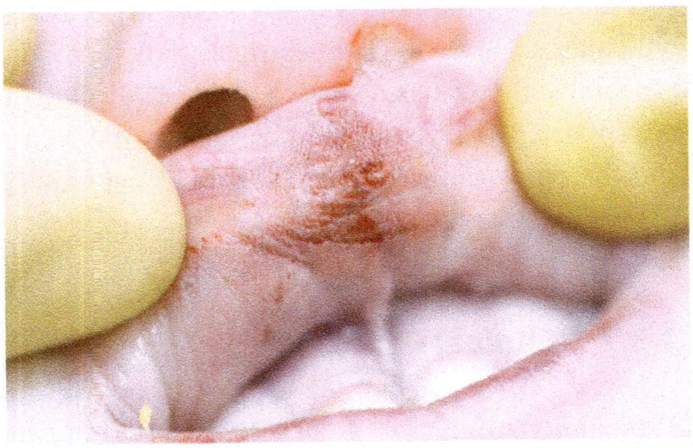

Fig. 3.94 Same child: injury on the inside of the upper lip as sign of the smothering

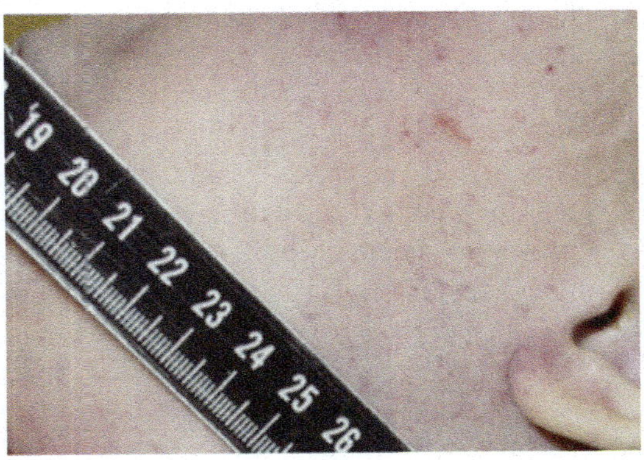

Fig. 3.95 Extensive petechiae in the face of a strangled child (= Fig. 2.4)

which petechiae may be seen. These conditions range from harmless to life-threatening. The differential diagnosis of petechiae includes:

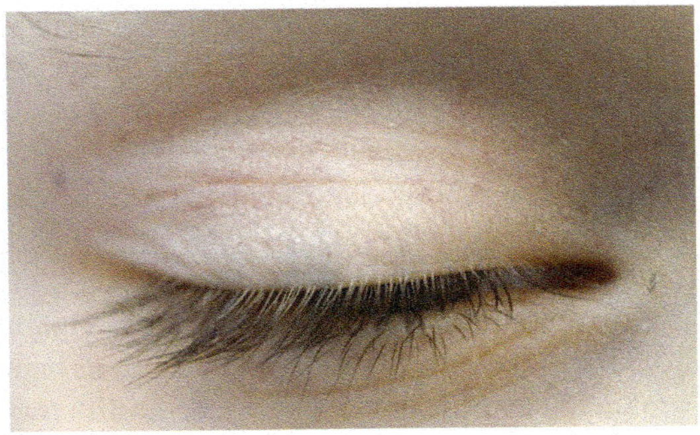

Fig. 3.96 Petechiae in the eyelids of the right eye of a smothered child

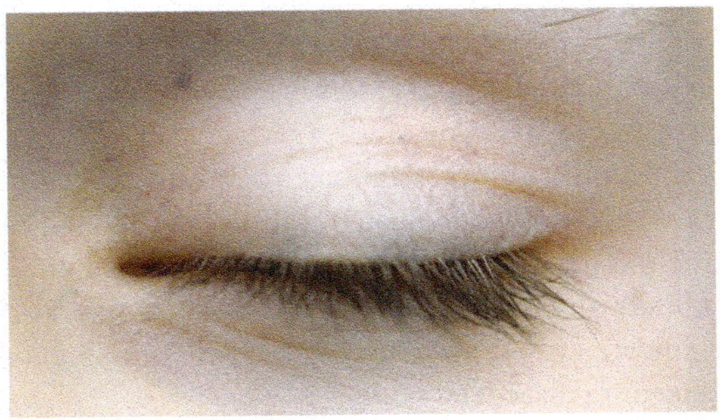

Fig. 3.97 Same child as in Fig. 3.96: petechiae in the eyelids of the left eye

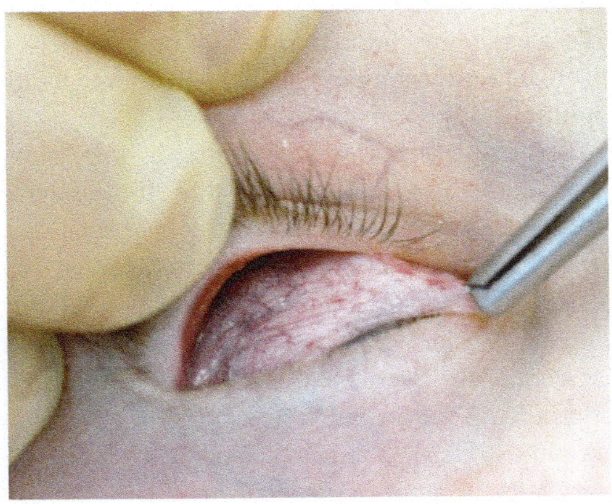

Fig. 3.98 Same child as in Fig. 3.96: petechiae on the inside of the upper eyelid of the right eye

- Hemostatic defects, such as platelet disorders (e.g., idiopathic thrombocytopenic purpura) or other coagulation disorders (e.g., disseminated intravascular coagulopathy)

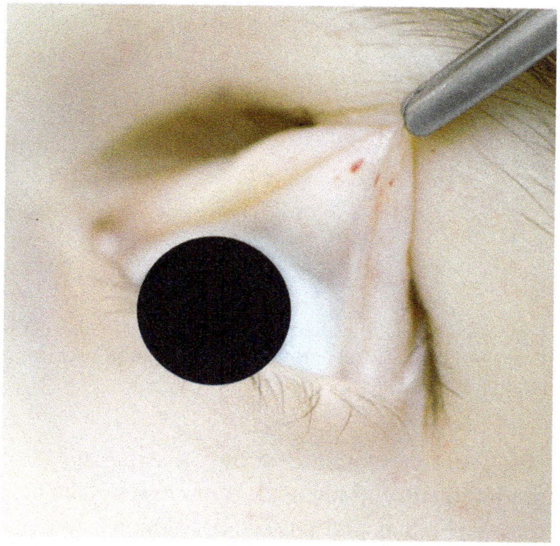

Fig. 3.99 Same child as in Fig. 3.96: petechiae on the inside of the upper eyelid of the left eye

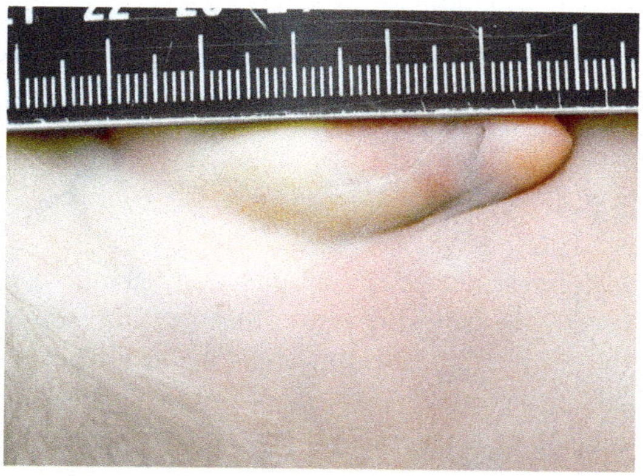

Fig. 3.100 Same child as in Fig. 3.96: petechiae behind the right ear

- Bacterial (sepsis – Fig. 3.102) and viral infections and live-virus vaccinations (e.g., measles and varicella)
- Autoimmune disorders (e.g., allergic vasculitis/Henoch-Schönlein purpura – Chaps. 5 and 6)
- Allergic reactions
- Use of medication (anticoagulants, like warfarin, heparin, or aspirin; some antibiotics and anticonvulsants; chemotherapy) (Chap. 5)
- Radiation
- Trauma (accidental and inflicted)
- Malignancies (leukemia and other bone marrow malignancies)
- Other rare causes

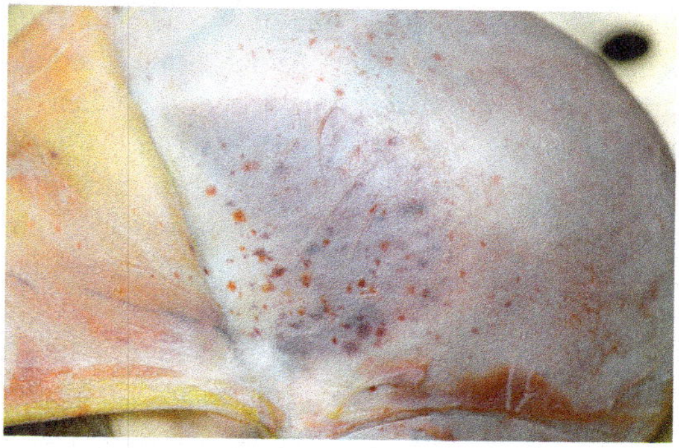

Fig. 3.101 Same child as in Fig. 3.96: petechiae in and under the scalp

Fig. 3.102 Petechiae in a person with sepsis

A patch of localized petechiae can be caused by moderate pressure, impact, or suction on the skin (see 2.3.3) (Saukko and Knight 2004a, b).

Petechiae can be found in healthy children. In healthy newborns after a vaginal delivery, a few petechiae in the face are likely caused by the trauma of passing through the birth canal. However, newborns with diffuse petechiae should be evaluated further. Downes et al. (2002) did find one or more petechiae in almost 30% of 116 babies under the age of 12 months, who visited child health surveillance clinics; 8.6% had two or more petechiae; and 2.6% of the children had three or more petechiae: one child had three petechiae, one child had nine, and the third child twenty (found in association with eczema).

Downes concluded that one or two petechiae are common and that without other clinical indications, their presence should not be taken as pathological.

In infants and older children, petechiae may develop on the face as the result of severe coughing, for example, in pertussis. Obstruction of the upper most part of the airways may be present but is not necessary to develop petechiae in these situations. Sometimes, petechiae are seen after prolonged and severe vomiting (Thomas 2004; Lee 2008; Minford and Richards 2010). In straining, petechiae can be found in the skin of the abdominal wall.

Griest and Zumwalt (1989) and Somers et al. (2008) describe the development of periorbital and conjunctival petechiae as a result of accidental drowning in children.

3.3.3 Suction Petechiae

Suction petechiae result from the applying negative pressure (suction) on the skin. Suction petechiae are nearly always caused by human actions, whether the petechiae are caused by "kissing, sucking, and sometimes biting (lovebite or hickey)" or, for example, by using an implement such as a vacuum cleaner or during "cupping."

The classical lovebite is caused by firm application of the lips, which form an airtight seal against the skin (Fig. 3.103) (Saukko and Knight 2004c). Sucking then leads to negative pressure over the area encircled by the lips and to extravasation of blood from the venules in the superficial layers of the skin. If enough pressure is applied, the petechiae will merge. Additional bruising can result from pressure by the tongue, pushing the skin against the palate, which sometimes creates an imprint of the inner side of the teeth or the palatineal rugae in the bruise (Kellogg 2005).

The classic lovebite tends to have a circular or an ovoid shape and is of uniform color because over the area of suction, the negative pressure applied to the skin is similar (Payne-James 2003). Lovebites are often multiple and found in the neck.

In children, suction petechiae are generally the result of voluntary actions (for fun, self-induced/self-inflicted, predominantly on the arms) or interactions (during kissing and sex, predominantly in the neck, sometimes elsewhere like the breasts and buttocks). Suction petechiae are also seen in sexual assault (bitemarks as well as suction petechiae) (Chap. 8).

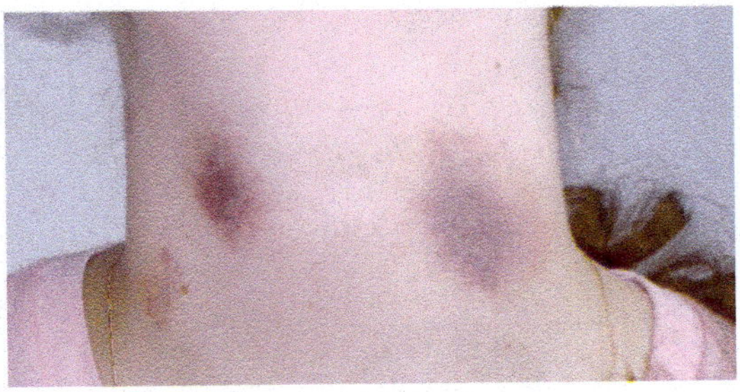

Fig. 3.103 Suction petechiae: lovebite (Janek 2008. From Wikipedia 2011 http://en.wikipedia.org/wiki/Lovebite) (= Fig. 8.21)

A another type of suction petechiae can be found intraorally on the soft palate as a result of negative intraoral pressure, for example, during fellatio (Damm et al. 1981).

3.3.4 Vibices

In forensic medicine and pathology, the term is used to describe tiny, most often spot-like, sometimes merging, oval-to-round, bluish-blackish hemorrhages of postmortem origin exclusively limited to areas of livor mortis (Tsokos 2005) (Figs. 3.104 and 3.105). According to Tsokos (2005), vibices result from the postmortem mechanical rupture of subcutaneous capillaries and smaller vessels (predominantly veins), which is caused by an increase in intravascular pressure resulting from pooling of erythrocytes in these vessels under the influence of gravity during the formation of livor mortis. Vibices, just like petechiae, do not blanch under diascopy.

During postmortem examination, vibices should be differentiated from petechiae resulting from traumatic asphyxia or other conditions. Differentiation is possible because the appearance, intensity, and extent of the vibices are positively correlated with that of livor mortis (Tsokos 2005). Vibices are only found in areas of livor mortis. However, sometimes it is difficult or even impossible to differentiate between vibices and

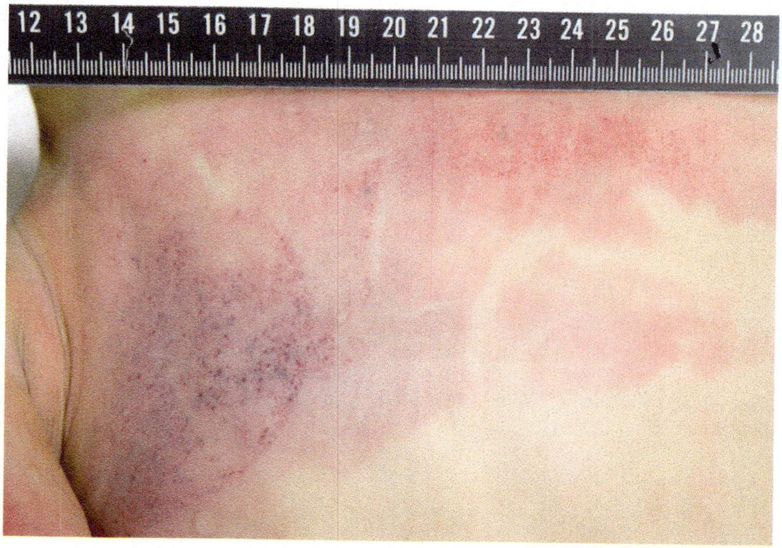

Fig. 3.104 Vibices

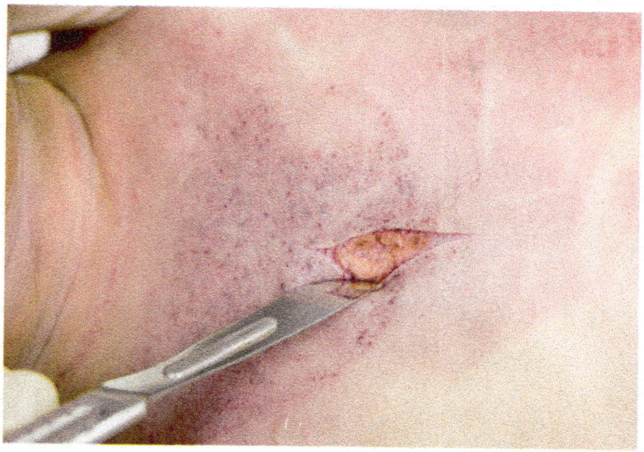

Fig. 3.105 Vibices

petechiae, for example, in deceased children who were found in a prone position which is a common position in sudden unexplained death in infancy. This may lead to an unjustified suspicion of suffocation or choking.

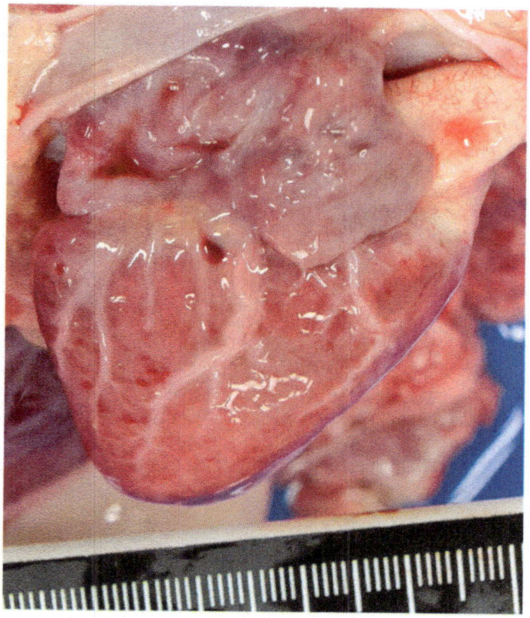

Fig. 3.106 Tardieu's spots in SIDS: subepicardial petechiae

3.3.5 Tardieu's Spots

Using the term Tardieu's spots (also known as Tardieu's petechiae or Tardieu's ecchymosis) in forensic medicine, without defining these specific spots properly, is confusing. Some do use the term as a synonym for petechial hemorrhages in general (Jain et al. 2001) or for vibices more specifically (e.g. DiMaio and DiMaio 2001a, c). Some authors restrict the use only to subpleural and subepicardial petechiae (Yamamoto et al. 2000). To prevent confusion, one should limit the use of this term to the classical meaning as described by Tardieu in 1870: subpleural and subepicardial petechiae or ecchymoses (or both) (Figs. 3.106, 3.107, 3.108, 3.109, 3.110, and 3.111), as can observed in the tissues of persons who are victims of mechanical asphyxia

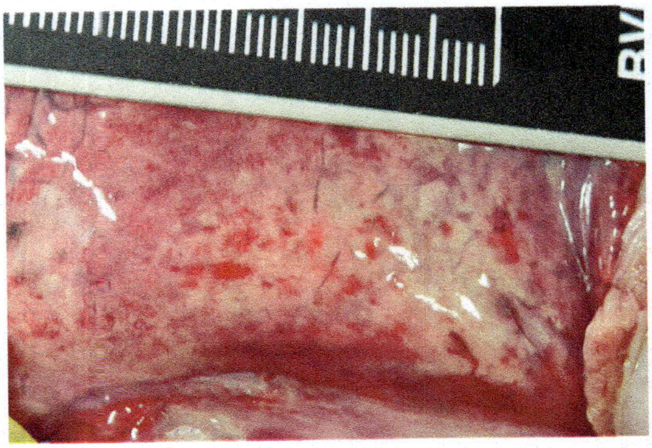

Fig. 3.107 Tardieu's spots in SIDS: subpleural petechiae

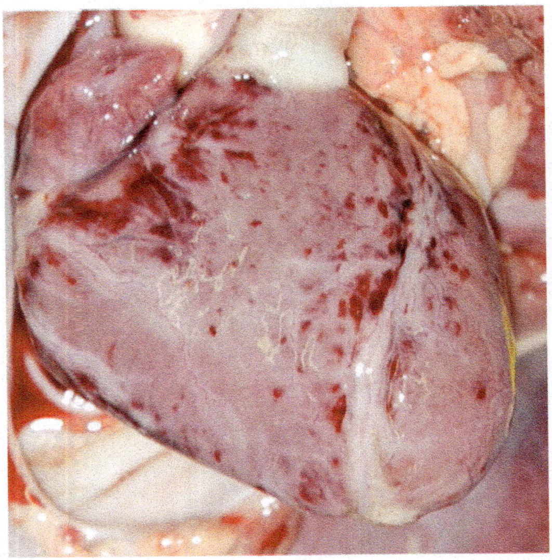

Fig. 3.108 Tardieu's spots in SIDS: extensive subepicardial petechiae

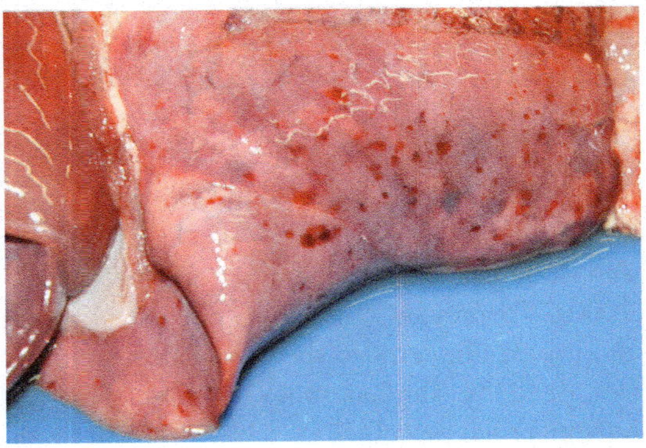

Fig. 3.109 Tardieu's spots in SIDS: extensive subpleural petechiae

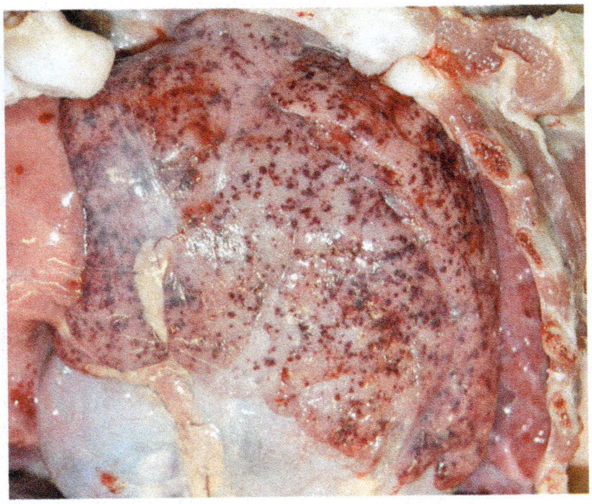

Fig. 3.110 Tardieu's spots in SIDS: extensive thymic petechiae

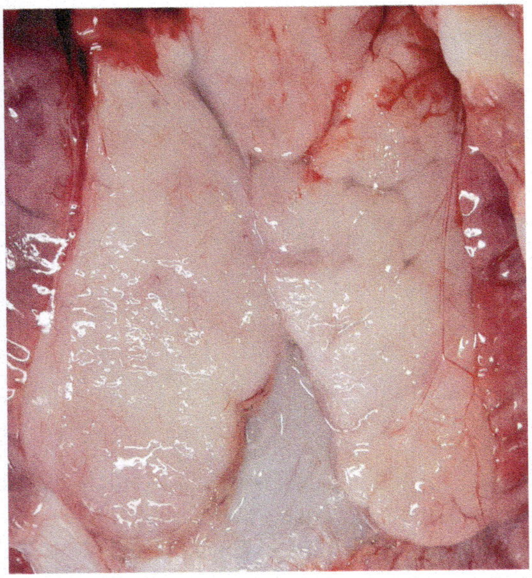

Fig. 3.111 Normal thymic surface in a victim of abusive head trauma

(e.g., strangulation, suffocation, or choking) but also in sudden unexplained infant death (Tardieu 1870; Ellis 1997).

3.3.6 Dating of Petechiae

Dating of petechial bleeding is not possible. Petechiae are an intravital reaction and vanish quickly in a living person, as long as there is no confluencing of petechiae. Parturitional petechiae in the mother, for example, vanish within 12 h or less (Purdue 2000). Petechiae may vanish in a living person within 1–3 days after a strangulation incident (Plattner et al. 2005). After death, petechiae are preserved for relatively long periods of time (Purdue 2000).

3.3.7 Petechiae and Child Abuse

As stated before, petechiae can result from mechanical asphyxiation. Asphyxiation can be the result of a true accident (e.g., traffic accidents, accidental hanging, drowning), a suicide-related act, an incident related to neglect and pure abusive acts (e.g., attempted suffocation or strangulation). In adolescents, traumatic asphyxia is sometimes the result of autoerotic asphyxiation. Petechiae, if present, are always found above the level of obstruction, mainly on the face, particularly around the eyes, on the inside of the lips and the nose, and behind the ears.

Patterned bruising in abused children may be accompanied by petechiae (Nayak et al. 2006). According to Nayak, bruising together with petechiae is found more commonly in abused children than in non-abused children with accidental injuries.

Non-accidental petechiae should be differentiated from petechiae in children with thrombocytopenia or thrombocytopathy, which often can be reproduced in the arm after a tourniquet is tied for venipuncture or in the face after crying (Lee 2008).

References

Bariciak ED, Plint AC, Gaboury I et al (2003) Dating of bruises in children: an assessment of physician accuracy. Pediatrics 112(4):804–807

Becker S, Schneider W, Kreuz W et al (1999) Post-trauma coagulation and fibrinolysis in children suffering from severe cerebro-cranial trauma. Eur J Pediatr 158(Suppl 3):S197–S202

Brenner JC (2004) Forensic science, an illustrated dictionary. CRC Press, Boca Raton

Busuttil A (2004) Wonden en verwondingen. In: Cohen BAJ, Holtslag H, Smitshuijzen RPh (eds) Forensische geneeskunde, raakvlakken tussen geneeskunst, gezondheidszorg en recht. Van Gorcum, Assen, pp 247–268

Busuttil A (2009) Chapter 16. Asphyxial death in children. In: Busuttil A, Keeling JW (eds) Paediatric forensic medicine & pathology. Hodder Arnold, London, pp 329–335

Carpenter RF (1999) The prevalence and distribution of bruises in babies. Arch Dis Child 80(4):363–366

Crimescope (2003). http://www.crimescope.com/march%2015/Applications.htm. Accessed on 2010

Damm D, White D, Brinker M (1981) Variations of palatal erythema secondary to fellatio. Oral Surg Oral Med Oral Pathol 52(4):417–421

David TJ (2004) Avoidable pitfalls when writing medical reports for court proceedings in cases of suspected child abuse. Arch Dis Child 89(9):799–804

David TJ (2005) Child abuse and paediatrics. J R Soc Med 98(5):229–231

Davis HW, Carrasco MM (2002) Child abuse and neglect. In: Zitelli BJ, Davis HW (eds) Atlas of pediatric physical diagnosis. Mosby, St Louis, pp 153–222

DiMaio VJ, DiMaio D (2001a) Chapter 2. Timing of death. In: DiMaio VJ, DiMaio D (eds) Forensic pathology, 2nd edn. CRC Press, Boca Raton, pp 21–41

DiMaio VJ, DiMaio D (2001b) Chapter 4. Blunt trauma wounds. In: DiMaio VJ, DiMaio D (eds) Forensic pathology, 2nd edn. CRC Press, Boca Raton, pp 91–116

Dimaio VJ, Dimaio D (2001c) Chapter 8. Asphyxia. In: Dimaio VJ, Dimaio D (eds) Forensic pathology, 2nd edn. CRC, Boca Raton, pp 229–277

Downes AJ, Crossland DS, Mellon AF (2002) Prevalence and distribution of petechiae in well babies. Arch Dis Child 86(4):291–292

Ellis PSJ (1997) The pathology of fatal child abuse. Pathology 29(2):113–121

Ely SF, Hirsch CS (2000) Asphyxial deaths and petechiae: a review. J Forensic Sci 45(6):1274–1277

Feldman KW (1992) Patterned abusive bruises of the buttocks and the pinnae. Pediatrics 90(4):633–636

Gavin L, Lanz M, Leung D (1997) Chronic subungual hematomas: a presumed immunologic puzzle resolved with a diagnosis of child abuse. Arch Pediatr Adolesc Med 151(1):103–104

Gilbert-Barnes E, Debich-Spicer DE (2005) Chapter 20. Pediatric forensic pathology. In: Gilbert-Barnes E, Debich-Spicer DE (eds) Handbook of pediatric forensic pathology. Humana Press, Totowa, pp 471–498

Glasgow JFT, Graham HK (1997) Chapter 4. Bruising and abrasions. In: Glasgow JFT, Graham HK (eds) Management of injuries in children. BMJ Publishing Group, London, pp 89–112

Griest KJ (2010) Timing of death and injuries in infants and young children. In: Griest KJ (ed) Pediatric homicide, medical investigation. CRC Press, Boca Raton, pp 197–228

Griest KJ, Zumwalt RE (1989) Child abuse by drowning. Pediatrics 83(1):41–46
Hammond H (2009) Chapter 1. Clinical assessment in suspected child abuse cases. In: Busutill A, Keeling JW (eds) Paediatric forensic medicine & pathology. Hodder Arnold, London, pp 1–23
Harris TL, Flaherty EG (2011) Chapter 29. Bruises and skin lesions. In: Jenny C (ed) Child abuse and neglect – diagnosis, treatment and evidence. Elsevier Saunders, St. Louis, pp 239–251
Herrmann B, Dettmeyer R, Banaschak S et al (2008) Kapitel 4. Hautbefunde. In: Herrmann B, Dettmeyer R, Banaschak S et al (eds) Kindesmisshandlung, Medizinische Diagnostik, Intervention und rechtliche Grundlagen. Springer Medizin Verlag, Heidelberg, pp 51–71
Hobbs CJ, Hanks HGI, Wynne JM (1999a) Chapter 4. Physical abuse. In: Hobbs CJ, Hanks HGI, Wynne JM (eds) Child abuse and neglect – a clinician's handbook, 2nd edn. Churchill Livingstone, London, pp 63–104
Hobbs CJ, Hanks HGI, Wynne JM (1999b) Chapter 9. Clinical aspects of sexual abuse. In: Hobbs CJ, Hanks HGI, Wynne JM (eds) Child abuse and neglect – a clinician's handbook, 2nd edn. Churchill Livingstone, London, pp 191–272
Hymel KP, Abshire TC, Luckey DW, Jenny C (1997) Coagulopathy in pediatric abusive head trauma. Pediatrics 99(3):371–375
Jain V, Ray M, Singhi S (2001) Strangulation injury, a fatal form of child abuse. Indian J Pediatr 68(6):571–572
Jenny C, Reece RM (2009) Cutaneous manifestations of child abuse. In: Reece RM, Christian CW (eds) Child abuse, medical diagnosis and management, 3rd edn. American Academy of Pediatrics, Elk Grove Village, pp 18–51
Johnson CF (1996) Physical abuse: accidental versus intentional trauma in children. In: In the APSAC handbook on child maltreatment. Sage Publications, Thousand Oaks, pp 206–226
Johnson CF, Showers J (1985) Injury variables in child abuse. Child Abuse Negl 9(2):207–215
Kaplan JM (1986) Pseudoabuse – the misdiagnosis of child abuse. J Forensic Sci 31(4):1420–1428
Kellogg N (2005) American Academy of Pediatrics/American Academy of Pediatric Dentistry – clinical report: oral and dental aspects of child abuse and neglect. Pediatrics 116(6):1565–1568
Knottenbelt JD (1994) Traumatic rhabdomyolysis from severe beating–experience of volume diuresis in 200 patients. J Trauma 37(2):214–219
Kornberg AE (1992) Skin and soft tissue injuries. In: Ludwig S, Kornberg AE (eds) Child abuse – a medical reference, 2nd edn. Churchill Livingstone, New York, pp 91–104
Kos L, Shwayder T (2006) Cutaneous manifestations of child abuse. Pediatr Dermatol 23(4):311–320
Kuban K, Winston K, Bresnan M (1983) Childhood subgaleal hematoma following minor head trauma. Am J Dis Child 137(7):637–640
Kumar V, Abbas AK, Fausto N et al (2007) Robbins basic pathology, 8th edn. Saunders, Philadelphia, p 86
Langlois NEI, Gresham GA (1991) The ageing of bruises: a review and study of the colour changes with time. Forensic Sci Int 50(2):227–238
Lee ACW (2008) Bruises, blood coagulation tests and the battered child syndrome. Singapore Med J 49(6):445–450
Leung A, Robson L (1987) Myoglobinuria from child abuse. Urology 29(1):45–46
Maguire S, Mann MK, Sibert J et al (2005a) Can you review bruises accurately in children? Arch Dis Child 90(2):187–189
Maguire S, Mann MK, Sibert J et al (2005b) Are there patterns of bruising in childhood which are diagnostic or suggestive of abuse? A systematic review. Arch Dis Child 90(2):182–186
Merck Manuals Online Medical Library (2007) Blunt injuries to the eye. http://www.merckmanuals.com/home/injuries_and_poisoning/injuries_to_the_eye/blunt_injuries_to_the_eye.html. Accessed on 2010
Minford AMB, Richards EM (2010) Excluding medical and haematological conditions as a cause of bruising in suspected non-accidental injury. Arch Dis Child Educ Pract Ed 95(1):2–8
Mukherji SK, Siegel MJ (1987) Rhabdomyolysis and renal failure in child abuse. Am J Roentgenol 148(6):1203–1204
Munang LA, Leonard PA, Mok JY (2002) Lack of agreement on colour description between clinicians examining childhood bruising. J Clin Forensic Med 9(4):171–174
Nathanson M (2006) Chapter 11. The physically and emotionally abused child: In Mason JK, Purdue BN. The Pathology of Trauma, 3rd edn. Arnold, London, pp 155–175
Nayak K, Spencer N, Shenoy M et al (2006) How useful is the presence of petechiae in distinguishing non-accidental from accidental injury? Child Abuse Negl 30(5):549–555
Newson J, Newson E (1986) Findings on use of physical punishment on 1, 4, 7 and 11 year old children, together with some sequelae in later life. Child Development Research Unit. University of Nottingham, Nottingham (cited from Hobbs, 1999)
Pascoe JM, Hildebrandt HM, Tarrier A et al (1979) Patterns of skin injury in nonaccidental and accidental injury. Pediatrics 64(2):245–247
Payne-James J (2003) Chapter 36. Assault and injury in the living. In: Payne-James J, Busuttil A, Smock W (eds) Forensic medicine: clinical and pathological aspects. Greenwich Medical Media Ltd, San Francisco, pp 543–564
Pediatric Care Online (2009). http://www.pediatriccare-online.org/pco/ub/view/Point-of-Care-Quick-Reference/397100/1.2/Petechiae_and_Purpura. Accessed on 2011
Peebles J, Losek JD (2007) Child physical abuse and rhabdomyolysis: case report and literature review. Pediatr Emerg Care 23(7):474–477

Plattner T, Bolliger S, Zollinger U (2005) Forensic assessment of survived strangulation. Forensic Sci Int 153(2):202–207

Purdue BN (2000) Chapter 15. Asphyxial and related death. In: Mason JK, Purdue BN (eds) The pathology of trauma, 3rd edn. Arnold, London, pp 230–252

Raimer BG, Raimer SS, Hebeler JR (1981) Cutaneous signs of child abuse. J Am Acad Dermatol 5(2): 203–214

RCPCH (Royal College of Paediatrics and Child Health) (2008a) The physical signs of child sexual abuse – an evidence-based review and guidance for best practice. RCPCH, London, pp 14–89

RCPCH (Royal College of Paediatrics and Child Health) (2008b) The physical signs of child sexual abuse – an evidence-based review and guidance for best practice. RCPCH, London, pp 153–157

Reece RM, Grodin MA (1985) Recognition of nonaccidental injury. Pediatr Clin North Am 32(1):41–60

Robertson I (1957) Antemortem and postmortem bruises of the skin: their differentiation. J Forensic Med 4:2–10

Robinson S (2000) Chapter 10. The examination of the adult victim of assault. In: Mason JK, Purdue BN (eds) The pathology of trauma, 3rd edn. Arnold, London, pp 140–154

Rosenberg HK, Gefter WB, Lebowitz RL et al (1983) Prolonged dense nephrograms in battered children. Suspect rhabdomyolysis and myoglobinuria. Urology 21(3):325–330

Roy D, Al Saleem BM, Al Ibrahim A et al (1999) Rhabdomyolysis and acute renal failure in a case of child abuse. Ann Saudi Med 19(3):248–250

Saukko P, Knight B (2004a) Chapter 4. The pathology of wounds. In: Saukko P, Knight B (eds) Knight's Forensic pathology, 3rd edn. Arnold Publications, London, pp 136–173

Saukko P, Knight B (2004b) Chapter 14. Suffocation and 'asphyxia'. In: Saukko P, Knight B (eds) Knight's forensic pathology, 3rd edn. Arnold, London, pp 352–367

Saukko P, Knight B (2004c) Chapter 26. Forensic dentistry for the pathologist. In: Saukko P, Knight B (eds) Knight's forensic pathology, 3rd edn. Arnold Publications, London, pp 527–540

Schmitt BD (1987) The child with nonaccidental trauma. In: Helfer RE, Kempe RS (eds) The battered child, 4th edn. University of Chicago Press, Chicago, pp 178–196

Schwartz AJ, Ricci LR (1996) How accurately can bruises be aged in abused children? Literature review and synthesis. Pediatrics 97(2):254–257

Schwengel D, Ludwig S (1985) Rhabdomyolysis and myoglobinuria as manifestations of child abuse. Pediatr Emerg Care 1(4):194–197

Simpson CK (1979) Forensic medicine, 8th edn. Edward Arnold, London

Somers GR, Chiasson DA, Taylor GP (2008) Presence of periorbital and conjunctival petechial hemorrhages in accidental pediatric drowning. Forensic Sci Int 175(2–3):198–201

Speight N (1997) Non-accidental injury. In: Meadow R (ed) ABC of child abuse, 3rd edn. BMJ Publishing Group, London, pp 5–8

Stephenson T, Bialas Y (1996) Estimation of the age of bruising. Arch Dis Child 74(1):53–55

Sugar NF, Taylor JA, Feldman KW (1999) Bruises in infants and toddlers: those who don't cruise rarely bruise. Arch Pediatr Adolesc Med 153(4):399–403

Sussman SJ (1968) The battered child syndrome. Calif Med 108(6):437–439

Tardieu (1870) Etude medico-legale sur la pendaison, la strangulation, et la suffocation. Bailliere et fils. Paris

Thomas AE (2004) The bleeding child: is it NAI? Arch Dis Child 89(12):1163–1167

Tsokos M (2005) Postmortem changes and artifacts occurring during the early postmortem interval. In: Tsokos M (ed) Pathology reviews, vol 3. Humana Press, Totowa, pp 183–238

Vanezis P (1997) Ageing of bruises by colour photometry. Lecture at the autumn symposium of the association of police surgeons (quoted from Robinson 2000)

Vogeley E, Pierce MC, Bertocci G (2002) Experience with Wood lamp illumination and digital photography in the documentation of bruises on human skin. Arch Pediatr Adolesc Med 156:265–268

Vu TT, Guerrera MF, Hamburger EK (2004) Subgaleal hematoma from hair braiding: case report and literature review. Pediatr Emerg Care 20(12):821–823

Watson AA (1990) Letsels en verwondingen. Uit Cohen BAJ, Leliefeld HJ (eds) Inleiding tot de Forensische geneeskunde, 2e druk. Kerckebosch BV Zeist, pp 279–96

Wheeler DM, Hobbs CJ (1988) Mistakes in diagnosing non-accidental injury, 10 years' experience. Br Med J 296(6631):1233–1236

Wilson EF (1977) Estimation of the age of cutaneous contusions in child abuse. Pediatrics 60(5):750–752

Wynne J (2003) Chapter 30. The physical and emotional abuse of children. In: Payne-James J, Busuttil A, Smock W (eds) Forensic medicine, clinical and pathological aspects. Greenwich Medical Media Ltd, San Francisco, pp 469–485

Yamamoto K, Hayase T, Yamamoto Y et al (2000) Application of the term 'Tardieu's Spots' to postmortem developed petechiae. A literature survey. Res Pract Forensic Med 43:386–392

4 Accidental Trauma

4.1 Introduction

Accidents are the most prevalent cause of bruising in children, especially when they start to become more mobile. Therefore, accidents are the most important differential diagnosis in bruising in children.

In evaluating the differential diagnosis between abuse and accident, one should always take into account the history from both parents and child (Sect. 2.8.2), the age and developmental stage of the child, and the shape, size, number, and location of the bruises.

4.2 Trauma: Accidental Versus Non-accidental Trauma

4.2.1 Age and Developmental Level

Bruises are the most common injury in children, despite the circumstances (accidental or abusive). Accidental bruising may be the result of everyday activities, including sports and play (Figs. 4.1, 4.2, 4.3, 4.4, 4.5, 4.6, 4.7, 4.8, 4.9, 4.10, 4.11, and 4.12), or of (traffic) accidents (Figs. 4.13, 4.14, 4.15, and 4.16). In other words, bruising is strongly related to physical activities and therefore to the level of mobility of the child. Bruising in a nonmobile child is rarely found. Once a child is able to move independently, the child may sustain injuries.

Wedgwood (1990) found that the older the child, the more bruises are found, particularly on the shins and knees: in this study, 17% of children in the crawling stage showed 1–5 bruises, while 52% of children who could walk had 1–27 bruises.

In a prospective study, Sugar et al. (1999) found similar results in 973 children <3 years old,

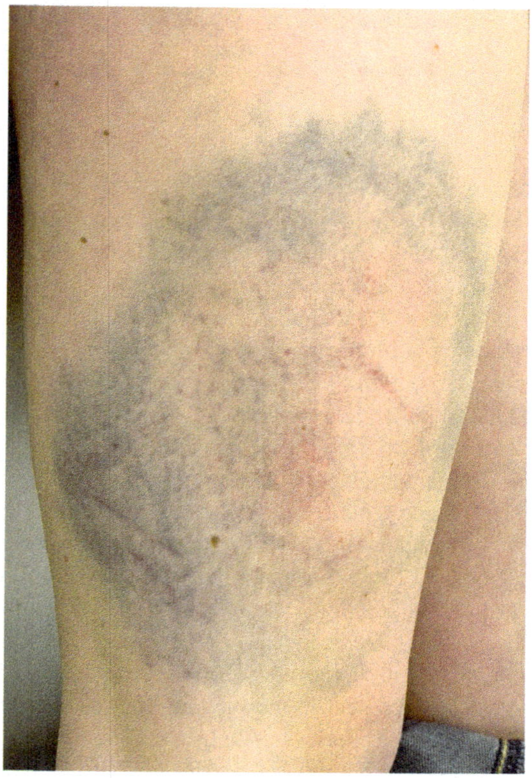

Fig. 4.1 Sports: bruising after being hit by a soccer ball – day 2

R.A.C. Bilo et al., *Cutaneous Manifestations of Child Abuse and Their Differential Diagnosis*,
DOI 10.1007/978-3-642-29287-3_4, © Springer-Verlag Berlin Heidelberg 2013

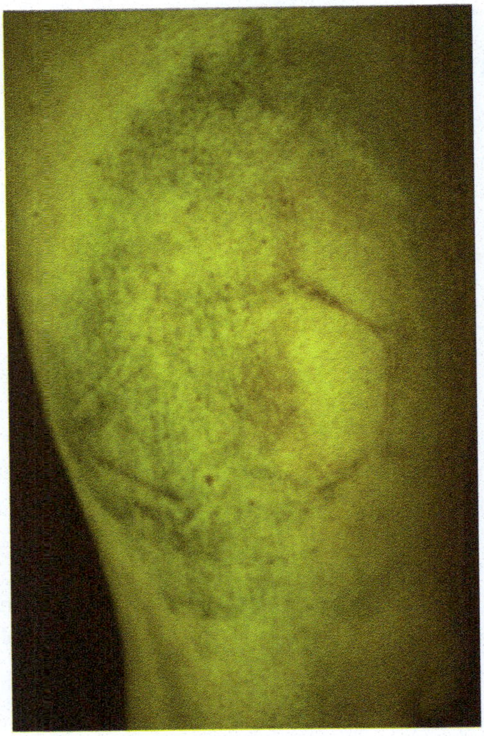

Fig. 4.2 Bruising after being hit by a soccer ball – day 2 (forensic light)

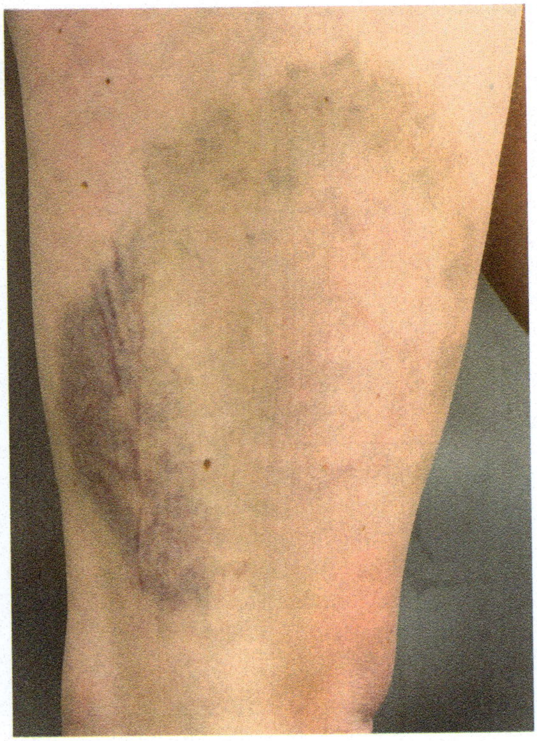

Fig. 4.3 Healing bruise after being hit by a soccer ball – day 10

examined during well-child visits. She found that bruises were rare in non-abused children of up to 1 year old and in nonmobile children. She saw a clear increase in the number of bruises in mobile children and "walkers." According to Sugar, child abuse should be considered when bruises are found in children of less than 9 months old or in nonmobile children: "Those who don't cruise rarely bruise."

Carpenter (1999) prospectively documented size, shape, and color of bruises related to the mobility status in 177 children between the ages of 6 and 12 months, examined during well-child visits. Bruises were present in 12% of the children, and all were located on bony prominences on the front of the body. Bruises on the shins were only present in mobile children. Carpenter found bruising in less than 1% of non-crawling, non-abused children. The main conclusion that was drawn from this study was that doctors should take into account the developmental level of the child when deciding whether a bruise is the result of an accident or has been inflicted.

Labbé and Caouette (2001) prospectively studied the presence of skin injuries in normal children to establish whether there was a possible relationship between the number of injuries, the age of the child, and the time the injury was sustained (time of year) in a temperate climate. In total, 2,040 physical examinations in children between 0 and 17 years were evaluated. Most children of 9 months and older had one or more recent injuries (bruises, abrasions, lacerations, incised wounds, burn wounds). During the summer, injuries were more prevalent and were found on every part of body but predominantly on the extremities. A suspicion of child abuse or a clotting disorder was justified in cases where the bruising was in an unusual location, the presence of >15 injuries, an age of <9 months, and in the cold seasons injuries in locations other than the extremities.

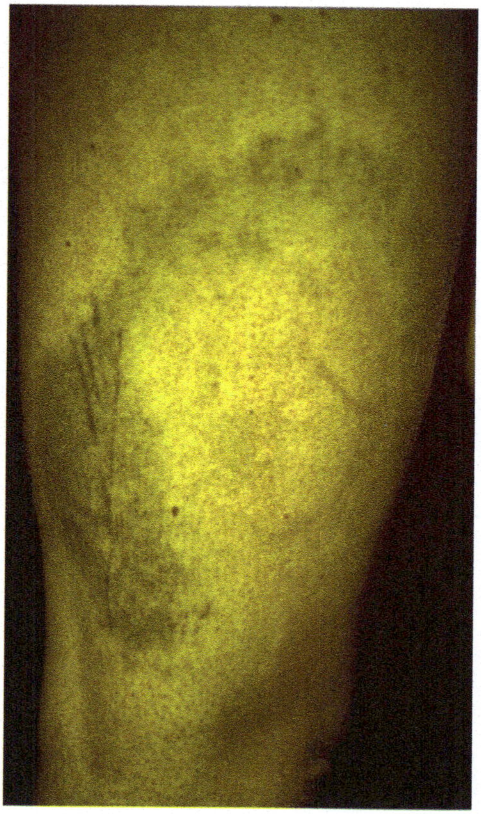

Fig. 4.4 Healing bruise after being hit by a soccer ball – day 10 (forensic light)

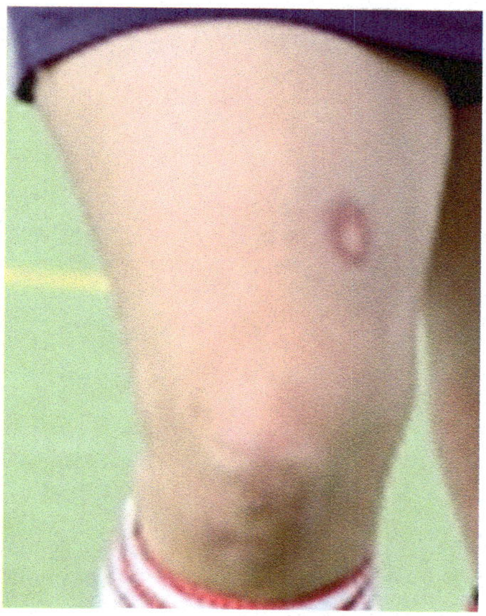

Fig. 4.5 Sports: bruising directly after being hit by a field hockey ball on the inside of the right thigh

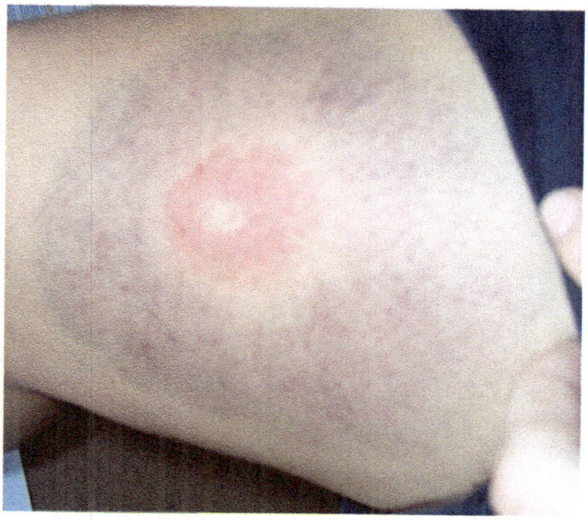

Fig. 4.6 Same field hockey player as in Fig. 4.5, bruising 3–4 days after being hit by the ball

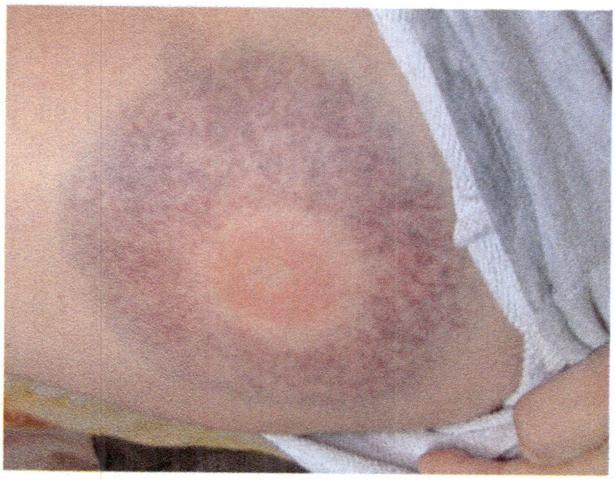

Fig. 4.7 Same field hockey player as in Fig. 4.5, other incident: bruising some days after being hit by a field hockey ball on the outside of the left thigh

Maguire et al. (2005) reviewed the medical literature comprehensively on data regarding bruising in children (1951–2004; all language search). Ultimately, 23 studies suitable for further evaluation were found (7 studies in non-abused children, 14 studies in abused children, and 2 studies in either group). In the non-abused group, the prevalence, number, and location of the bruises depended on the level of mobility of the child. In nonmobile babies, bruising turned out to be very rare (<1%). Bruising was present in 17% of children who were starting to become mobile (e.g., walking by holding on to furniture) and in up to 53% of children

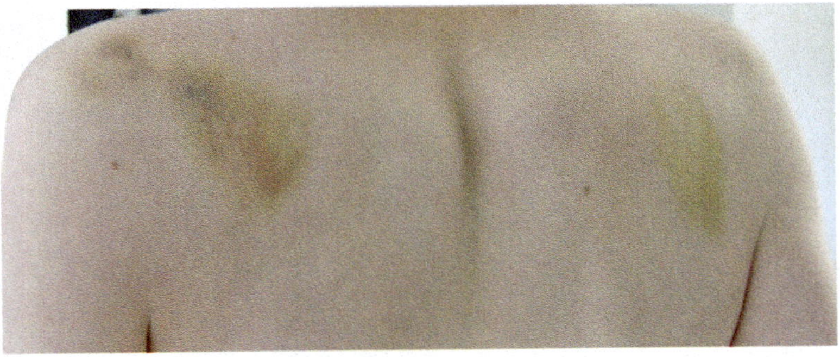

Fig. 4.8 Bruises due to break dancing

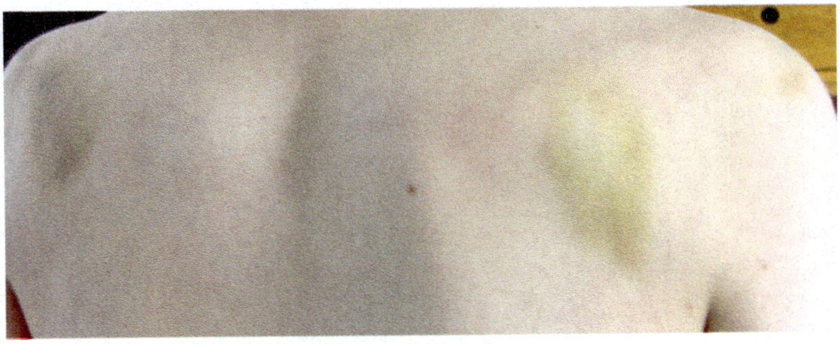

Fig. 4.9 Same boy: bruises due to break dancing

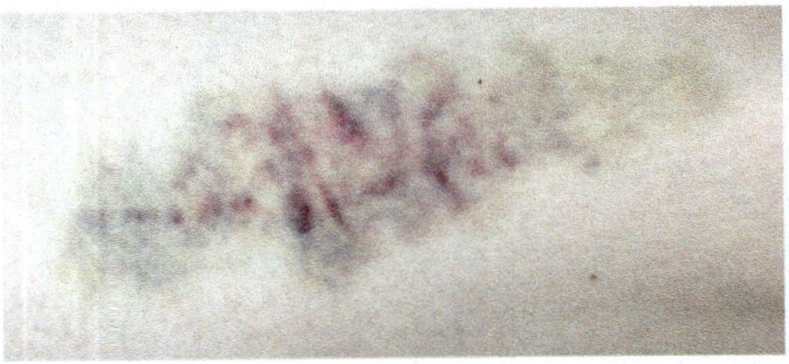

Fig. 4.10 Healing bruise caused by a climbing rope

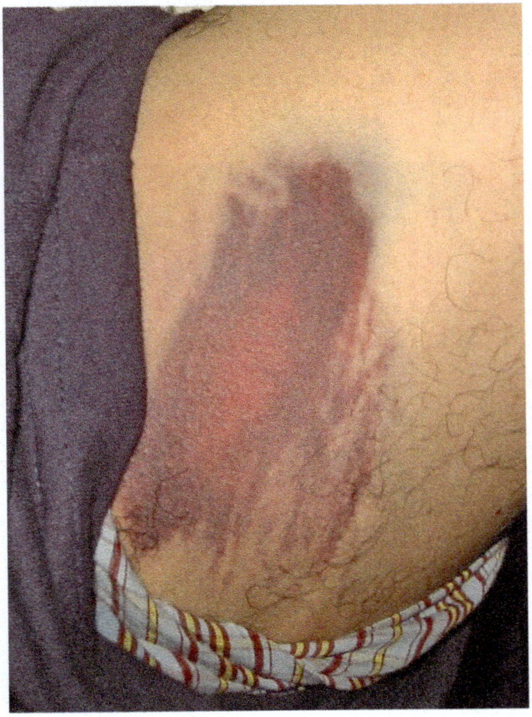

Fig. 4.11 Bruising caused by handrail skateboarding (a.k.a. grinds) (Nherdboi 2006 from Wikimedia Commons 2011: Severebruise.jpg)

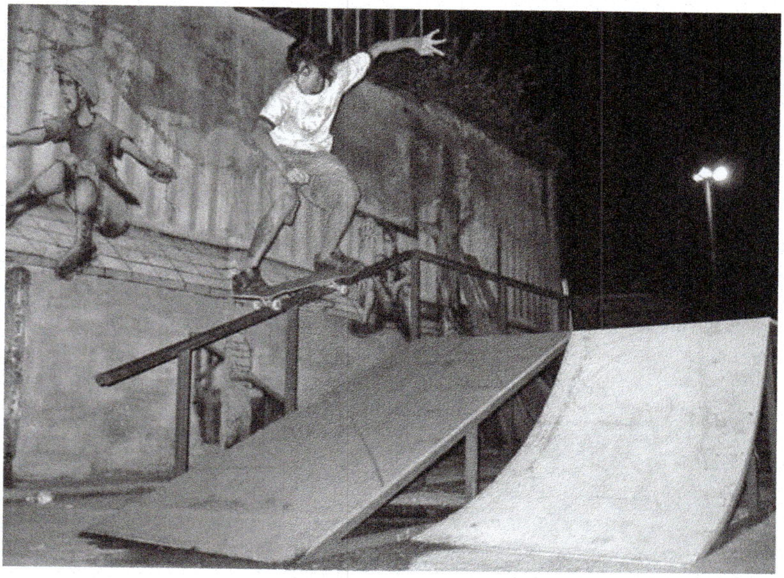

Fig. 4.12 Handrail skateboarding. Telanjanggmail, 2006 from Wikimedia Commons, 2011: Reno-Backside50-50Grind.jpg

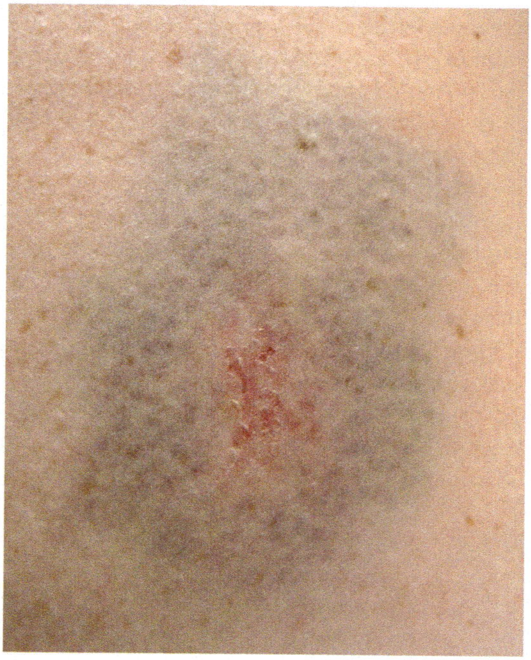

Fig. 4.13 Bruise from bicycle accident, in the center a grade 1 abrasion (see Sect. 7.3.1) (Ksuel 2007 from Wikimedia Commons 2011: Bruise from bicycle accident.jpg)

who walked by themselves. Bruises were seen in the vast majority of school-aged children.

4.2.2 Gender

There are no significant differences in frequency, pattern, and extent in bruising of any cause between girls and boys as revealed by several studies (Johnson and Showers 1985; Labbé and Caouette 2001; Wedgwood, 1990).

4.2.3 Shape, Size, and Number

Bruises in non-abused children are generally small and located on the front of the body, mainly on bony prominences (Maguire et al. 2005). The presence of multiple bruises with a uniform shape/size or recognizable form or pattern (Sect. 3.2.5) justifies a suspicion of child abuse (Chap. 3). Inflicted bruises tend to be larger than accidental bruises. Usually, inflicted bruises are multiple and found in clusters. Often, they are seen

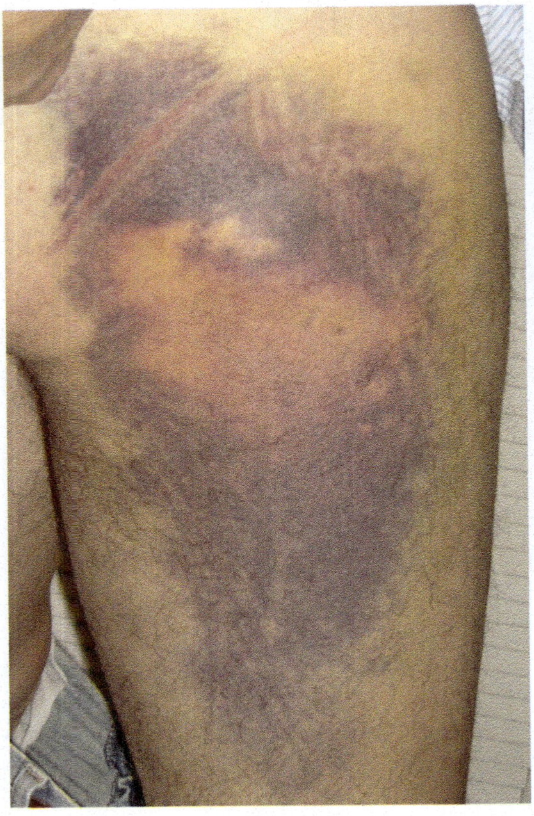

Fig. 4.14 Large hematoma of the right thigh after an accidental fall downstairs (Martinkidgell 2007 from Wikimedia Commons 2011: Hematoma Feb 07.jpg)

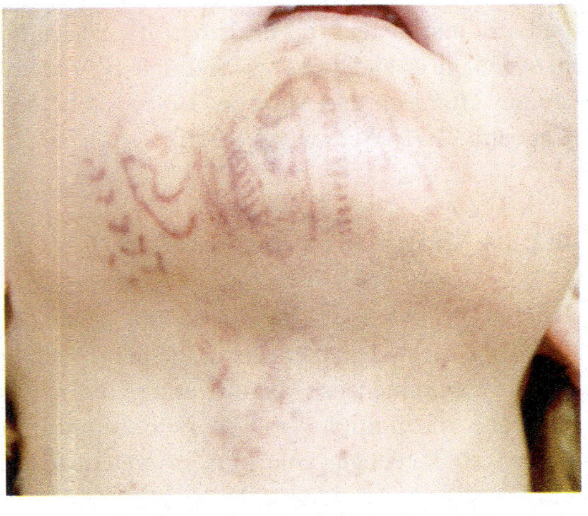

Fig. 4.15 Shoe imprint, due to being overrun in a crowd

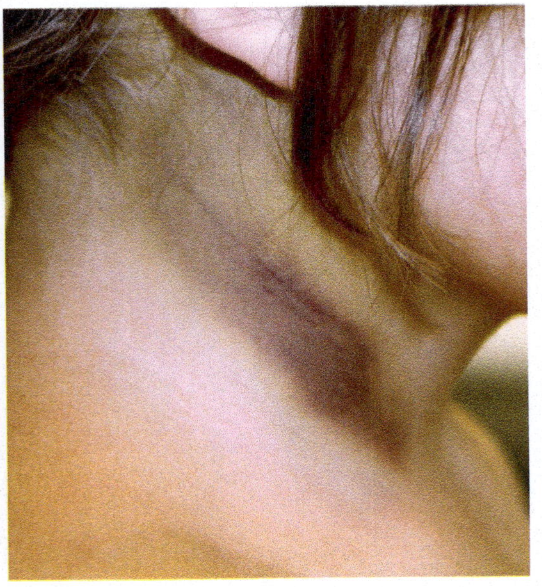

Fig. 4.16 Bruising in the neck (observed accident – cycling child versus car)

combined with other types of recent and older injuries, such as scars from burns or healing abrasions. Abused children tend to have more bruises than non-abused children (Labbé and Caouette 2001; Maguire et al. 2005).

Pierce et al. (2010) showed that the total number of bruises in abused children of less than 4 years old is significantly different from the total number of bruises in non-abused children ($P < .0005$): the abused children had up to 25 bruises (median 6 bruises) and children who had sustained an accidental trauma had 4 bruises or less (median 1.5 bruises) (see also Sect. 4.2.5).

4.2.4 Location

4.2.4.1 Accidental Bruising

Slips, trips, and falls are frequent events, especially in young mobile children. Slips and trips are more often seen in toddlers. Falls tend to happen more frequently in children of <1 year old (Chang and Tsai 2007) (see also Table 4.1). Craniofacial injuries are seen more often in slips and trips than in falls. Generally, these events will take place head first and as such may lead to craniofacial injuries. Once the child has learned to walk or climb adequately, the child generally lands on the front of the head (Pascoe et al. 1979). For that reason, most injuries will be found on the face, often in a T-shaped distribution (forehead and periorbital area, nose, upper lip, and chin). When a bruise develops after a fall on the forehead, it may relocate to the periorbital area, and particularly to the lower eyelid, probably due to the influence of gravity and sometimes leading to "raccoon" eyes. This will mostly happen in case of a substantial injury and a hematoma in the deeper tissues. It is less likely in case of superficial bruising. Sometimes, the child will fall backward and "land" on the buttocks or on the back of the head. This will almost never lead to bruising of the buttocks but may lead to bruising of the impact area, predominantly the posterior area of the head (Chang and Tsai 2007). In case of slips, trips, and falls, only 5% of accidental bruising is found on the cheeks and about 6% around the eyes (Chang and Tsai 2007).

In older mobile children, the most prevalent locations of bruising are the shins, the knees, the elbows, the forehead, and the cheekbone, reflecting normal daily activities.

As shown above, accidental bruising will be found predominantly on the front of the body in locations where the skin lies almost directly above the bone (the so-called bony prominences) (Wedgwood 1990; Sugar et al. 1999). Most frequently, only a single bruise is seen or in uncomplicated accidental slips, trips, and falls a few bruises. The explanation provided by the caretaker for the injury is usually sufficient.

In accidental trauma, bruising is only rarely seen on certain parts of the body, like the cheeks, ears, and neck; parts of the trunk (back, buttocks, abdomen, or hip); and on the extremities (hand, forearm, upper arm, posterior part of the leg, foot) (Figs. 4.16, 4.17, 4.18, 4.19, and 4.20) (Wedgwood 1990; Carpenter 1999; Sugar et al. 1999; Dunstan, 2002; Chang and Tsai 2007). Figure 4.21 shows an often used overview of locations in which accidental bruising

Table 4.1 Typical age-related falls in childhood

Age (years)	Falls
0–1	Arms of caretakers
	Furniture (baby bouncers, sofas, beds, and tables)
	Stairs (including using baby walkers)
	Prams and supermarket trolleys
1–4	From static standing position or during running
	Stairs
	Windows and balconies
	Furniture (e.g., tables, couches, other furniture)
5–9	Bicycles, horses, playground equipment, fences, and trees
10–14	Bicycles, horses, playground equipment, fences, and trees
	Sports and adventurous play

After Glasgow and Graham (1997) and Warrington and Wright (2001)

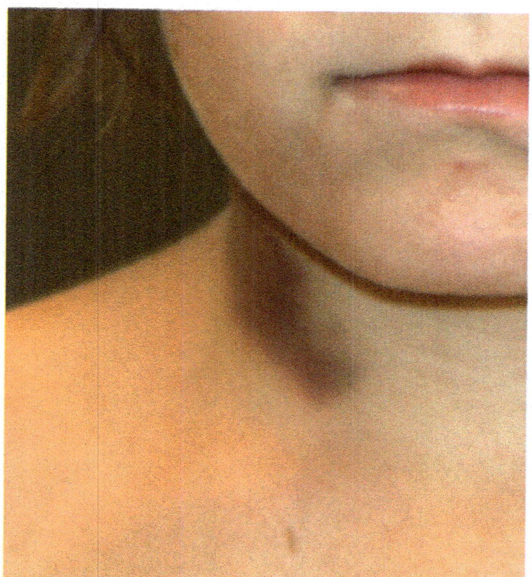

Fig. 4.17 Same child: bruising in the neck (observed accident – cycling child versus car)

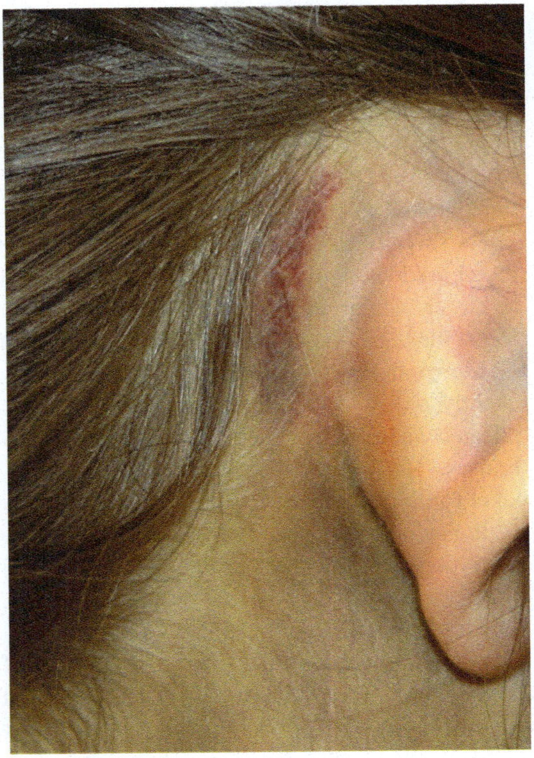

Fig. 4.18 Same child: bruising behind the ear (observed accident – cycling child versus car)

is more common and in which bruises are less common accidentally or suspicious for inflicted bruising.

4.2.4.2 Non-accidental Bruising

Bruises from child abuse may be found on any part of the body, but the part of the body that is most commonly bruised in child abuse is the face, followed by other areas of the head/neck region, including ears, cheeks, and the neck. Other commonly bruised areas include the trunk (abdomen, back, and buttocks) and the arms and legs. According to Schmitt (1987), the simultaneous appearance of injuries on multiple body planes in young children merits a suspicion of physical abuse.

Non-accidental bruising often occurs on soft-tissue areas such as the cheeks and the thighs (Naidoo 2000). Bruises on the neck are rarely of accidental origin (Figs. 4.16 and 4.17). If bruising is encountered on the neck, an (attempted) strangulation must be considered.

Defensive injuries (Sect. 2.7.2) may occur when the child assumes a defensive position during the assault. These injuries can be found on the arms (upper arm and forearm), on the lateral side of the upper leg, or on the back, sometimes reflecting a fetal-like defensive position.

Bruises in the anogenital area, on the inner sides of the upper and lower arms and the thighs (e.g., "fingertip bruising"), or in the armpits may indicate sexual abuse. Bruises in the anogenital area and on the buttocks may also indicate an assault related to problems regarding toilet/potty training (Hobbs et al. 1993).

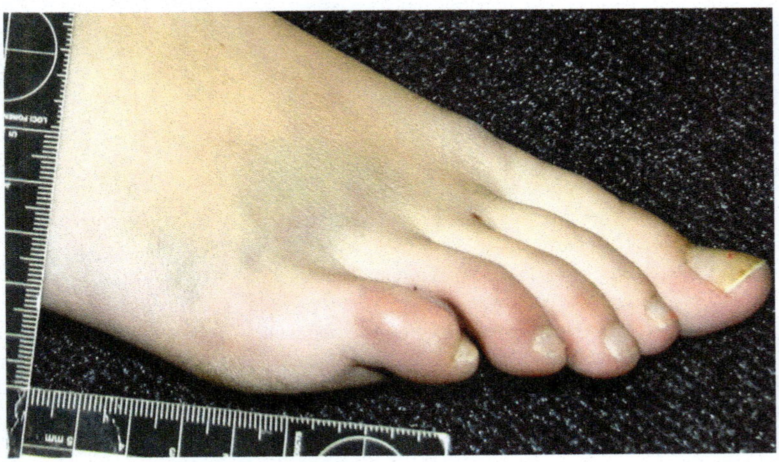

Fig. 4.19 Bruising of foot, caused during a motor vehicle accident (foot overrun by car tire)

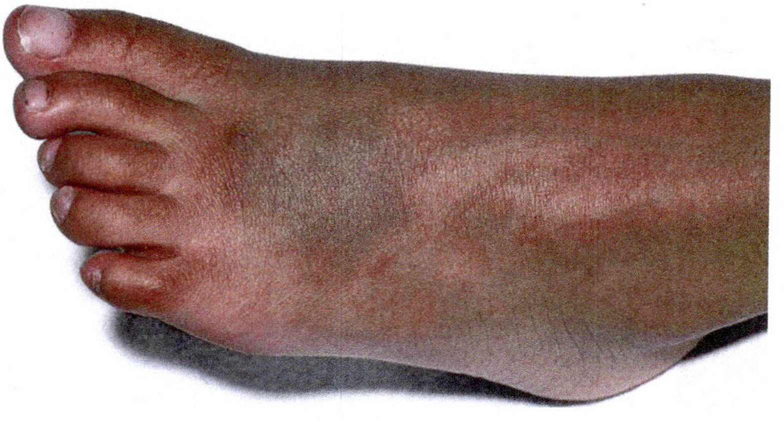

Fig. 4.20 Bruising of foot, caused by stamping on the foot by the child's parent

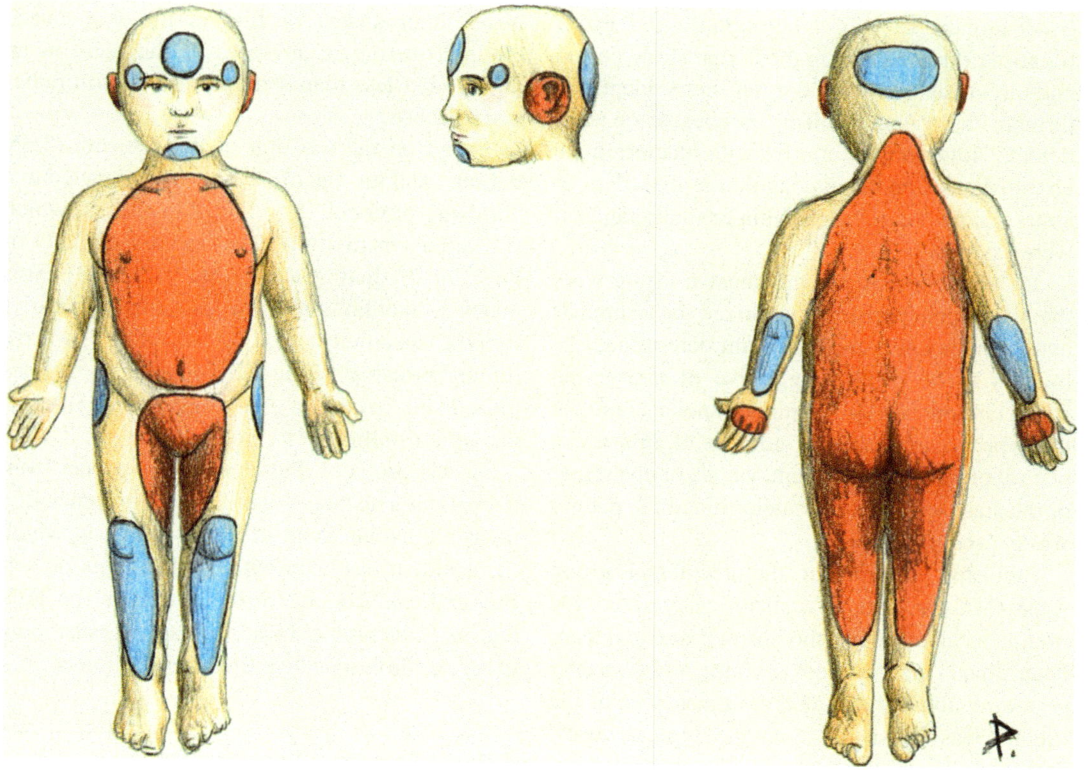

Fig. 4.21 Overview: in *blue*, more common locations for accidental bruises; in *red*, less common locations for accidental bruises or locations suspicious for inflicted bruises

Sometimes, the bruise shows a recognizable pattern or imprint – a so-called telltale injury (Sect. 3.2.5). Patterned bruising in abused children may be accompanied by petechiae (Nayak et al. 2006). According to Nayak, bruising together with petechiae is found more frequently in abused children than in non-abused children with accidental injuries.

4.2.5 Pierce's Study on Discriminating Bruising Characteristics

Pierce's study was aimed at identifying characteristics which would enable the differentiation between inflicted and accidental bruises. The study was also aimed at developing a more or less evidence-based screening tool for high-risk children. For that reason, she evaluated the data of 95 children of 0–48 months of age (retrospective, casecontrolled study of patients with abusive or accidental trauma: 42 victims of physical abuse and 53 children with accidental trauma). Children in the accidental trauma group were age-matched as closely as possible to the children in the group with abusive trauma. Inclusion criteria were 0–48 months of age, admission to the PICU because of trauma during the 2-year study period and circumstances related to an injury identified through the trauma registry as abusive or accidental. Children with injuries with indeterminate circumstances and/or a coagulation disorders or abnormalities (e.g., hemophilia or malignancies) were excluded.

Inclusion criteria for the abusive group were that the trauma registry categorized the trauma as abuse; the hospital medical team determined the injuries to be highly suggestive of abuse; the stated circumstances of injury did not account for the type, severity, and/or number of injuries; a history of trauma was absent, vague, or changing; or the state social services determined the patient was abused.

Inclusion criteria for the accidental group were that the trauma registry categorized the trauma as an accident; the hospital medical team determined the injuries to raise no concerns regarding abuse; the stated circumstances of the trauma was consistent with the type, severity, and/or number of injuries; the history was detailed, thorough, and consistent; and no indicators of abuse were found during skeletal survey, social service assessment, and/or forensic team evaluations.

Skin findings did not play any role in determining whether the child was categorized as belonging to the abusive or accidental group. Categorization occurred before any data analysis.

Table 4.2 TEN (Torso, ear, neck) body regions

Torso	Chest
	Abdomen
	Back
	Buttocks
	Genitourinary area
	Hip
Ear	
Neck	

Pierce et al. (2010)

Seventy-one children showed bruises (33 victims of abuse; 38 children with accidental trauma). Characteristics predictive of abuse were bruising on the torso, ear, or neck (TEN region, see Table 4.2). Bruises on the torso, ear, or neck were either absent or rare in the non-abused group. Bruising in any area of the body in an infant aged less than 4 months was also predictive of abuse.

Based on the location of the bruising (TEN regions) and the age of the child, the data led to a "bruising protocol" for clinical decisions, which showed a sensitivity of 97% and a specificity of 84% for predicting abuse (see Table 4.3). This means a likelihood ratio of just over 6 (sensitivity/(100-specificity) = 6,07); in other words, finding bruising in the TEN regions is 6 times more likely in case of abuse than in case of accidental/non-inflicted circumstances.

In this protocol, Pierce uses one aspect from the patient's history: the absence or presence of a plausible explanation for the accident, in which the accident has been witnessed in a public setting and can account for the bruises in the TEN region. If the protocol leads to a serious suspicion of abuse, further evaluation will be required.

4.3 Trauma: Insufficient or Inadequate Supervision

In situations where there is a lack of supervision, the risk of injuries in children is high. Children who are growing up in a negligent environment sustain accidental injuries more frequently than children who are living in a more protective environment. These injuries do not result from active

Table 4.3 Clinical-decision protocol for bruising: differentiating between accidental and inflicted bruising in children ≤4 years of age

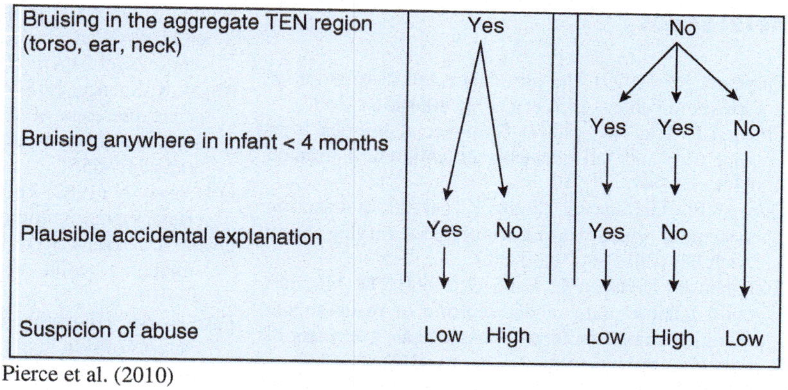

Pierce et al. (2010)

abusive acts by parents or caregivers but from a lack of protection or supervision. The characteristics of these injuries are similar to those of "normal" accidental injuries.

When injuries are found that result from a lack of supervision, it should lead to further evaluation because inadequate supervision may lead to serious or even life-threatening accidents such as falls from heights, playing with fire, poisoning, or drowning.

If it is suspected that the injury (or the death) of the child is the result of a lack of supervision, the following questions should be answered:

1. Was the injury accidental or inflicted?
2. If the injury was accidental, could it have been prevented by adequate supervision?
3. Was the accident part of an established pattern of inadequate supervision?

A lack of supervision may happen once or may be chronic. If it happens once, the child may die as a result of a sudden and unexpected life-threatening situation. The postmortem examination will reveal no further evidence of child abuse. Death in chronically negligent circumstances is often the result of an accumulation of problems (Ewigman et al. 1993; Zuravin 1991). Death may be related to a repeated pattern of inadequate and poor parenting, untreated or severe illness, including infection and malnutrition and preventable non-intentional injury. In the postmortem examination, one will often find evidence of neglect and other forms of child abuse (physical violence, sexual abuse).

4.4 Trauma: Bruising in Children with a Coexistent Disease

Excessive bruising as a result of trauma can be found in various disorders, many of them congenital in nature. The parents prior to the diagnosis being made may not be able to provide an adequate explanation. This may result in suspected child abuse. In these conditions, the distribution of the bruising can be similar to the bruising that is seen after an accident, although it is often more extensive.

Descriptions of children with coexistent disorders include, for example, children with bleeding disorders (Chap. 5) and collagen vascular disorders, for example, Ehlers-Danlos syndrome (Sect. 5.4.1 and Chap. 6), in which the findings during the physical examination may lead to suspected maltreatment (Owen and Durst 1984).

Also, children with the very rare disorder of congenital indifference/insensitivity to pain (MIM #243000) may be a cause of confusion (O'Doherty 1982; Makari et al. 1994; Mendelian Inheritance in Man 2010). These children will have painless injuries as early as infancy. There may be injuries without the child having any noticeable hindrance. This may lead to an accumulation of various kinds of trauma at various anatomical locations. There may even be recurrent fractures without adequate recovery (Spencer and Grieve 1990).

References

Carpenter RF (1999) The prevalence and distribution of bruises in babies. Arch Dis Child 80(4):363–366

Chang LT, Tsai MC (2007) Craniofacial injuries from slip, trip, and fall accidents of children. J Trauma 63(1):70–74

Dunstan FD, Guildea ZE, Kontos K et al (2002) A scoring system for bruise patterns: a tool for identifying abuse. Arch Dis Child 86(5):330–333

Ewigman B, Kivlahan C, Land G (1993) The Missouri child fatality study: underreporting of maltreatment fatalities among children younger than five years of age, 1983 through 1986. Pediatrics 91(2):330–337

Glasgow JFT, Graham HK (1997) Chapter 1. Epidemiology of accidents and patterns of injury, healing and recovery. In: Glasgow JFT, Graham HK (eds) Management of injuries in children. BMJ Publishing Group, London, pp 1–27

Hobbs CJ, Hanks HGI, Wynne JM (1993) Physical abuse. In: Hobbs CJ, Hanks HGI, Wynne JM (eds) Child abuse and neglect – a clinician's handbook. Churchill Livingstone, London, pp 47–75

Johnson CF, Showers J (1985) Injury variables in child abuse. Child Abuse Negl 9(2):207–215

Labbé J, Caouette G (2001) Recent skin injuries in normal children. Pediatrics 108(2):271–276

Maguire S, Mann MK, Sibert J et al (2005) Are there patterns of bruising in childhood which are diagnostic or suggestive of abuse? A systematic review. Arch Dis Child 90(2):182–186

Makari GS, Carroll JE, Burton EM (1994) Hereditary sensory neuropathy manifesting as possible child abuse. Pediatrics 93(5):842–844

Mendelian Inheritance in Man (2010) (MIM#243000) http://www.ncbi.nlm.nih.gov/entrez/dispomim.cgi?id=243000

Naidoo S (2000) A profile of the oro-facial injuries in child physical abuse at a children's hospital. Child Abuse Negl 24(4):521–534

Nayak K, Spencer N, Shenoy M et al (2006) How useful is the presence of petechiae in distinguishing non-accidental from accidental injury? Child Abuse Negl 30(5):549–555

O'Doherty N (1982) The battered child – recognition in primary care. Bailliere Tindall, London

Owen SM, Durst RD (1984) Ehlers-Danlos syndrome simulating child abuse. Arch Dermatol 120(1):97–101

Pascoe JM, Hildebrandy HM, Tarrier A et al (1979) Patterns of skin injury in nonaccidental and accidental injury. Pediatrics 64(2):245–247

Pierce MC, Kaczor K, Aldridge S et al (2010) Bruising characteristics discriminating physical child abuse from accidental trauma. Pediatrics 125(1):64–71

Schmitt BD (1987) The child with nonaccidental trauma. In: Helfer RE, Kempe RS (eds) The battered child, 4th edn. University of Chicago Press, Chicago, pp 178–196

Spencer JA, Grieve DK (1990) Congenital indifference to pain mistaken for non-accidental injury. Br J Radiol 63(748):308–310

Sugar NF, Taylor JA, Feldman KW (1999) Bruises in infants and toddlers: those who don't cruise rarely bruise. Arch Pediatr Adolesc Med 153(4):399–403

Warrington SA, Wright CM (2001) Accidents and resulting injuries in premobile infants: data from the ALSPAC study. Arch Dis Child 85(2):104–107

Wedgwood J (1990) Childhood bruising. Practitioner 234(1490):598–601

Zuravin S (1991) Research definitions of child abuse and neglect: current problems. In: Starr R, Wolfe D (eds) The effects of child abuse and neglect: issues and research, 1st edn. Guilford Press, New York

5 Coagulation Disorders

5.1 Introduction

> Whenever the presence of blood serves as evidence of inflicted trauma, coagulopathy must be considered. (Hymel and Boos 2009)

5.1.1 Child Abuse or Coagulation Disorder?

Second to accidental injuries, coagulation disorders are the most important differential diagnosis of non-accidental bruising, although these disorders in general are much less common than accidents or child abuse. Coagulation disorders are always prominently mentioned as a possible pitfall, but there are only a relatively small number of case reports described in medical literature (Table 5.1).

Many clotting problems are first recognized because of externally visible bruising. This applies to both congenital and acquired problems. Only a small proportion of the most common clotting disorders in childhood, especially in neonates and children under the age of 1 year, will lead to intracranial bleeding (see Table 5.1). Intracranial bleeding however is only rarely an isolated finding in children with a coagulation disorder. Usually one will find bruises, petechiae, and mucosal bleeding prior to or simultaneous with the intracranial bleeding (Hennes et al. 2001).

According to Lee (2008), child abuse generally can be diagnosed on clinical grounds alone, and most victims do not require laboratory testing to exclude bleeding disorders. If testing is done, the purpose mostly will be to exclude or provide proof of a coexistent bleeding disorder. In case of a bleeding disorder, a suspicion of child abuse may arise because of the unexplained and sometimes life-threatening bruising or bleeding. Misdiagnosis however should be rare when these children are evaluated in a systematic manner (Lee 2008).

5.1.2 Child Abuse and Coagulation Disorder

In evaluating the differential diagnosis between child abuse and a coagulation disorder, one should always keep in mind that an abnormal coagulation test does not exclude child abuse (O'Hare and Eden 1984; Sibert 2004; Khair and Liesner 2006; Lee 2008; Olivieri et al. 2009; Minford and Richards 2010). O'Hare and Eden (1984) routinely tested 50 children with bruising in whom child abuse was suspected. Abnormalities in the results of the clotting tests were present in 8 (16%) children. Child abuse was excluded with certainty in only one child. Simultaneous occurrence of a coagulation disorder and abuse-related bruising was found in the remaining seven children. Children with these disorders who are also physically abused seem to be at greater risk of severe bleeding as a result of the abuse (O''Hare and Eden 1984; Thomas 2004; Minford and Richards 2010).

R.A.C. Bilo et al., *Cutaneous Manifestations of Child Abuse and Their Differential Diagnosis*,
DOI 10.1007/978-3-642-29287-3_5, © Springer-Verlag Berlin Heidelberg 2013

Table 5.1 Overview of disorders with bleeding/bruising mistaken for child abuse

	Author and year	Main clinical manifestation
Disorders with increased fragility of the vessels		
Ehlers-Danlos syndrome	Owen and Durst (1984)	Bruising
	Roberts et al. (1984)	Bruising
	Wardinsky et al. (1995)	Bruising
	de Paepe and Malfait (2004)	Bruising
Vasculitis allergica	Brown and Melinkovich (1986)	Bruising
	Menter (1987)	Bruising
	Daly and Siegel (1998)	Bruising
Osteogenesis imperfecta	Ganesh et al. (2004)	Subdural hematoma and retinal hemorrhages
Vitamin C deficiency	Mimasaka et al. (2000)[a]	Bruising
Platelet disorders		
Immune thrombocytopenic purpura	Wheeler and Hobbs (1988)	Bruising
	Harley (1997)	Bruising
Leukemia and thrombocytopenia	McClain et al. (1990)	Bruising
	Nadjem and Sutor (1991)	Bruising
Glanzmann thrombasthenia	Taylor (1982)	Bruising Nosebleeds
Hermansky-Pudlak syndrome	Russell-Eggitt et al. (2000)[b]	Theoretically bruising and subdural hemorrhage
Hemophagocytic lymphohistiocytosis (HLH)	Rooms et al. (2003)[c]	Microscopic intracranial hemorrhages
Clotting factor deficiency		
Von Willebrand disease	Stray-Pedersen et al. (2011)[c]	Subdural hemorrhage
Hemophilia	Taylor (1982)	Bruising
	Schwer et al. (1982)[d]	Bruising
	O''Hare and Eden (1984)	Bruising
	Wheeler and Hobbs (1988)	Bruising
	Harley (1997)	Bruising
	Bach et al. (2001)	Subdural hemorrhage
	Pinto et al. (2003)	Epidural hemorrhage
	Vorstman et al. 2003	Intracranial hemorrhage
	Feldman (2009)	Bruising
Vitamin K deficiency (hemorrhagic disease of the newborn)	Lane et al. (1983)	Intracranial hemorrhage
	Wheeler and Hobbs (1988)	Bruising
	Wetzel et al. (1995)	Intramuscular bleeding
	Rutty et al. (1999)	Subdural hemorrhage
	Fenton et al. (2000)	Intracranial hemorrhage
	Demirören et al. (2004)[c]	Subdural hemorrhage
	Brousseau et al. (2005)	Intracranial hemorrhage and bruising
Disease-related vitamin K deficiency	Carpentieri et al. (1978)[e]	Bruising
	Vorstman et al. (2003)[f]	Subdural hemorrhage
Factor II	Strijks et al. (1999)	Intracranial hemorrhage
Factor V	Bach et al. (2001)	Intracranial hemorrhage
Factor XIII	Newman et al. (2002)	Subdural hemorrhage
Afibrinogenemia	Vorstman et al. (2003)	Intraventricular hemorrhage

(continued)

Table 5.1 (continued)

	Author and year	Main clinical manifestation
Coagulopathy due to infection		
Disseminated herpes simplex virus infection	Fenton et al. (2000)	Intracranial hemorrhage
Disseminated intravascular coagulation due to meningitis	Kirschner and Stein (1985)	Intracranial injuries and bruising
Purpura fulminans	Kirschner and Stein (1985)	Bruising

[a]Bruising resulted from vitamin C deficiency, caused by severe abusive malnutrition
[b]Misdiagnosis of child abuse described as a theoretical possibility because of bruising or intracranial hemorrhage in children with HPS
[c]Unclear from the case reports, whether child abuse was excluded effectively. It can also not be excluded that the disease and child abuse were coexisting
[d]The 10-month-old child had severe bruising over the whole body and a healing clavicular fracture. There was no explanation for the fracture
[e]Vitamin K deficiency due to cystic fibrosis
[f]Vitamin K deficiency in alpha 1 antitrypsin deficiency and in Alagille syndrome

Abnormal findings in the results of clotting tests can also be caused in child physical abuse by the extent of the bruising and bleeding, for example, in inflicted intracranial or intra-abdominal bleeding. Bruising and bleeding will lead to activation of coagulation and to subsequent loss of coagulation factors (coagulopathy caused by consumption) (Hymel et al. 1997). Furthermore, (abusive or negligent) malnutrition can result in deficiencies (deficiency coagulopathy, malnutrition deficiency) (Lee 2008; Olivieri et al. 2009). Finally, child abuse-related coagulopathies can be found in pediatric condition falsification (Munchausen syndrome by proxy) (e.g., warfarin poisoning, phenolphthalein poisoning) (White et al. 1985; Babcock et al. 1993; Mason 2010).

5.2 Bruising and Bleeding: Hemostasis

Bruising and bleeding result from the extravasation of blood from blood vessels into the skin or mucous membranes. Therefore, bruising does not blanch under pressure (Leung and Chan 2001). Whatever causes bleeding or bruising, after the occurrence of the damage, hemostasis starts. Hemostasis involves three major processes:

- Contraction of blood vessels (leading to restricting of blood flow to the damaged area)
- Activation of platelets (leading to platelet aggregation)
- Activation of clotting factors (forming of a fibrin clot) (Leung and Chan 2001)

Disease-related bruising and bleeding in children result from congenital or acquired disorders with increased fragility of the vessels, platelet dysfunction, and/or dysfunction of blood clotting factors. If clotting is excessive, thrombosis and its complications occur (Montgomery and Scott 2003).

5.3 Diagnosis

5.3.1 Introduction

Although unexplained bruising or the claim by a parent of "easy bruising" is often mentioned as a sign of child abuse, they are not pathognomonic of child abuse. This is also seen in bleeding disorders, whether the disorder is mild or severe. Also significant or multiple bruises, bruises of apparently different ages without a history of trauma or a history inconsistent with the severity of the injury, are seen in both child abuse and coagulation disorders (Thomas 2004; Minford and Richards 2010). When in doubt, one should always consult a pediatric hematologist to obtain an accurate diagnostic approach and a correct diagnosis.

A thorough diagnostic approach to bruising and bleeding disorders is based on three elements: a carefully taken and comprehensive medical history, a thorough physical examination, and finally laboratory tests (Sham and Francis 1994; Vora and Makris 2001; Montgomery and Scott 2003; Lee 2008; Minford and Richards 2010). According to Leung and Chan (2001), in most cases the diagnosis can be established on the basis of a careful history and physical examination and a few key laboratory tests (complete blood cell count with platelet count, peripheral blood smear, prothrombin time, and activated partial thromboplastin time). Lee (2008) even states that coagulation tests in the differential diagnosis of abusive bruising are only indicated when a bleeding diathesis is suspected on clinical grounds or when a pattern of bleeding remains unexplained after initial evaluation.

5.3.2 Medical History

A comprehensive medical history provides the most useful information for hemostatic disorders, whether they are hemorrhagic or thrombotic (Table 5.2). The medical history will indicate whether a bleeding disorder exists and what kind of bleeding disorder could be responsible for the bruising. Special attention should be paid to (Vora and Makris 2001; Montgomery and Scott 2003; Lee 2008):

- The age of onset of symptoms and the developmental level at the age of onset (nonmobile/mobile).
- Previous bruising and bleeding in the child (acute, chronic, or recurrent pattern of bleeding).
- "Spontaneous" or posttraumatic bleeding.
- Severity and duration of the bleeding.
- Site(s) of bleeding.
- Medication used by the child (current medications and medication in the past). One should also inform which medication is present in the home and whether the child could have had access to this medication (accidental ingestion).

Table 5.2 Signs and symptoms in the medical history suggestive for bleeding disorders

During infancy
Prolonged bleeding after heel prick
Excessive bleeding immediately after separation of umbilical cord, later umbilical cord bleeding
Excessive or prolonged bleeding/swelling after vaccination or intramuscular vitamin K injection given after birth
Breastfeeding without vitamin K supplementation
Prolonged bleeding after circumcision
Cephalhematoma
All ages
Unexplained skin bleeding, ongoing instead of isolated episodes
Prolonged bleeding during or after surgery, tooth extraction, injury, or wound suturing
Recurrent epistaxis or gum bleeding
Unexplained joint or muscle bleeding/swelling
Recurrent bloody diarrhea or hematemesis
Bleeding requiring surgical intervention, transfusion, or replacement therapy
Coexisting gastrointestinal, liver, or renal disorders
Recent intake of drugs like acetylsalicylic acid, valproic acid, or antibiotics
Poisoning, e.g., with superwarfarin (Babcock et al. 1993)
During adolescence
(Hyper)menorrhagia resulting in significant anemia
Family bleeding history
Bleeding tendency, including menorrhagia, postpartum bleeds, and bleeding during or after surgery, including circumcision
Proven bleeding disorders (always complete workup)
Consanguinity

Vora and Makris (2001); Montgomery and Scott (2003); Khair and Liesner (2006); Lee (2008); Ballas and Kraut (2008); Olivieri et al. (2009)

- Recent infections.
- The existence of an increased bleeding tendency in the family.

Hereditary bleeding disorders will present early, usually when a child is starting to ambulate. Hereditary disorders will have more often a positive family history (Lee 2008). Delayed or slow healing of superficial injuries may suggest a hereditary bleeding disorder (Montgomery and Scott 2003). A clinically significant hereditary bleeding disorder usually can be excluded if the child has undergone surgery (e.g., tonsillectomy, major dental extractions, or appendectomy) without (excessive, prolonged, or delayed) bleeding (Montgomery and Scott 2003). According to Jenny and Reece (2009), a child with a bleeding disorder will have ongoing problems with bruising rather than just an isolated episode with bruising.

5.3.3 Physical Examination

The physical examination should be thorough with complete documentation of all physical findings. The examination should focus on:

- The presence of pattern injuries
- The age and development of the child
- The distribution of the bruising and bleeding and the finding of other signs and symptoms
- The size and severity of the bruising and bleeding

5.3.3.1 Pattern Injuries

If identifiable and/or specific patterns of bruises/bruising are recognized, for example, bruising caused by a slap in the face or grip marks on the upper arm or trunk, the bruising should be considered to be a non-accidental injury, until proven otherwise, regardless of the presence or absence of a coagulation disorder (Vora and Makris 2001; Thomas 2004; Olivieri et al. 2009; Minford and Richards 2010). Also the presence of multiple bruises with the same shape is indicative of abuse (Maguire et al. 2005). One should, however, always keep in mind that, for example, fingertip bruising can be seen in children with a bleeding disorder from normal physical activities (Thomas 2004).

5.3.3.2 Age and Developmental Stage

Comparing the pattern of distribution, the size, and severity of the bruises to the child's history and stage of development is essential in the differential diagnosis between accidental bruising and the "sudden and unexplained" bruising, which can happen in abuse as well as in coagulation disorders. Normal accidental bruising is mobility related and starts as the child has developed enough motor skills to move independently (cruising). Bruising in nonmobile babies is very uncommon (<1%) (Maguire et al. 2005). Mobility-related bruising is common after the age of 1 year (in 17% of infants starting to mobilize, 53% in walkers, majority of schoolchildren) (Maguire et al. 2005). Accidental bruising of the head is not rare in toddlers who just started to walk, although it is very uncommon in preambulatory children and in school children. Mobility-related bruises generally are small, usually over bony prominences and on the front of the body, for example, knees, chins, and forehead and in general associated with petechiae or mucosal bleeding, except in case of a coexisting coagulation disorder (Thomas 2004; Maguire et al. 2005; Minford and Richards 2010). They are normally not found on unexposed area (Thomas 2004).

Further evaluation of bruising is indicated in case of (Vora and Makris 2001; Thomas 2004; Maguire et al. 2005; Khair and Liesner 2006; Lee 2008; Minford and Richards 2010):

- Nonmobile children with bruising. This may indicate abuse or a bleeding disorder.
- Children with bruising all over the body, often away from the bony prominences and (especially in young children) over soft tissue areas. In physical abuse, the commonest sites are the head and neck (particularly the face – cheeks) followed by the buttocks, trunk, and arms, although any part of the body is vulnerable (Maguire et al. 2005). The bruises are usually large, commonly multiple, and may occur in clusters (Maguire et al. 2005). The bruising in abuse is often combined with other bruises or abrasions that may be older. In coagulation disorders, one also may find bruising on any part of the body, sometimes related to minor trauma. Usually one will not find any without other injury types or older injuries, except older bruises.
- Children with bruising in unusual sites, especially the ears, the genitalia, or soft parts of the body, for example, the cheeks or the inside of the thighs, because these areas are rarely injured during play or accidents (Labbe and Caouette 2001; Maguire et al. 2005; Swerdlin et al. 2007; Minford and Richards 2010).
- Children with bruising of the abdominal wall. Accidental bruising of the abdominal wall is rare. When bruising is present, it indicates a strong impact (Wood et al. 2005) (see also Sects. 2.5.2.9 and 3.2.2.1).

Table 5.3 Differentiating between defects in the platelet/blood vessel interaction and clotting factor deficiencies by using physical findings

Disorder	Failure in	Principle symptoms
Defects in the platelet/blood vessel interaction, e.g., Von Willebrand disease, platelet disorders, leukemia	Primary hemostasis	Mucocutaneous bleeding Mucous membrane bleeding (gum and nosebleeds, menorrhagia, hematuria, gastrointestinal bleeding), often recurrent or prolonged Petechiae of skin and mucous membranes Small bruises
Clotting factor deficiencies, e.g., hemophilia A and B	Secondary hemostasis	Deep bleeding Bleeding in deeper tissues: Muscles Joints (hemarthrosis) Internal cavities More extensive bruising and bruises with thick, round, indurated centers

Davis and Carrasco (2002); Montgomery and Scott (2003); Lee (2008); Minford and Richards (2010)

5.3.3.3 Distribution and Other Physical Findings

The physical examination should also include an evaluation whether symptoms are primarily associated with the mucous membranes or skin (mucocutaneous bleeding) or the muscles and joints (deep bleeding) (Montgomery and Scott 2003). This may indicate either a defect in the platelet/blood vessel interaction or a clotting factor deficiency (Table 5.3).

Finding other signs and symptoms may be helpful in differentiating between bruising caused by a bleeding disorder or physical abuse:

- Children may show bruising and persistent bleeding or epistaxis (often bilateral) in addition to bruising, which might indicate thrombocytopenia or Von Willebrand disease.
- Children may show excessive blood loss after hemostatic stress: tooth extractions, minor surgery, and circumcision, which is characteristic of hemostatic disorders. The absence of this symptom does exclude a significant coagulation abnormality (Vora and Makris 2001).

5.3.3.4 Size and Severity of the Bruising

Size and severity of the bruising (and bleeding) should be evaluated properly. If there is a clear mechanism of injury, which is consistent with the configuration but not severity of the bruising, one should think of a bleeding disorder (Davis and Carrasco 2002). In case of significant bruising or bleeding without a history of trauma or a history that is not consistent with the severity of the injury, one should consider child abuse, but also a bleeding disorder because the same can account for a child with bleeding disorder in the initial presentation (Thomas 2004).

Nosek-Cenkowska et al. (1991) compared the bruising patterns of 31 children with a bleeding disorder (Von Willebrand disease and/or platelet function defects) with the pattern in children without a bleeding disorder. The results of this study is given in Table 5.4. The study shows that especially bruises on more than one part of the body and frequent large bruises are rare in children without a bleeding disorder and much more common in children with a bleeding disorder (Figs. 5.1, 5.2, 5.3, and 5.4), just like in physically abused children (see Chaps. 3 and 4). In other words, finding bruises on more than one part of the body and frequent large bruises in a child may indicate a bleeding disorder as well as physical abuse.

5.3.4 Laboratory Testing

Laboratory testing includes both screening tests and more specific diagnostic tests depending on the results of the screening tests and the clinical findings (Minford and Richards 2010). Testing and interpretation of the results should always be

Table 5.4 Differences in severity of bleeding patterns between children without and with a bleeding disorder

Bleeding disorder	No (%)	Yes (%)
Easy bruising	24	67
Bruises at least once a week	36	68
Nosebleeds	39	69
Bruises on more than one body part	4.9	38.5
Frequent large bruises	3.5	29.6

Nosek-Cenkowska et al. (1991)

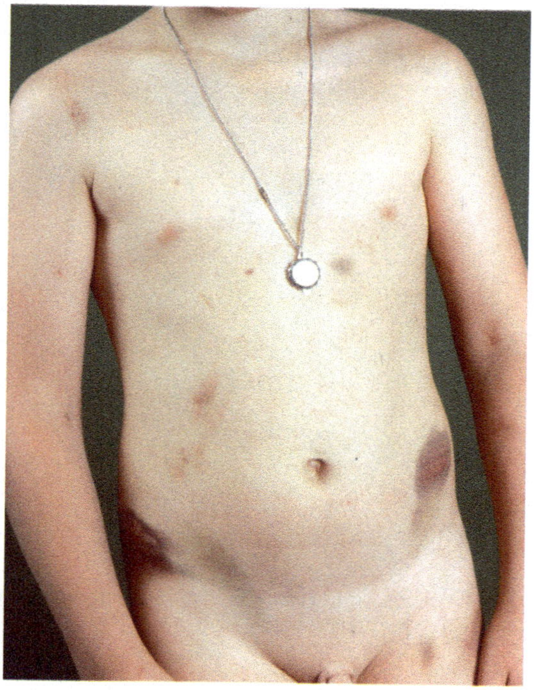

Fig. 5.1 Bruises on more than one part of the body and large bruises in a boy with a bleeding disorder (idiopathic thrombocytopenic purpura)

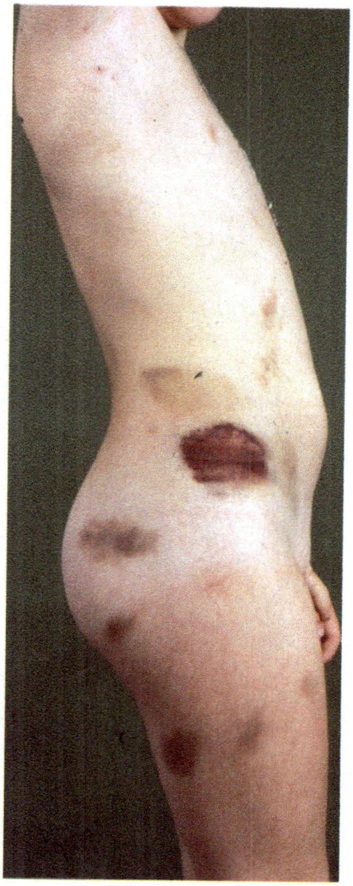

Fig. 5.2 Same child as in Fig. 5.1

done in case of doubt and in consultation with an experienced pediatrician or a (pediatric) hematologist. Minford and Richards (2010) adapted the screening tests proposed by the Royal College of Paediatrics and Child Health (2006) (see Table 5.5). Minford advises, just like Thomas (2004), to add, in the initial screening, tests for Von Willebrand disease because it is the most common inherited bleeding disorder and the APTT is often normal. Minford also advises to add screening for hemophilia A and B because the APTT may be normal or only slightly prolonged.

Any abnormal result found in the initial screening should be repeated after consulting a pediatric hematologist (Tables 5.6, 5.7, and 5.8). More specific tests and evaluation of the results should always be done by a pediatric hematologist. A factor XIII assay should be considered, for example, in case of an intracranial bleeding in the neonatal period (Newman et al. 2002; Minford and Richards 2010).

It is important to interpret the results of clotting screening tests in relation to age-related normal ranges (Vora and Makris 2001). The levels of several clotting factors are considerably lower in healthy full-term infants at birth when compared to adults (Khair and Liesner 2006). Infant values are approaching adult values at the age of 6 months (Khair and Liesner 2006). There is also

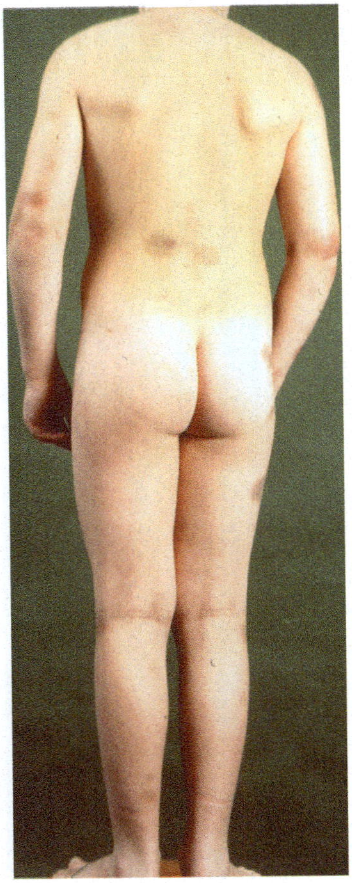

Fig. 5.3 Same child as in Fig. 5.1

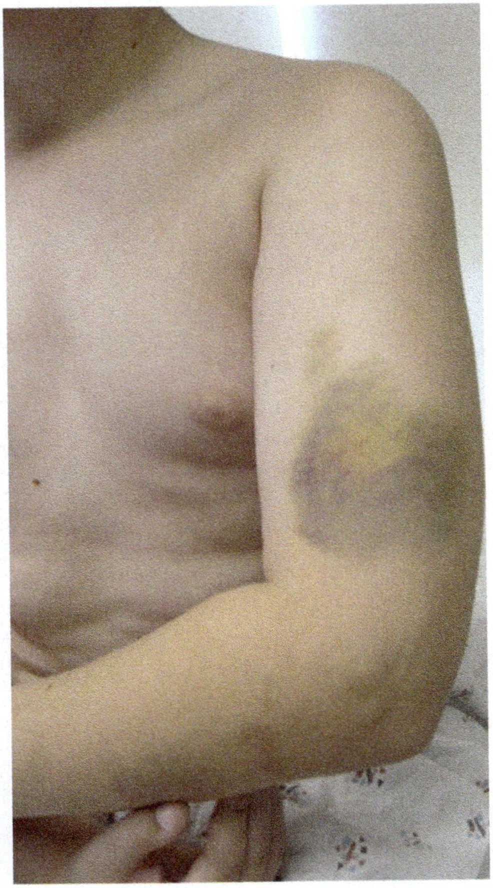

Fig. 5.4 Large posttraumatic bruise in an adolescent with a coagulation disorder

Table 5.5 Screening tests for coagulation disorders

Royal College of Paediatrics and Child Health (2006)
Full blood count, examination of blood film, measurement of mean platelet volume
Tests of liver and renal function
Prothrombin time
Activated partial thromboplastin time
Thrombin time and Clauss fibrinogen concentration
Plus (added by Minford and Richards 2010)
Factor VIII and factor IX assays
Von Willebrand factor antigen, ristocetin cofactor, and blood group
Factor XIII assay, platelet membrane glycoproteins (in certain situations – see text)
Platelet function analyzer-100 (if available)

Thomas (2004); RCPCH (2006); Minford and Richards (2010)

an apparent hypofunction of the platelets in newborns (Khair and Liesner 2006).

A normal result of laboratory testing excludes "spontaneous" bruising or bleeding and it also excludes that the bruising or bleeding was caused by a minor trauma (Vora and Makris 2001). Full blood count and the usual screening tests however do not detect all bleeding disorders (Table 5.8).

Laboratory testing is rarely indicated for the differentiation between abusive bruises and bruising caused by bleeding disorders. In general, even children with mild coagulation disorders will be noted previously during well baby visits, school visits, or hospital visits. According to Schmitt (1987), screening for bleeding

Table 5.6 Indicative diagnostic value of the results of screening tests

Screening test	Indicative diagnostic value
Blood count and film	Anemia, leukemia, disseminated intravascular coagulation
Platelet count	Thrombocytopenia
Bleeding time	Test of platelet-vessel wall interaction
Isolated aPTT prolongation	Von Willebrand disease Deficiency of factors VIII, IX, XI, and XII Heparin contamination
Isolated PT prolongation	Vitamin K deficiency (early) Acquired Vitamin K deficiency due to liver failure (early) Deficiency of factors I, II, V, VII, and X Warfarin ingestion
PT and aPTT prolonged with normal fibrinogen	Vitamin K deficiency (severe) Prothrombin deficiency Deficiency of factor II, V, and X Combined deficiency of factor V and VIII Warfarin ingestion Overdose of heparin
Prolonged PT and aPTT, decreased fibrinogen, normal or low platelets	Liver failure (severe) Disseminated intravascular coagulation, including meningococcal sepsis Afibrinogenemia or dysfibrinogenemia
Thrombin time prolonged (or low/absent fibrinogen)	Hereditary or acquired fibrinogen abnormalities (hypofibrinogenemia or dysfibrinogenemia) Heparin Elevated fibrin/fibrinogen degradation products (e.g., in DIC)

Vora and Makris (2001); Hampton and Preston (2003); Thomas (2004); Khair and Liesner (2006); Minford and Richards (2010)

Table 5.7 Indicative diagnostic value of combined findings in screening tests

Disease	Platelet count	Bleeding time	PT	aPTT
Idiopathic thrombocytopenic purpura	Low	Normal	Normal	Normal
Von Willebrand disease	Normal	Prolonged	Normal	Normal/prolonged
Factor VIII, IX, XI deficiency	Normal	Normal	Normal	Prolonged
Factor I, II, V, VII, X deficiency	Normal	Normal	Prolonged	Normal
Vitamin K deficiency	Normal	Normal	Prolonged	Normal/prolonged
Diffuse intravascular coagulation	Low	Prolonged	Prolonged	Prolonged

Hymel et al. (1997); Wynne (2003); Khair and Liesner (2006)

disorders is not indicated for differentiation if bruising is confined to only one specific anatomical location, such as the buttocks, or show a clearly recognizable shape, for example, a belt or a hand imprint. In this situation, testing is only indicated if a simultaneous existence of a bleeding disorder is suspected on other grounds. Testing is also indicated when nonspecific bruising is found and the parents state that the child develops bruising easily and quickly (Vora and Makris 2001).

5.4 Disorders with Increased Fragility of the Vessels

5.4.1 Genetic Disorders

Vascular integrity is essential for primary hemostasis (Vora and Makris 2001). In children with genetic or acquired disorders, in which the integrity of the vessel wall is compromised, the trauma needed to damage the vessel is less severe than in children with normal vessels. The symptoms of

Table 5.8 Hemostatic disorders which may present with normal results in full blood count and coagulation screening tests

Platelet disorders	Mild platelet function disorders Glanzmann thrombasthenia Platelet storage pool disease Platelet release defect

Factor deficiencies	Mild subtypes of Von Willebrand disease
	Mild congenital factor deficiencies:
	  Hemophilia A, B, and C
	Rare congenital factor deficiencies:
	  Single factor deficiencies
	  Factor XIII deficiency

Others, including collagen disorders	Classical Ehlers-Danlos syndrome Osteogenesis imperfecta Marfan syndrome Henoch-Schönlein purpura (Sect. 6.3.3) Alpha 2 antiplasmin deficiency (extremely rare) Plasminogen activation inhibitor-1 deficiency Vitamin C deficiency

Vora and Makris (2001); Hampton and Preston (2003); Thomas (2004); Khair and Liesner (2006); Olivieri et al. (2009)

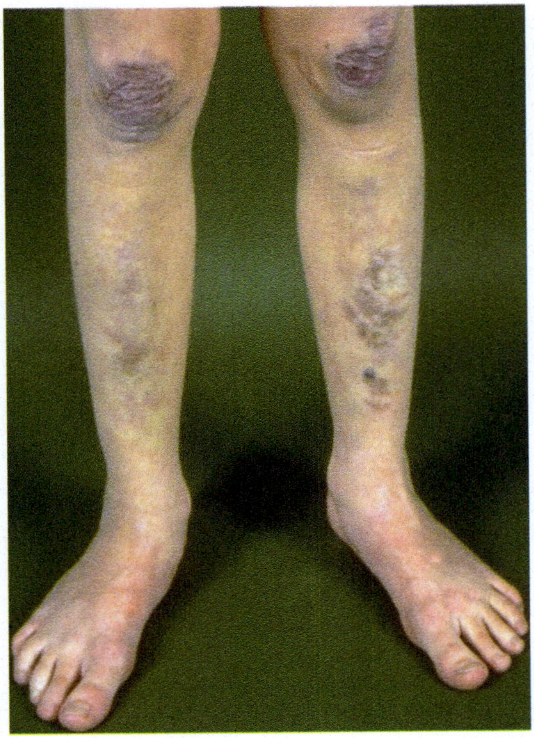

Fig. 5.5 Characteristic findings in classical type Ehlers-Danlos syndrome (type I and II): extensive bruising and cigarette paper tissue scars (= Fig. 6.72)

these disorders may resemble the symptoms of thrombocytopenia or dysfunctional platelets (Vora and Makris 2001). Examples of genetic disorders with increased fragility of the vessels are Ehlers-Danlos syndrome, Rendu-Osler-Weber syndrome, Marfan syndrome, and osteogenesis imperfecta. In all these syndromes, child abuse may be suspected.

5.4.1.1 Ehlers-Danlos Syndrome

In Ehlers-Danlos syndromes (EDS), not only the integrity of the connective tissue is compromised but also of the vessels (Leung and Chan 2001; de Paepe and Malfait 2004). This makes the vessels (capillaries) more prone to damage and the subcutaneous tissue more prone to easy and more extensive bruising. In persons with classical type EDS (types I and II), the disease may mimic child abuse because of symptoms of connective tissue fragility, skin hyperextensibility, joint hypermobility, and cigarette paper tissue scars (Lee 2008)(Figs. 5.5, 5.6, and 5.7). Symptoms may already be present in infancy but usually more prominent at toddlers age. Referral to a specialized (pediatric) dermatologist is advocated in suspected cases.

Ehlers-Danlos Syndrome and Suspicions of Child Abuse

Misdiagnosis of child abuse has been described several times in children with classical type EDS (type I and II) (Owen and Durst 1984; van Oostrom et al. 1984; Wardinsky et al. 1995; Oranje, own observations) and once in a child with type IV (vascular type of EDS) (Roberts et al. 1984).

5.4.1.2 Osteogenesis Imperfecta

Osteogenesis imperfecta (OI) is a genetic disorder caused by a defect in the synthesis of type I collagen. There are different types of OI with clinical

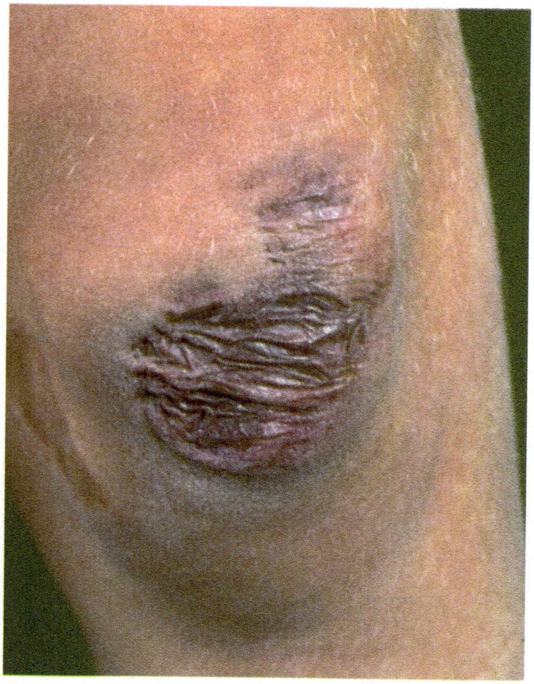

Fig. 5.6 Characteristic findings in classical type Ehlers-Danlos syndrome (type I and II): cigarette paper tissue scar (= Fig. 6.73)

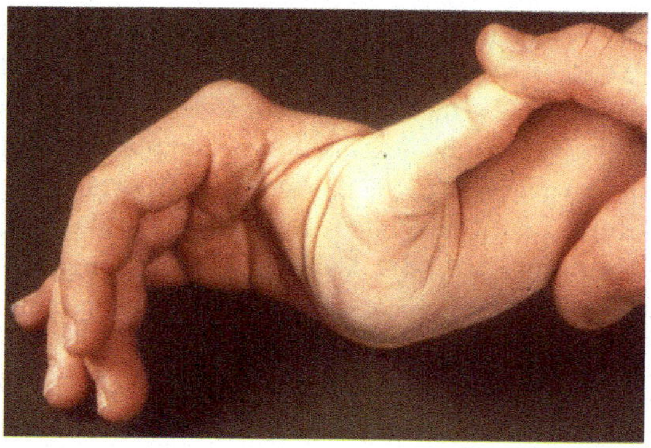

Fig. 5.7 Characteristic findings in classical type Ehlers-Danlos syndrome (type I and II): joint hypermobility (= Fig. 6.74)

differences. Type I collagen is an important protein in the extracellular matrix of many tissues. In the bones, a defect in the synthesis of type I collagen will lead to osteoporosis, which makes it possible for minimal trauma to cause multiple fractures. The protein is also present in ligaments, teeth, sclera, and blood vessels. Consequently, the symptoms can occur to a higher or lesser degree in all these systems (Bilo et al. 2010). Clinically suspect are blue sclerae, triangular face, loose joints, muscle weakness, and multiple spontaneous fractures of the bones. About 50% of all people with OI bruise more easily than normal. In about 25% of the tested patients, blood and clotting problems will be detected, but the condition is usually mild (Swedish Information Centre for Rare Diseases 2011). Patients with normal tests may bleed more than normal during surgery. This may be the result from a failure of the platelets to interact adequately with the abnormal collagen in the vascular walls (Swedish Information Centre for Rare Diseases 2011).

Osteogenesis Imperfecta and Suspicions of Child Abuse

In young nonmobile children, osteogenesis imperfecta (OI) is the most common cause next to child abuse for the presence of multiple fractures, often at various stages of healing, and without a plausible explanation (Bilo et al. 2010). If there are also unexplained bruises, a suspicion of child abuse will be enforced. Another possible pitfall could be the finding of a subdural hematoma and/or retinal hemorrhages in a young child without a plausible explanation (Ganesh et al. 2004; Groninger et al. 2005). In most cases, the differential diagnosis between OI and child abuse is based on (family) history, physical examination, and radiological imaging. Specialist expertise (geneticist, pediatric radiologist) should be asked for. Even if OI provides a plausible explanation for the physical findings that correspond with the minimal trauma recorded in the medical history, one should still consider abuse. Knight and Bennet (1990) described a child with OI in whom child abuse could only be confirmed after facial injuries were found that proved that the child had been beaten.

5.4.2 Acquired Disorders

Examples of acquired diseases in which the integrity of the vessels is affected are vitamin C deficiency, autoimmune disorders, and allergic vasculitis/Henoch-Schönlein purpura (Sect. 6.3.3 – Figs. 5.8 and 5.9).

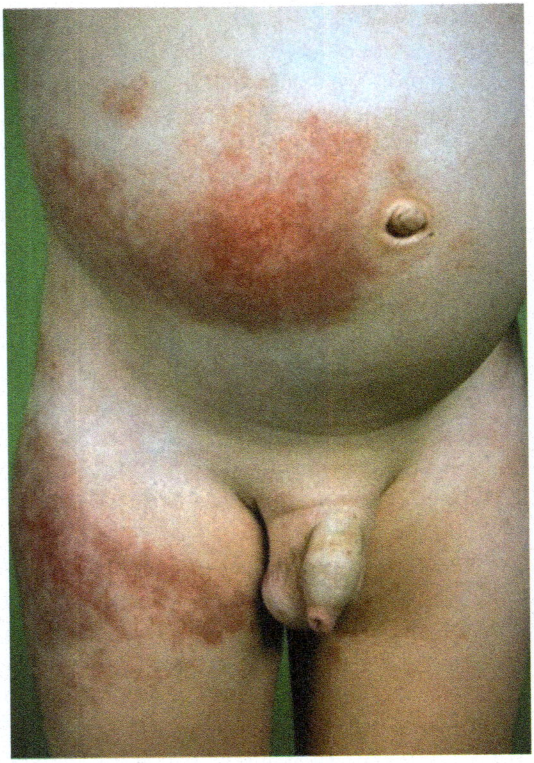

Fig. 5.8 Atypical Henoch-Schönlein purpura (= Fig. 6.37)

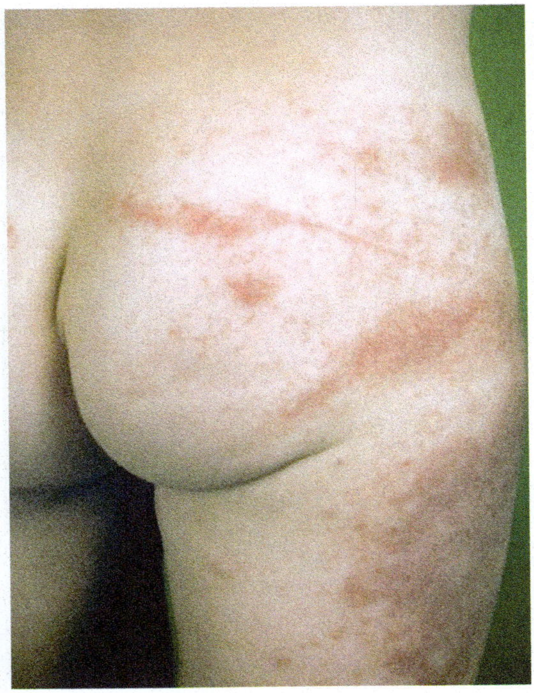

Fig. 5.9 Same child as in Fig. 5.8 (= Fig. 6.38)

5.4.2.1 Vitamin C Deficiency (Scurvy) and Bruising/Bleeding

Vitamin C (ascorbic acid) is a water-soluble vitamin. Vitamin C in the form of fresh fruits, vegetables, or vitamin supplements is an essential nutrient in the human diet (Weinstein et al. 2001). It is necessary for synthesizing collagen, reducing free radicals, and aiding in iron absorption (Burk and Molodow 2007). If the formation of collagen is disturbed, it will lead to many of the classical symptoms of scurvy: poor wound healing, increased capillary fragility, and osteoporosis. Iron deficiency anemia is another common finding in scurvy. This anemia may be secondary to coexisting other dietary deficiencies but also to the bleeding/bruising and decreased iron absorption due to the vitamin C deficiency (Weinstein et al. 2001). The anemia will lead to complaints of malaise. Untreated vitamin C deficiency can be fatal (Weinstein et al. 2001; Mimasaka et al. 2000).

Scurvy has become very rare in the Western world. However, it may frequently be misdiagnosed because the symptoms mimic many other disorders (e.g., rheumatological diseases or complex regional pain syndrome (CRPS)) (Ratanachu-Ek et al. 2003; Kumar and Choudhury 2009; Kumar et al. 2009; Popovich et al. 2009; Vitale et al. 2009). This may lead to many unnecessary diagnostic procedures (Popovich et al. 2009).

The earliest manifestations are usually skin related with perifollicular petechiae and bruising (often multiple and scattered), hyperkeratosis, and corkscrew hairs (Hodges 1980). In the next stage, the gingiva is affected with swelling, bruising, inflammation, and loosening of the teeth, also secondary to blood vessel fragility. Symptoms of bone disease, including fractures around the growth plates and arthritis/hemarthrosis, are frequently seen in children. Severe bone pain is caused by subperiosteal hemorrhaging (Weinstein et al. 2001). Also skeletal muscle degeneration can be seen in children with scurvy. The bone and muscle abnormalities will lead to weakness and difficulties in walking (painful gait) or even inability to walk (Tamura et al. 2000; Ratanachu-Ek et al. 2003). Other clinical signs of scurvy include cardiac hypertrophy, diminished adrenal and bone marrow function, psychological changes, poor wound healing, edema, and alopecia (Weinstein et al. 2001).

Children most at risk for a vitamin C deficiency are those who are only fed evaporated or boiled milk, in which ascorbic acid is destroyed by heat and the vitamin C intake is not replaced by eating of fresh fruit or other sources of vitamin C. The second group at risk is children with unusual eating habits or severely restricted diets. Dietary restrictions may stem from:

- Psychiatric or developmental disorders of the child itself (Weinstein et al. 2001; Vitale et al. 2009)
- Self-chosen restrictive eating pattern (Bari et al. 2009) or extremely limited food preferences (Weinstein et al. 2001)
- Vitamin C-deficient diet, for example, a ketogenic diet in children with difficult-to-control epilepsy (Willmott and Bryan 2008) or a highly restricted diet in an autistic child (Duncan et al. 2007)
- Restricted diet secondary to religious practices, for example, a diet recommended by the Church of Scientology that included a boiled mixture of organic whole milk, barley, and corn syrup devoid of fruits and vegetables (Burk and Molodow 2007)

Vitamin C Deficiency and Suspicions of Child Abuse

Vitamin C deficiency has been mentioned as possible cause of clinical symptoms that can be seen in abusive head trauma (Clemetson 2002; Clemetson 2004). A deficiency would induce a coagulopathy, which according to Clemetson could cause a subdural hematoma. Fung and Nelson (2004) concluded, based on an extensive literature review, that there is no sound scientific proof for this hypothesis.

Mimasaka et al. (2000) reported a fatal case of scurvy in a 6-year-old girl in which a vitamin C deficiency-related bleeding tendency led to the suspicion of physical abuse. During autopsy, many bruises were seen in the face, trunk, and lower extremities. The gums were swollen and some teeth were missing. Subperiosteal bleeding was found on the humerus, tibia, and femur. The findings during the autopsy could be explained as resulting from a severe and long-lasting vitamin C deficiency. Mimasaka concluded that the fatal course was not the result of physical violence but of severe neglect because the child was not taken care of and fed properly by the parents.

5.5 Platelet Disorders

5.5.1 General Aspects of Platelet Disorders

Platelet disorders are caused by rare congenital/inherited or much more common acquired disorders (Jurk and Kehrel 2007). Platelet disorders can be divided into quantitative platelet disorders (decreased production or increased consumption or destruction – thrombocytopenia) and qualitative platelet disorders (defective platelet function, platelet dysfunction). Platelet counts within reference ranges do not exclude qualitative disorders (Jurk and Kehrel 2007; Olivieri et al. 2009). Platelet disorders (quantitative and qualitative) belong to the most common coagulation disorders (Sharathkumar and Shapiro 2008). Thrombocytopenia, whether congenital/inherited or acquired, is the most common coagulation disorder (Culvert and Norris 2006).

Children with thrombocytopenia or thrombocytopathy will often present with (muco)cutaneous bleeding, like bruising, gum bleeds, nosebleeds and menorrhagia, and bleeding after hemostatic stress during minor surgery (e.g., tonsillectomy or dental extraction) or (rarely) postpartum (Sharathkumar and Shapiro 2008). Petechial hemorrhages are also common (Lee 2008). These petechial hemorrhages can often be reproduced by applying a tourniquet around the arm, for example, during a venepuncture. Petechiae may also be found in the area of the superior vena cava drainage, for example, in the face after vigorous crying or a severe bout of coughing or vomiting, even in children without a bleeding disorder (Thomas 2004; Lee 2008; Minford and Richards 2010). Petechiae in the same region (head and neck) also occur in attempted strangulation. According to Minford and Richards (2010), the petechiae in the case of strangulation will be more profuse.

5.5.2 Inherited Platelet Disorders

5.5.2.1 Introduction

According to the United Kingdom Haemophilia Centre Doctors' Organisation (2006), inherited platelet disorders can be categorized in five subcategories (Table 5.9). The group of inherited thrombocytopenias is a heterogenous group of uncommon conditions that result in early-onset thrombocytopenia. The thrombocytopenia is either an isolated finding or associated with other abnormalities. Many of these disorders are very rare, although these disorders may have been underdiagnosed in the past (Bolton-Maggs et al. 2006).

5.5.2.2 Inherited Thrombocytopenias and Suspicions of Child Abuse

Child abuse may only be suspected in the initial phase before physical examination or laboratory testing in most of the inherited thrombocytopenias. Other congenital disorders are often seen as part of these disorders. Only a few of these disorders have been described in medical literature as pitfalls in case of suspicion of child abuse: Glanzmann thrombasthenia and Hermansky-Pudlak syndrome.

Table 5.9 Classification of the heritable platelet disorders as suggested by the UKHCDO

	Estimated number of cases worldwide
Defects in platelet numbers	
MYH9 disorders	
May-Hegglin anomaly	<1,000
Sebastian syndrome	
Fechtner syndrome	
Epstein syndrome	
Congenital amegakaryocytic thrombocytopenia	<100
Amegakaryocytic thrombocytopenia with radioulnar synostosis	<100
Thrombocytopenia absent radius syndrome	<100
X-linked thrombocytopenia with dyserythropoiesis	<100
Severe disorders of platelet function	
Wiskott-Aldrich syndrome	<1,000
Glanzmann thrombasthenia	<1,000
Bernard-Soulier syndrome	<1,000
Disorders of receptors and signal transduction	
Platelet cyclooxygenase deficiency	<100
Thromboxane synthase deficiency	<100
Thromboxane A2 receptor defect	<100
ADP receptor defect (P2Y12)	<100
Collagen receptor defects	<10
Disorders of the platelet granules	
Hermansky-Pudlak syndrome	>1,000
Chediak-Higashi syndrome	<1,000
Idiopathic dense-granule disorder (delta-storage pool disease)	<1,000
Gray platelet syndrome	<100
Paris-Trousseau/Jacobsen syndrome	<100
Idiopathic alpha- and dense-granule storage pool disease	<1,000
Disorders of phospholipid exposure	
Scott syndrome	<10

Bolton-Maggs et al. (2006)

5.5.2.3 Glanzmann Thrombasthenia (Normal Platelet Count)

Glanzmann thrombasthenia is a rare autosomal recessive disorder, with over 500 cases of thrombasthenia reported in the medical literature (Chang 2011). It is characterized by a deficiency or functional defect of platelet GPIIb/IIIa (Bolton-Maggs et al. 2006). This results in defective platelet adhesion and aggregation (Liesner and Machin 2003). The incidence is higher in communities in which consanguineous partnerships are frequent (Bolton-Maggs et al. 2006).

Most clinical symptoms present before the age of 5 years. Often the first symptoms are noted during the neonatal period. In neonates, the symptoms usually are not as severe as in early childhood. The most prevalent symptom in the neonatal period is nonsevere bruising and sometimes petechiae. Occasionally, more severe bleeding, for example, hematemesis, may occur (Bolton-Maggs et al. 2006). Intracranial bleeding in the neonatal period is not described in the study of George (1990). In early childhood, when the child becomes more mobile, the most significant finding is excessive bruising. Epistaxis is the most common manifestation of serious bleeding and is more severe in childhood than on other ages. Other symptoms in childhood and adolescence are purpura; gingival bleeding, especially in poor dental hygiene; and menorrhagia (Bolton-Maggs et al. 2006). Changing of the primary teeth to permanent teeth may lead to serious bleeding. Gastrointestinal hemorrhage may occur, especially in young children. Severe bleeding may happen after trauma or surgical procedures, like a circumcision or dental extractions. Iron deficiency anemia is common in children. In general, the severity of bleeding will diminish with age (menorrhagia and pregnancy excluded) (Bolton-Maggs et al. 2006).

George (1990) evaluated the "bleeding spectrum" of 177 patients with Glanzmann thrombasthenia. In these patients, menorrhagia, easy bruising, and epistaxis were most common. The age of the included patients ranged from young children with symptoms in the neonatal period up to the age of 60 years and older. From the study of George (1990), it is not clear whether spontaneous hemarthrosis, intracranial hemorrhage, or visceral (intrahepatic) hematomas do occur. George states: "*Spontaneous, unprovoked bleeding is actually uncommon in Glanzmann's thrombasthenia. Severe bleeding typically occurred in association with physiologic or pathologic conditions that cause bleeding in normal subjects.*"

Glanzmann thrombasthenia cannot be distinguished on clinical grounds from other severe platelet defects or from severe Von Willebrand disease (Thomas 2009). In these and similar circumstances, a specialized pediatric hematologist should be consulted.

Glanzmann Thrombasthenia and Suspicions of Child Abuse

Although Glanzmann thrombasthenia is almost always mentioned as a coagulation disorder in the differential diagnosis of non-accidental bruising, there is only one case description in the medical literature. This concerned a girl in which a suspicion of child abuse arose before adequate laboratory testing was done and the final diagnosis was made (Taylor 1982).

5.5.2.4 Hermansky-Pudlak Syndrome (HPS)

Hermansky-Pudlak syndrome consists of a group of at least eight autosomal recessive multisystem disorders (Gahl 2010). HPS is rare worldwide (just over 1,000 known patients worldwide); however, the syndrome is very common in Puerto Rico (a prevalence of 1 in 800 and more than 500 known cases). Furthermore, there are clusters described in Switzerland (Valais), the Netherlands (Southern Holland), Japan, and the UK (residents of Turkish origin) (Bolton-Maggs et al. 2006). Common symptoms to all forms are:

- A bleeding disorder/platelet dysfunction caused by platelet dense-granule defects (leading to easy bruising and bleeding): bleeding after circumcision, tooth extraction, and other surgeries, frequent nosebleeds, bleeding gums, and frequent/easy bruising.
- Oculocutaneous albinism.
  - Hypopigmentation of the skin and hair: skin color ranging from white to olive and hair color ranging from white to brown
  - Ocular findings: reduced iris and retinal pigment, photophobia, strabismus, nystagmus, reduction of visual acuity, and cataract

In some types, there are additional clinical findings: a ceroid deposition in bone marrow (leading to neutropenia and possibly a mild immunodeficiency), lung (leading to pulmonary fibrosis), and the intestinal macrophages (leading to a granulomatous colitis) (Izquierdo et al. 1995; Kugler 2005; Bolton-Maggs et al. 2006; Walker et al. 2007; Gahl 2010).

Hermansky-Pudlak Syndrome and Suspicions of Child Abuse

There is only one case description of a 7-week-old infant in which symptoms of HPS could have been theoretically misdiagnosed as resulting from inflicted traumatic brain injury: "…. There *were no signs of external injury…. There was no suggestion on history or examination that this was a case of shaken-baby syndrome. A skeletal survey was normal*" (Russell-Eggitt et al. 2000).

5.5.3 Acquired Platelet Disorders

5.5.3.1 Categories

According to Leung and Chan (2001), simple bruising strongly indicates the presence of a qualitative or quantitative platelet disorder.

Acquired Quantitative Platelet Disorders: Decreased Platelet Production

Acquired platelet disorders, resulting in decreased production of thrombocytes, are the most common cause of thrombocytopenia. It is seen in leukemia (e.g., acute lymphoblastic leukemia), aplastic anemia, viral infections (e.g., HIV/AIDS, infectious mononucleosis), and other infections (e.g., malaria) (Liesner and Machin 2003). Viral infections are the most common cause of mild transient thrombocytopenia (Liesner and Machin 2003).

Acquired Quantitative Platelet Disorders: Increased Platelet Consumption/Destruction

Examples of acquired disorders resulting in increased consumption or destruction are idiopathic thrombocytopenic purpura (ITP), thrombocytic thrombocytopenic purpura (TTP), hemolytic uremic syndrome (HUS), and disseminated intravascular coagulation (DIC). It is also seen in hypersplenism and splenomegaly. Acquired platelet dysfunction is seen, for example, in liver disease, myeloproliferative disorders, and massive blood transfusions.

Acquired Qualitative Platelet Disorders

Acquired qualitative platelet disorders are classified as primary ("autonomous" disease) or secondary (associated with an underlying disease) platelet dysfunctions (Jurk and Kehrel 2007) (Table 5.10). The group of secondary dysfunctions can be divided in those caused by defects that are intrinsic to the platelets and those caused by defects which are extrinsic to the platelets (Sharathkumar and Shapiro 2008).

5.5.3.2 Idiopathic (or Immune) Thrombocytopenic Purpura

Idiopathic (or immune) thrombocytopenic purpura (ITP) is defined as isolated thrombocytopenia with normal bone marrow and the absence of other causes of thrombocytopenia (Silverman 2011). ITP is by far the most common etiology of thrombocytopenia in childhood (Leung and Chan 2001). ITP usually is a benign, self-limiting disorder (Medeiros 2003). According to Kuhne et al. (1998), ITP is caused by the development of IgG autoantibodies to platelet membrane antigens as a result of an unbalanced response to an infectious agent or autoimmunity. There are two different clinical syndromes, namely, an acute disorder, which is seen in younger children, and a chronic disorder, which is seen in adults and older children, mainly adolescents (Silverman 2011). Acute ITP can be preceded by an acute (viral) infection, especially an upper respiratory tract infection, or a live virus vaccination (Medeiros and Buchanan 2000; Leung and Chan 2001; Lee 2008; Silverman 2011).

Clinical Features

The characteristic presentation is an abrupt onset of mucocutaneous bruising/bleeding and petechiae (often of the extremities) (Figs. 5.10, 5.11, and 5.12) in a child who is otherwise in excellent health (Leung and Chan 2001; Lee 2008). Mucocutaneous bruising and bleeding include gingival bleeding, epistaxis, menorrhagia, and

Table 5.10 Acquired qualitative platelet disorders

Primary: "autonomous" disease	
Antiplatelet antibodies	Immunothrombocytopenia [idiopathic thrombocytopenic purpura (ITP)]
Drugs/medication	Section 5.7
Food, spices, additives, and herbal medicine	Clove
	Cumin
	Feverfew
	Garlic in large amounts
	Ginger (not dried ginger)
	Ginkgo biloba
	Ginseng (Asian)
	High saturated (omega-3) fatty acids, fish oil
	Onion extract
	Saw palmetto (Serenoa repens)
	Turmeric
	Vitamin E
	Willow bark
Secondary: associated with an underlying disease (systemic disorders or surgery)	
	Chronic myeloproliferative disorders
	Myelodysplastic syndrome/leukemias
	Uremia
	Liver dysfunction
	Paraproteinemia
	Disseminated intravascular coagulation
	Hypothermia

Jurk and Kehrel (2007); Sharathkumar and Shapiro (2008); Schulman (2006)

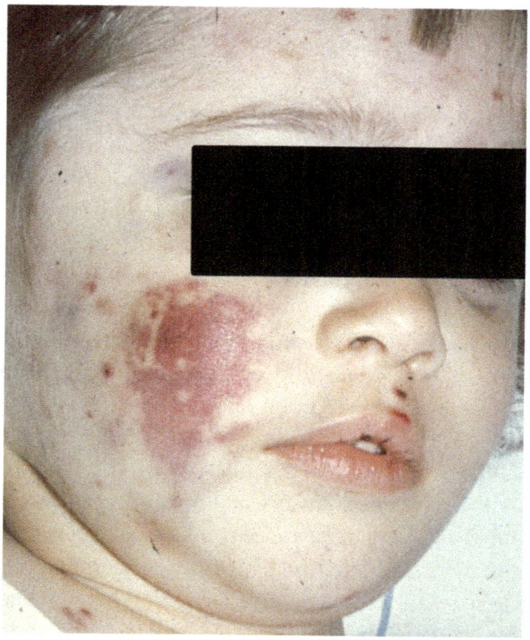

Fig. 5.10 Facial bruising in a child with idiopathic thrombocytopenic purpura

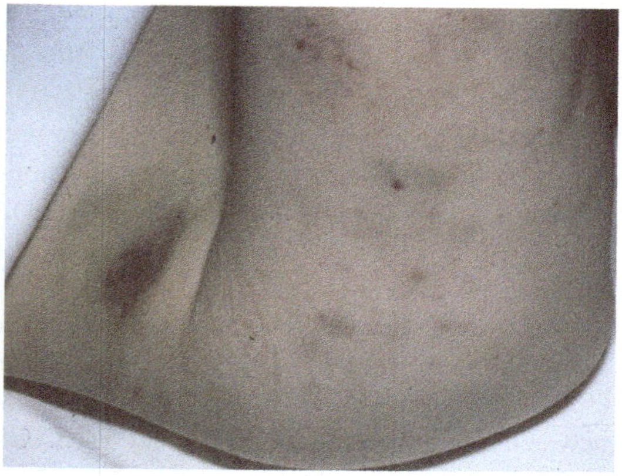

Fig. 5.11 Same child as in Fig. 5.10

hemorrhagic bullae on mucous membranes (Silverman 2011). Also gastrointestinal bleeding after abdominal trauma, intracranial hemorrhage, and retinal hemorrhages are described (Silverman 2011). ITP-related petechiae can be reproduced in the arm after applying a tourniquet, for example, for venepuncture (Lee 2008). They can also

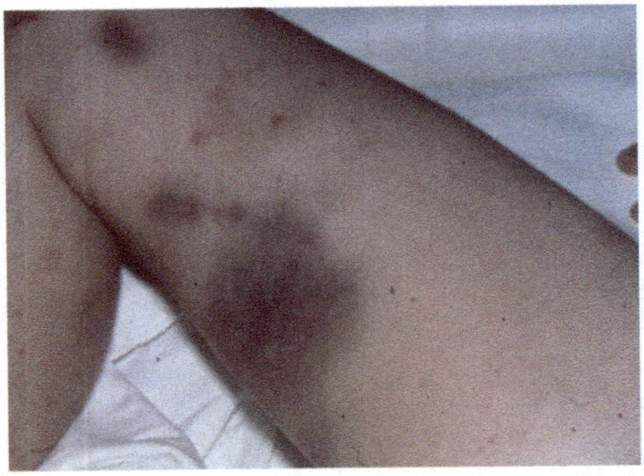

Fig. 5.12 Same child as in Fig. 5.10

be found in the face of a child with ITP after crying (Lee 2008). Resolution of the bleeding symptoms in an untreated child usually happens within 3–10 days after the diagnosis, regardless of the platelet count (Medeiros 2003).

ITP can be asymptomatic, although a very low number of thrombocytes will lead to visible symptoms (bruising) or spontaneous bleeding (Silverman 2011). Other symptoms, like fever, lethargy, weight loss, bone pain, joint pain, pallor, lymphadenopathy, and hepatosplenomegaly, are characteristically absent (Leung and Chan 2001). A minimal splenomegaly is found in about 5–10% of symptomatic children (Souid and Sadowitz 1995). This finding does not have any diagnostic value because it is about the same percentage as in non-ITP children (12% in children) (Silverman 2011).

Epidemiology of ITP

Idiopathic thrombocytopenic purpura (ITP) is the most common cause of thrombocytopenia in children (Leung and Chan 2001). The peak age is between 2 and 4 years of age (Leung and Chan 2001). Both genders are equally affected (Leung and Chan 2001).

Spontaneous remission occurs in 80–90% of cases in children, usually within a few weeks, although it may take 6–12 months (George et al. 1996). Recurrence of the ITP may occur. Silverman mentioned one study with a 6% prevalence of recurrence with most patients (69%) having only one recurrence. In one-third of the patients, the recurrence happened within 3 months.

Laboratory Studies

An isolated thrombocytopenia in the CBC and peripheral blood smear is the key finding. The platelets tend to be large. The leukocyte count and hemoglobin concentration typically are normal, unless severe hemorrhage has occurred. Coagulation studies are normal (Medeiros 2003).

ITP and Intracranial Bleeding

Intracranial bleeding can occur in children with ITP (Kolluri et al. 1986; Medeiros and Buchanan 1998). This concerns mainly intracerebral or subarachnoid bleedings although (chronic) subdural bleedings have been described (Medeiros and Buchanan 1998; Seçkin et al. 2006). Intracranial bleeding can occur immediately after the ITP has been diagnosed or it may take up to 8 years before intracranial bleeding occurs (median time of 32 days) (Butros and Bussel 2003). In almost 75%, intracranial bleeding takes place within 6 months after the diagnosis. According to Butros and Bussel (2003), the risk is higher when there is a very low number of thrombocytes, but Butros states that the low number is not the only or most important contributing factor. Because the occurrence of intracranial bleeding cannot be predicted based on the number of thrombocytes alone, one should always consider a CT scan if concerns exists regarding intracranial hemorrhage (Silverman 2011).

According to Lilleyman (1994), intracranial bleeding is less frequent than one should expect in children with ITP. Lilleyman found intracranial hemorrhages in about 0.1% of children of ITP. This low figure is conformed in later studies (<1% of children with ITP). Medeiros and Buchanan (1998) found intracranial bleeding in 2 out of more than 300 children with ITP. Both children recovered completely.

ITP and Suspicions of Child Abuse

Although ITP is always mentioned in the list of misdiagnoses, there are only a few case reports in the medical literature. This only concerned children with cutaneous bruising (Wheeler and Hobbs 1988; Harley 1997). Misdiagnosis of child abuse in case of intracranial bleeding, especially in subdural hematoma, has not been described probably because of the immediate and extensive laboratory investigations in children with intracranial bleeding, which in case of ITP will show the typical findings.

5.5.3.3 Leukemia, Thrombocytopenia, and Misdiagnosis of Child Abuse

In the medical literature, several case reports are found concerning bruises due to leukemia-related thrombocytopenia, which initially were misdiagnosed as child abuse (Nadjem and Sutor 1991; McClain et al. 1990). In both cases, hematological evaluation could have prevented the misdiagnosis.

5.5.3.4 Disseminated Intravascular Coagulation and Purpura Fulminans

Severe infections may result in complications such as disseminated intravascular coagulation (DIC) and purpura fulminans.

DIC is a complex systemic thrombohemorrhagic disorder involving the generation of intravascular fibrin and the consumption of procoagulants and platelets. The resultant clinical condition is characterized by intravascular coagulation and hemorrhage (Becker 2011). Intravascular coagulation will lead to the formation of small clots which will disrupt normal blood flow to organs, resulting in malfunction or even multiorgan failure. Hemorrhage may occur from the skin, the gastrointestinal tract, and the respiratory tract. DIC is not an illness in itself but always a complication resulting from a variety of disorders (Matsuda 1996). DIC is most commonly observed in patients with severe sepsis and septic shock (Levi and Ten Cate 1999).

Purpura fulminans is a nonthrombocytopenic purpura, which is seen mainly in children, including infants. It is an acute, often lethal syndrome of disseminated intravascular coagulopathy (Leung and Chan 2001). It may develop because of a severe bacterial infection/sepsis, notably meningococcal disease, or because of protein C or S deficiency (Smith and White 1999). According to Leung and Chan (2001), the skin lesions are rapidly progressive and characterized by microvascular thrombosis in the dermis, which ultimately results in perivascular hemorrhage and necrotic gangrene with minimal inflammation. Often the skin lesions are symmetrically located on the lower limbs (Figs. 5.13 and 5.14). There is a sharp demarcation between the cutaneous lesions and the normal skin. Other clinical symptoms include fever, vomiting, shock, oliguria/hematuria, and anemia. Adrenal hemorrhages may occur (Figs. 5.15 and 5.16).

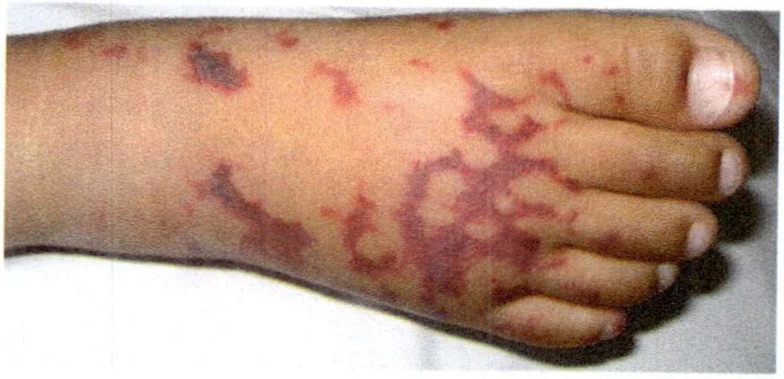

Fig. 5.13 Mild manifestation of purpura fulminans: vasculitis due to intravascular coagulation

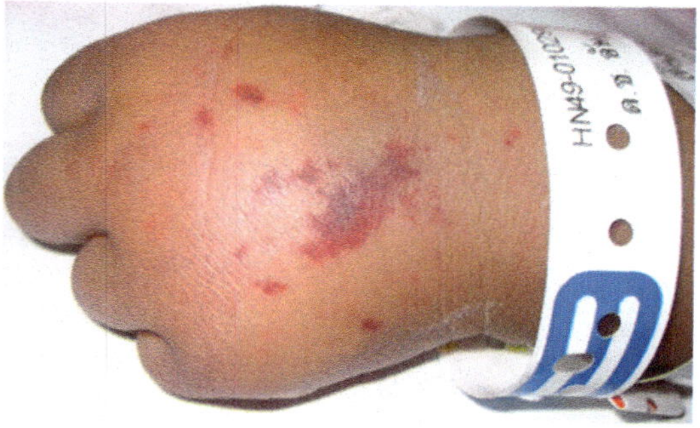

Fig. 5.14 Same child as in Fig. 5.13

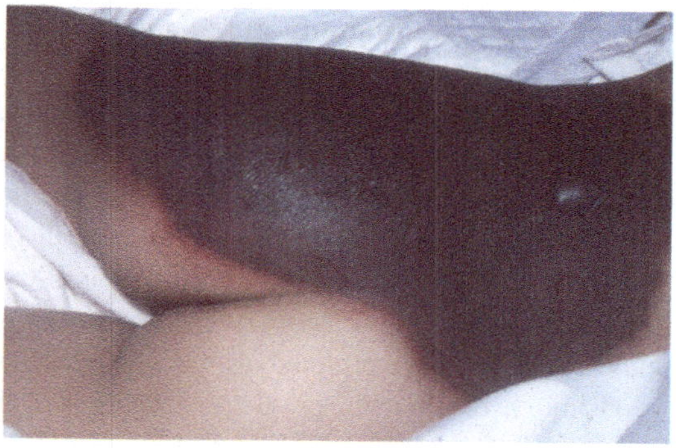

Fig. 5.15 Purpura fulminans in a child with Waterhouse-Friderichsen syndrome

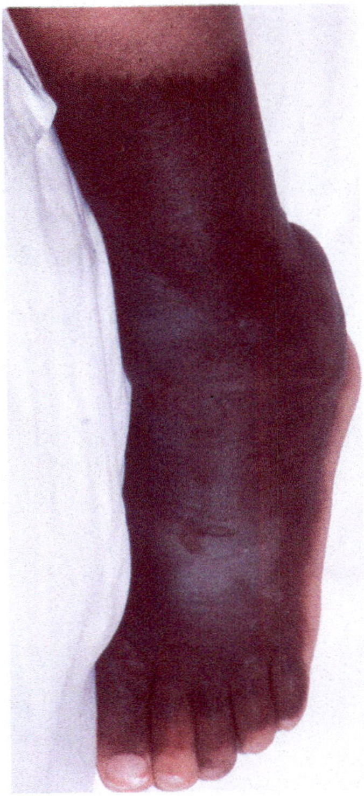

Fig. 5.16 Same child as in Fig. 5.15

DIC or Purpura Fulminans and Suspicions of Child Abuse
Because the child usually is severely ill and because of the presence of other symptoms, one would not expect misdiagnosis in a child which is hospitalized in time. If a child is hospitalized terminally ill or found dead, misdiagnosis may occur, as is illustrated by Kirschner and Stein (1985). In two cases, children were misinterpreted as having inflicted head injury, resulting in progressive lethargy and coma, but in fact had died from meningitis and DIC. In a 2-year-old boy, the severe bruising on the buttocks and lower extremities, according to the father of the boy, developed acutely and without any explanation, was misinterpreted as abusive bruising but turned out to be due to purpura fulminans.

5.6 Clotting Factor Deficiencies

5.6.1 General Aspects of Clotting Factor Deficiencies

Congenital disorders of coagulation factors result from deficiency or dysfunctioning of clotting factors. Acquired disorders are caused by impaired production, increased consumption, or rarely the formation of autoantibodies against clotting proteins (Hampton and Preston 2003). Acquired disorders mostly result from liver disease, often combined with spleen dysfunctioning, or from side effects of medication. The severity of the (bruising and) bleeding depends on the levels of remaining activity of the deficient or dysfunctioning factor(s) (Table 5.11) (Canadian Hemophilia Society 2008).

Table 5.11 Bleeding severity in factor deficiencies

Factor deficiency	Bleeding severity
I	Usually mild, except with complete absence of fibrinogen
II	Usually mild
V	Usually mild
V + VIII	Usually mild
VII	Severe when factor VII levels are low
VIII	Severe when factor VIII levels are below 1%
IX	Severe when factor IX levels are below 1%
X	Moderate to severe when factor X levels are below 10%
XI	Mild to moderate when factor XI levels are below 15%
XIII	Severe

Canadian Hemophilia Society (2008)

5.6.2 Von Willebrand Disease

Von Willebrand disease results from a quantitative or qualitative defect in Von Willebrand factor. Von Willebrand factor binds to factor VIII and mediates platelet aggregation (Ballas and Kraut 2008). Typical presentation of the disease is mucocutaneous bleeding (Thomas 2004): easy bruising, nosebleeds (often recurrent), or bleeding after tooth extraction, tonsillectomy, or other surgery.

Von Willebrand disease is the most common inherited bleeding disorder (Ballas and Kraut 2008). Werner found a prevalence of 1.3% in a multiethnic group of 600 healthy children between the age of 2 and 18 years (Werner et al. 1993). Culver mentions that Von Willebrand disease occurs in the USA in approximately 1 in 90 persons (1.10% or three million people – male and female) (Culvert and Norris 2006).

Most of the people affected by Von Willebrand disease will never be diagnosed (Culvert and Norris 2006) probably because the hemorrhagic tendency varies from hardly any bleeding to repeated and significant bleeding (Thomas 2004). This depends on the type and severity. Although males and females in theory should be affected equally, in practice more females are diagnosed with the disease because it often causes menorrhagia (Khair and Liesner 2006).

Three types with subtypes are distinguished. In type 1, the Von Willebrand factor is quantitatively reduced but not absent; in type 2, the factor is qualitatively abnormal; and in type 3, the factor is absent (Montgomery and Scott 2003). Type 1 is the mildest and most common type, about 85% of all cases (Montgomery and Scott 2003). Bleeding will occur only after a hemostatic challenge (Hampton and Preston 2003). Type 3 usually presents in early infancy and will stay symptomatic through childhood with severe mucosal bleeding (nosebleeds and sometimes extensive bruising) (Khair and Liesner 2006). This type is extremely rare: approximately 1:500,000 individuals (Montgomery and Scott 2003). Type 2 is more severe than type 1 and less severe than type 3 (Khair and Liesner 2006).

The diagnosis of Von Willebrand disease, especially type 1, can be difficult because the disease can give normal results on screening tests (Hampton and Preston 2003). The diagnosis requires often involvement of a pediatric hematologist to determine the amount, structure, and function of the Von Willebrand factor (National Hemophilia Foundation 2006).

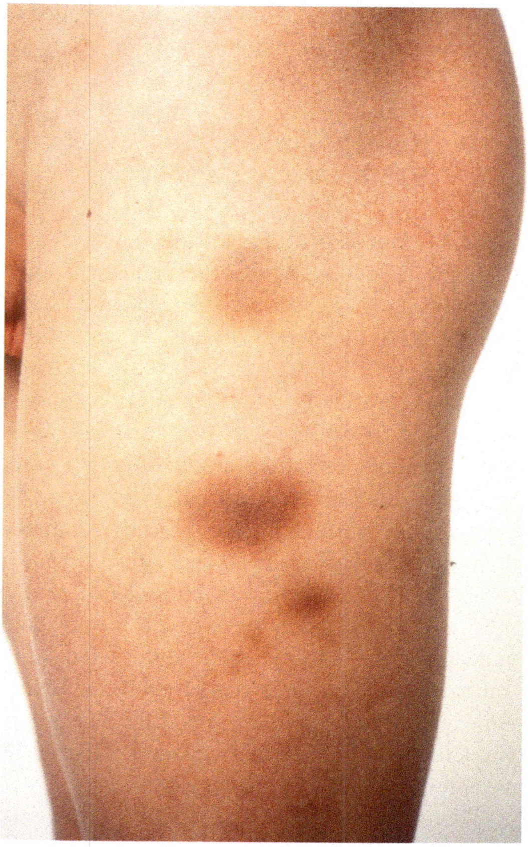

Fig. 5.17 Bruising in a child with Von Willebrand disease (type 1)

5.6.2.1 Von Willebrand Disease and Suspicions of Child Abuse

There are no reports found in the medical literature that Von Willebrand disease has been misdiagnosed as child abuse in children with bruising. According to O'Hare and Eden (1984), one needs to be cautious to attribute bruising in a child with suspected child abuse to low Von Willebrand factor levels if identified (Fig. 5.17).

Intracranial hemorrhages are only described in children with type 3 and always above the age of 1 year (Almaani and Awidi 1986; Montgomery and Scott 2003; Mishra et al. 2008) except for one neonate with a large intracranial bleeding because of severe Von Willebrand disease type 3 associated with sinus venous thrombosis (Wetzstein et al. 2006). Spontaneous intracranial bleeding in children with type 3 (bleeding caused by a minor or unnoticed trauma) is rare. Mostly these intracranial bleedings are trauma related. Stray-Pedersen et al. (2011) reported a massive subdural hematoma and bilateral retinal hemorrhages following an allegedly minor fall in an 11-month-old girl with mild Von Willebrand disease (type 1). However, from the report, it is not clear whether child abuse was excluded effectively during the evaluation or whether the disease was a coexisting disorder, which was "accidentally" diagnosed during the evaluation of suspected abusive head trauma and contributed to the severity of the subdural hematoma.

5.6.3 Hemophilia A, B, and C (Factor VIII, IX, and XI Deficiency)

5.6.3.1 Hemophilia A and B

Hemophilia A and B are the most common inherited clotting factor deficiencies. Hemophilia A (factor VIII deficiency, classic hemophilia) affects about 1 in 13,600 persons in the USA and worldwide 1 in 5,000 males (National Hemophilia Foundation 2006). Hemophilia A arises as a result of spontaneous mutation in about 30% of cases (Thomas 2004). Hemophilia B (factor IX deficiency, Christmas disease) is less common than type A and occurs in about 1 in 25,000 males (National Hemophilia Foundation 2006). About 30% of cases occur as result of a spontaneous gene mutation. A child with hemophilia, when injured, does not bleed harder or faster than a child without hemophilia. The child bleeds longer. Clinically, deficiencies of factor VIII and IX are indistinguishable (Thomas 2009).

There are different levels of severity of hemophilia: (Canadian Hemophilia Society 2008; National Hemophilia Foundation 2006; Hampton and Preston 2003):

- People with mild hemophilia (>5% up to 49% of factor VIII or IX) usually have problems with bleeding only after serious injury, significant trauma, or surgery. In many cases, mild hemophilia is not discovered until an injury or surgery or tooth extraction results in unusual bleeding. The first episode may not occur until adulthood.
- People with moderate hemophilia (up to 5% of factor VIII or IX), about 15% of the hemophilia population, tend to have bleeding episodes even after minor injuries. They may also experience occasional bleeding episodes without obvious cause ("spontaneous bleeding episodes").
- People with severe hemophilia (<1–2% of factor VIII or IX), about 60% of the hemophilia population, have bleeding following trauma and may have frequent spontaneous bleeding episodes, often into the joints and muscles.

Symptoms are found mostly in older children. The most common first symptoms are subcutaneous and mucosal bleeding. Small cuts or surface bruises are usually not a problem, but more traumatic injuries may result in serious problems and potential disability (called "bleeding episodes") (National Hemophilia Foundation 2006). Children with severe hemophilia may present with cutaneous bruising and intra-articular (tender swollen joints) or intramuscular bleeding (Lee 2008; Olivieri et al. 2009). Tender swollen joints may also be seen in Henoch-Schönlein purpura (see Sect. 6.3.3), acute leukemia, or neuroblastoma (Thomas 2004) and in some rare bleeding disorders (Table 5.13). In older children, one may find deformity of joints and muscle wasting (Lee 2008).

Symptoms in neonates are rare, although symptoms may be present in the first days of life (Newland and Evans 2003; Sirotnak 2006). Bleeding from the umbilical cord is rare (Newland and Evans 2003). Intracranial (subdural, subarachnoidal, and intracerebral) bleeding is also rare but has been described in hemophilia A and B (de Tezanos Pinto et al. 1992; Shih et al. 1993; Bach et al. 2001; Gedeit 2001; Newland and Evans 2003). These are either more or less spontaneous in children with severe hemophilia, for example, a minor or unrecognized trauma, or clearly trauma related (Yoshida et al. 1979). Mostly, these are found in children above the age of 6 months. In neonates, symptoms of intracranial bleeding are found mainly in the first week, and the situation is very rarely life-threatening (Franze and Forrest 1988; Venkateswaran et al. 1998). Hemophilia-related intracranial bleeding is very rare between the age of 2 weeks and 6 months (Ries et al. 1998; Myles et al. 2001). Nelson did find a prevalence of intracranial bleeding in 12% of 309 children with hemophilia and an incidence of intracranial hemorrhages of 2% per year (Nelson et al. 1999). Severe bleeding may occur at circumcision or when the child becomes more mobile (Newland and Evans 2003). There has never been described a causal relationship between mild hemophilia (factor VIII or IX deficiency) and spontaneous intracranial bleeding (Christian 2003). In moderate to severe hemophilia, however, spontaneous intracranial hemorrhage, including isolated subdural hemorrhage, may occur (Eyster et al. 1978; Bray and Luban 1987). Diagnosis is made certain by measuring the amount of factor VIII and factor IX in the blood (Canadian Hemophilia Society 2008). Patients with hereditary disorders in fibrinolysis like alpha 2 antiplasmin deficiency (extremely rare, around 20 cases reported) and plasminogen activation inhibitor-1 deficiency may clinically show the same symptoms as seen in patients with hemophilia (Lee 2008; Kozyreva 2009).

Hemophilia A and B and Suspicions of Child Abuse

Suspicions of child abuse may be present in almost 30% of the children with an undiagnosed hemophilia (Hazewinkel et al. 2003). Misdiagnosis mostly resulted from cutaneous bleeding and only rarely from intracranial bleeding (O'Hare and Eden 1984; Harley 1997).

5.6.3.2 Hemophilia C

Hemophilia C (factor XI deficiency, plasma thromboplastin antecedent deficiency, Rosenthal syndrome) is the most common type of factor deficiencies after hemophilia A and B. The disease affects about 1 in 100,000 persons. The disease is inherited as an autosomal recessive condition (men and women equally affected). Often there is no positive family history, unless there is consanguinity within the family (Thomas 2009).

Some people with hemophilia C may have milder symptoms than those of hemophilia, but clinical symptoms may vary in severity. Spontaneous bleeding is not likely. Bleeding normally occurs after a hemostatic challenge like a trauma or surgery, especially dental extractions, tonsillectomies, surgery in the urinary and genital tracts, and nasal surgery. Joint bleeds are uncommon. Patients are more prone to bruising, nosebleeds, or blood in the urine. Women may experience menorrhagia and prolonged bleeding after childbirth (National Hemophilia Foundation 2006).

Diagnosis is made through bleeding time test, platelet function tests, and prothrombin time (PT) and activated partial thromboplastin time (aPTT) tests. A specific factor XI assay is extremely useful in ruling out combined deficiencies (National Hemophilia Foundation 2006). The diagnosis should be made by a pediatric hematologist.

Hemophilia C and Suspicions of Child Abuse

There are no reports found in the medical literature that hemophilia C has been misdiagnosed as child abuse.

5.6.4 Deficiencies of Other Clotting Factors

Most deficiencies of clotting factors (excluding factor VIII and IX deficiency) are rare (Table 5.12) (International Registry of Rare Bleeding Disorders 2009). Almost all of these disorders are autosomal recessive (male and female equally affected), representing 3–5% of all the inherited factor deficiencies. The incidence in general population ranges from 1 in 500,000 to 1 in 2–5 million (International Registry of Rare Bleeding Disorders 2009; National Hemophilia Foundation 2006; Canadian Hemophilia Society 2008). In countries with high rates of consanguineous marriages, rare bleeding disorders (RBDs) occur more frequently and may even be 10–20 times higher than in countries with low rates of consanguineous marriages. Clinical symptoms vary from a mild bleeding tendency to potentially life-threatening hemorrhaging, for example, intracranial or intra-abdominal bleedings (Table 5.13). Even in major surgery, bleeding manifestations are extremely rare (International Registry of Rare Bleeding Disorders 2009; National Hemophilia Foundation 2006; Canadian Hemophilia Society 2008). Factor XII deficiency is not associated with clinical symptoms in children (Vora and Makris 2001).

Whenever one suspects a rare bleeding disorder, one should always consult a pediatric hematologist for the correct diagnostic procedures and a definitive diagnosis.

5.6.4.1 Rare Bleeding Disorders and Suspicions of Child Abuse

There are no reports found in the medical literature that cutaneous bruising caused by rare bleeding disorders has been misdiagnosed as child abuse, although theoretically it may happen in all RBDs

Table 5.12 Overview of rare bleeding disorders (RBDs)

Factor deficiency	Synonyms	Incidence/1,000,000 persons
I	Afibrinogenemia Hypofibrinogenemia Dysfibrinogenemia	1–2
II	Prothrombin deficiency	0.5–1
V	Parahemophilia Owren disease Labile factor deficiency Proaccelerin deficiency	1
V + VIII		1
VII	Alexander disease Stable factor deficiency Proconvertin deficiency	2
X	Stuart-Prower factor deficiency	1
XI	Hemophilia C	10
XII	Hageman factor deficiency	1
XIII	Fibrin stabilizing factor deficiency	0.2–0.5

International Registry of Rare Bleeding Disorders (2009); National Hemophilia Foundation (2006); Canadian Hemophilia Society (2008)

Table 5.13 Clinical symptoms of rare bleeding disorders (RBDs) (except factor XI deficiency)

Factor Symptom	I	II	V	V + VIII	VII	X	XII	XIII
Nosebleeding	+	+	+	+	+	+	–	+
Oral cavity bleeding	+	+	+	+	+	+	–	+
Cutaneous bleeding	+	?	+	+	+	+	–	+
Umbilical cord bleeding	+	+	–	–	0	+	–	+
Joint bleeding	+	+	0	0	+	+	–	+
Muscle bleeding	+	+	+	+	+	+	–	+
Intracranial bleeding	+	0	0	–	+	+	–	+
Gastrointestinal bleeding	+	+	+	–	+	+	–	+
Hematuria	–	0	–	–	0	+	–	+
Major surgery	+	+	+	+	+	+	–	–
Minor surgery, e.g., circumcision	+	+	+	+	+	+	–	+
Others	0	?	0	+	–	+	–	–

+ occasional or common, 0 rare, – absent, ? unknown
International Registry of Rare Bleeding Disorders (2009)

(Vora and Makris 2001; Thomas 2004). Misdiagnosis has been described in children with unexplained intracranial hemorrhages, including an acute subdural hematoma due to factor II and XIII deficiencies (Strijks et al. 1999; Newman et al. 2002).

5.6.5 Vitamin K Deficiency

Vitamin K is an essential, lipid-soluble vitamin that plays a vital role in the production of coagulation proteins (Patel 2008). Vitamin K controls the formation of coagulation factors II, VII, IX, and X in the liver (Merck Manual 2007). Other coagulation factors dependent on vitamin K are protein C, protein S, and protein Z (proteins C and S are anticoagulants) (Merck Manual 2007).

Vitamin K deficiency leads to decreased levels of the vitamin K–dependent coagulation factors, causing defective coagulation. Deficiency without bleeding may occur in as many as 50% of infants younger than 5 days (Patel 2008).

Table 5.14 Classification of vitamin K deficiency bleeding of the newborn (VKDB)

VKBD	Age	Incidence
Early onset	First 24 h postpartum	Rare
Classic onset	Between 24 h postpartum and 7 days, sometimes up to 1 month (overlapping late onset)	0.25–1.7/100 birth
Late onset	2–12 weeks up to 6 months (peak at 3–8 weeks)	4–7/100,000 birth

American Academy of Pediatrics (2003); Puckett and Offringa (2009); Nimavat (2009); Shearer (2009)

Deficiency leading to bleeding is rare, but potentially life-threatening: vitamin K deficiency bleeding of the newborn (VKDB), formerly known as hemorrhagic disease of the newborn (HDN) (Merck Manual 2007). The resulting coagulation disorder resembles the effect of warfarin ingestion (Hampton and Preston 2003).

Depending on the age of onset, vitamin K deficiency bleeding is classified by three different time periods after birth, which differ in incidence (Table 5.14), and in age-of-onset-related causes of the deficiency (see later). The severity of the clinical symptoms correlates with the severity of vitamin K deficiency. According to Rutty et al. (1999), bleeding caused by vitamin K deficiency usually is a self-limiting disease. Severe bleeding can be fatal (Patel 2008).

Serum PT and aPTT may be prolonged in infants with VKDB; however, aPTT may be normal. Platelet counts and fibrinogen levels are within the normal range for newborns. According to Nimavat (2009), direct blood measurement of vitamin K is not useful because levels normally are low in newborns. According to Patel (2008), the most sensitive marker is the high level of des-gamma-carboxy prothrombin (DCP), a protein induced by Vitamin K antagonism or absence (PIVKA). PIVKA measurements can confirm VKDB even several days after treatment. The diagnosis is confirmed if administration of vitamin K stops the bleeding and lowers the serum PT value (Nimavat 2009).

5.6.5.1 Vitamin K Deficiency Bleeding and Suspicions of Child Abuse

Vitamin K deficiency bleeding or its warning bleeds are often not recognized. Case histories of infants with VKDB regularly appear in the medical literature in which is described that bleeding, especially intracranial bleeding due to vitamin K deficiency, was wrongly diagnosed as child abuse (Lane et al. 1983; Wetzel et al. 1995; Rutty et al. 1999; Fenton et al. 2000; Brousseau et al. 2005). Cutaneous manifestations of VKDB, mistaken for child abuse, are also reported (Brousseau et al. 2005). Because of the routine administration of vitamin K prophylaxis immediately after birth, many doctors do not take into account the possibility of "late-onset VKDB" in an infant with bruising and bleeding.

5.7 Artificial Bruising and Bleeding

5.7.1 Introduction

Bruising and bleeding normally result from trauma or coagulation disorders but can also be "artificially" induced. Artificial bruising and bleeding (sometimes referred to as false bruising and bleeding – Chavali and Dasari 2011) are defined as any bruising or bleeding which is not trauma nor disease related, but self-inflicted and often intended. It can be induced by using several methods (cause – Table 5.15). A list of reports of drug-induced thrombocytopenia and thrombocytopenia related to food, spices, additives, and herbal medicine is available at "Platelets on the Web" (http://www.ouhsc.edu/platelets/index.html). It can happen under various circumstances (manner – Table 5.16).

5.7.2 Intended and Self-Inflicted Bruising and Bleeding: Malingering and Factitious Disorder (Munchausen Syndrome)

5.7.2.1 Malingering

According to the Diagnostic and Statistical Manual of Mental Disorders (APA 2000), malingering is the intentional and purposeful feigning

Table 5.15 The most common causes of nontraumatic or non-disease-related bruising and bleeding

Trauma	Methods		Effects
Nontraumatic	Ink, crayon, paint, or dyes (Sect. 6.7.3)		Discoloration of the skin
Mechanical	Pinching, rubbing, sucking		Traumatic extravasation of blood
Drug induced	Anticoagulants	Acetylsalicylic acid (aspirin) and other aspirin-containing drugs	Thrombocytopathy
		Quinidine	Thrombocytopenia (ITP): increased destruction
		Heparin	
		Acenocoumarol	Vitamin K deficiency
		Dicoumarol	
		Phenprocoumon	
		Warfarin	
	Rodenticide	Brodifacoum (superwarfarin)	Vitamin K deficiency
	Food, spices, additives, and herbal medicine	Clove	Thrombocytopathy
		Cumin	
		Feverfew	
		Garlic in large amounts	
		Ginger (not dried ginger)	
		Ginkgo biloba	
		Ginseng (Asian)	
		High saturated (omega-3) fatty acids, fish oil	
		Onion extract	
		Saw palmetto (Serenoa repens)	
		Turmeric	
		Vitamin E	
		Willow bark	
		EMLA[R] (de Waard-van der Spek and Oranje 1997)	

Schulman (2006); Sharathkumar and Shapiro (2008)

Table 5.16 Manner of artificial bruising and bleeding

Unintended	Side effect of prescribed and over-the-counter medication	
	Accidental ingestion	
Intended	Self-inflicted	Malingering
		Factitious disorder (Munchausen syndrome, painful bruising syndrome)
		Suicide
	Inflicted by other person	Pediatric condition falsification – fabricated/induced illness (Munchausen syndrome by proxy)
		Poisoning/manslaughter/murder

of an illness to achieve some recognizable goal. Malingering is seen in adults and in children (Dingle 2005; Walker 2011).

Symptoms may be fabricated or induced and can concern physical and mental symptoms or illnesses. Sometimes a malingerer may exaggerate the symptoms of an existing illness or the effect of an accident. In many cases, the deceit can be recognized easily by a physician, but it can take much longer because of the medical knowledge of the malingerer.

Malingering should be differentiated from a factitious disorder. Both are listed in the DSM-IV-TR, but factitious disorders are considered by the APA (2000) to be a mental disorder and malingering is not considered to be a mental disorder.

In a factitious disorder, just like in malingering, there is intentional production or feigning of signs or symptoms. However, the motivation is different. In a factitious disorder, the motivation for the behavior is a (probably unconscious) psychological need to assume the sick role. External incentives for the behavior are absent (Mehta and Bussing 1993; APA 2000; Pridmore 2009). Malingering is deliberate behavior motivated by external incentives, such as (APA 2000; Pridmore 2009; Bienenfeld 2010; Beach and Stern 2011; Chavali and Dasari 2011):

- Economic gain/financial compensation/disability payments
- Avoiding legal responsibility/criminal prosecution
- Avoiding school, work, or military duty
- Obtaining drug
- Improving physical well-being
- Extra attention, sympathy, or help from family, friends, or colleagues

The methods used to feign bruises and bleeding can be compared to those in a factitious disorder. Chavali and Dasari (2011) reported the use of dithranol by a prisoner to produce bruises with the purpose to bring a charge of torture/beating against the jail officials.

5.7.2.2 Factitious Disorder in Children and Adolescents

Several methods to simulate a factitious disorder are described in the medical literature. Factitious disorders are characterized by the intentional feigning or induction of signs and/or symptoms in order to assume the sick role (Stanziale et al. 1997). In a factitious disorder, the physical or psychological symptoms seem to be under voluntary control of the patient.

Factitious disorders in children and adolescents (also referred to as child and adolescent illness falsification) may go undetected for a long time (Libow 2000). In 2000, Libow found 42 cases of illness falsification in minors, described in the medical literature in a period of 30 years (mean age of 13.9 and a range from 8 to 18 years; 71% female; mean duration of falsification: 16 months). The most commonly reported falsified or induced conditions were fevers, ketoacidosis, bruises, and infections. The fabrications ranged from false symptom reporting to active injections, bruising, and ingestions.

Factitious bruising and bleeding disorders have been described in children as young as 9 years of age, although it is considered to be very rare in school-age children (White et al. 1966; Yamada et al. 2009). Factitious bruising and bleeding in children and adolescents are induced in many different ways, although there are no descriptions of the use of anticoagulants or other drugs in self-inflicted bruising and bleeding in minors. Sometimes, even after extensive investigations, one will not find a direct cause, but based on the circumstance, one can conclude it is a factitious disorder. Datta et al. (2009) described a 9-year-old girl with recurrent episodes of oozing of blood from the skin of both lower eyelids and lower periorbital areas along with bleeding from the tongue. The bleeding stopped spontaneously after a few minutes. There were no other findings like induration or edema at the bleeding sites. A coagulation disorder could be excluded. After psychotherapy, the symptoms did not recur.

Mostly suction is used to induce factitious bruising in older children and adolescents (White et al. 1966; Lovejoy et al. 1971; Brandrup 1990; Yates 1992; Landers and Schroeder 2004; Yamada et al. 2009) (Fig. 5.18). White described recurrent factitious bruising in a 9-year-old girl caused by skin suction, comparable to a hickey. Suction on the skin by creating a vacuum over the skin with a glass from which the air had been partially aspirated has been described by Lovejoy et al. (1971) in two girls, 10 and 14 years of age ("factitious purpura"); Brandrup (1990) in three children, 13–15 years of age (circular delimited petechial purpura around the mouth and chin); and Yates (1992) in an 11-year-old girl ("purpuric rash" on lips and chin). Landers and Schroeder (2004) described recurring bathtub suction-induced bruising in two girls, 9 and 14 years of age. According to the girls, the bruising occurred spontaneously on the lower back and in a U-shaped distribution. Histopathology showed extravasated erythrocytes and a sparse superficial inflammatory infiltrate. One girl admitted that the bruising was self-inflicted. In the other girl, the

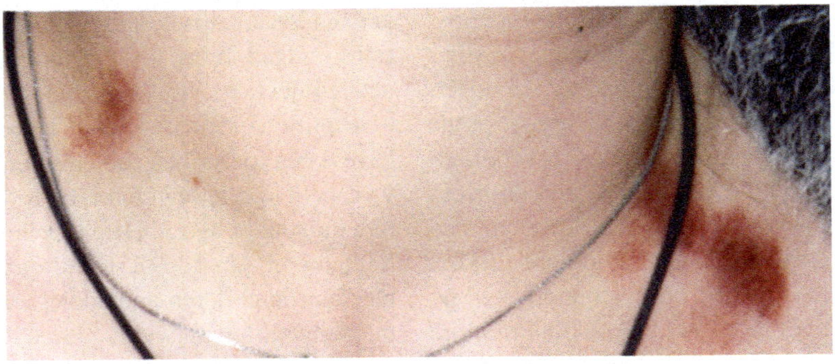

Fig. 5.18 Factitious purpura caused by suction in a false rape allegation: the girl initially stated that the lesions were grip marks. Then she stated that these were hickeys caused by the alleged perpetrator. Finally she admitted that she herself induced the suction marks

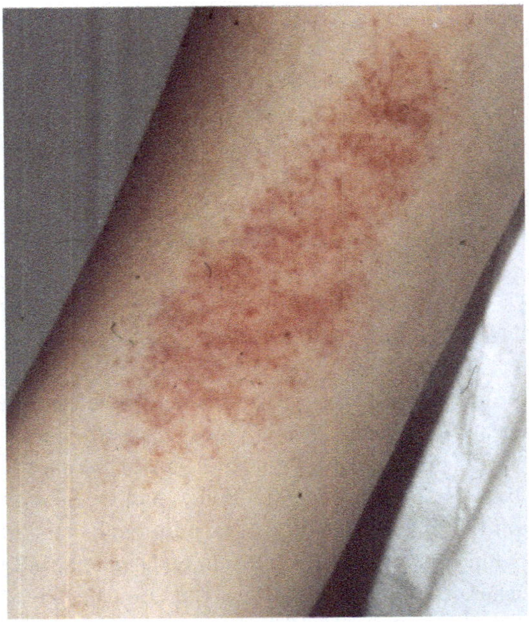

Fig. 5.19 Factitious purpura caused by rubbing

bruising improved when she stopped taking baths. Yamada described a 10-year-old girl with a bizarre bruising pattern, who was evaluated comprehensively. Coagulation disorders were excluded. Child abuse was suspected but ruled out because the bruising continued to develop after separation of the child from the family. Histologic examination of the skin lesions revealed disruption of collagen fiber bundles, which indicated the application of external force, most likely suction.

Pinching and rubbing may also be used (Fig. 5.19). Gil-Bistes et al. (2010) reported factitious bruising in a 12-year-old girl presenting as acute linear bruising on the right arm, suggestive for pinching or rubbing.

Sometimes dyes or ink is used to create "bruises" (Rogers et al. 2001; Bapat et al. 2011). Rogers described 32 patients aged 8–16 years (24 females, 8 males). Lesions were found on the head and neck in over 50% of the cases. The lesions were caused by scratching (grazing, erosions, and deep ulcers), chemical and thermal burns, hair cutting, and shaving and in four patients by skin painting. Bapat et al. (2011) described a 13-year-old girl with intermittent episodes of bruising on her extremities, face, and chin after little or no trauma. There were no findings consistent with a coagulation disorder. Eventually, a large bruise was noted on her left wrist. She complained of wrist pain and resisted examination. The wrist was cleansed for better inspection with an adhesive removal pad. The "bruise," which was caused by the application of blue pigments, resolved and the underlying skin was normal. In some cases there are skin lesions, which are self-inflicted with dyes or ink but cannot be seen as symptom of a factitious disorder. Cordell and Berry (2004) described two girls, 3 and 7 years of age, who were evaluated for a prominent macular rash, without showing any other symptoms, except excessive whispering, uncontrolled giggling, and avoidance of eye contact with their parents. The rash was most prominent on visible parts of the body, including the face and anterior neck. The two girls eventually confessed to marking each other with a colored pen to simulate a case of chickenpox they had recently seen on television.

Factitious cutaneous bleeding has been described by Tunnessen and Chessar (1984) in a 10½-year-old girl. The girl had a history of spontaneous episodes of nosebleeding and bleeding from the skin, eyes, and ears for almost a year. Medical evaluation led to the conclusion that the origin of the episodes was factitious. A gingivitis proved to be the source of blood for the bleeding. A similar case was described by Early and Lifschutz (1974) a 10½-year-old intensely religious Baptist girl who experienced religious stigmata periodically over a 3-week period immediately preceding Easter Sunday 1972. Early and Lifschutz (1974) was convinced that it was unlikely that the lesions were self-induced and concluded: "*The recently described entity, psychogenic purpura, strikingly demonstrates the reality of mentally induced bleeding*" (Sect. 5.7.3). Collard et al. (2008) reported factitious persistent bleeding and crusting of the lips in a 15-year-old girl in whom the diagnosis was made after excluding organic causes.

5.7.3 Painful Bruising Syndrome

Painful bruising syndrome (also known as psychogenic purpura, autoerythrocyte sensitization syndrome, or Gardner-Diamond syndrome) was first described in (1955) by Gardner and Diamond. The syndrome is characterized by the occurrence of recurrent painful bruising, usually located on the arms and legs and sometimes on the face and trunk. The bruises are ill defined, painful, swollen, and tender (James et al. 2006). The appearance of the bruises is often precipitated by an injury or surgical procedure in the weeks before the appearance or, more often, severe emotional stress (Ratnoff 1989; Hagemeier et al. 2011).

Painful bruising syndrome is mostly seen in young adult to middle-aged female, usually Caucasian, patients (Fey and Beck 1986; Archer-Dubon et al. 1998; Vun and Muir 2004; Geisler and Dezube 2011), although occasionally it has also been described in young adult males (Ingber et al. 1985) and in children or adolescents (Boxley and Wilkinson 1971; Campbell et al. 1983; Sorensen et al. 1985; Vaillant et al. 1986; Alvin 1988; Anderson et al. 1999; Chatterjee and Jaiswal 2002; Meeder and Bannister 2006).

The exact pathogenesis of this syndrome is still not known, although most research and most published cases do strongly indicate a psychosomatic or factitious origin (James et al. 2006; Harth et al. 2010). Because the exact pathogenesis is not known, the syndrome sometimes is referred to as Devil's pinches in the nonmedical literature. The majority of the described adult patients has psychiatric disorders (Clark 1984; Harth et al. 2010). As in adults, children and adolescents usually have a disturbed psychological background or a psychiatric disorder and seem to respond well to psychotherapy (Campbell et al. 1983; Sorensen et al. 1985).

According to Campbell et al. (1983), the typical skin lesion in the pediatric age group is a painful, erythematous bruise that starts after minor trauma or surgery. The lesion often involves an area away from the injury site. The skin manifestations can be debilitating and reappear unpredictably for an indefinite period. Some patients, even in the pediatric age group, report a premonition or are able to predict when lesions will occur because of prodromal symptoms like warmth and pain or a tingling, itching, or burning feeling at the future affected site (Meeder and Bannister 2006; Harth et al. 2008; Hagemeier et al. 2011). After these prodromal symptoms, edema and erythema can become visible within a few hours. Bruising usually will become visible within 24–48 h after the first symptoms (Chatterjee and Jaiswal 2002). Hagemeier et al. (2011) described three siblings (two girls, aged 12 and 9 years, and one boy, aged 10 years) with unexplained bruises, partly patterned, partly striped. The bruising in the children seemed to have occurred recently and almost simultaneously. The children reported, independently from each other, the same prodromal symptoms: itching of the affected skin, followed by a burning sensation and the appearance of bruises at the same site. The children all mentioned the same emotionally stressful event, namely, the death of their cat a week before the

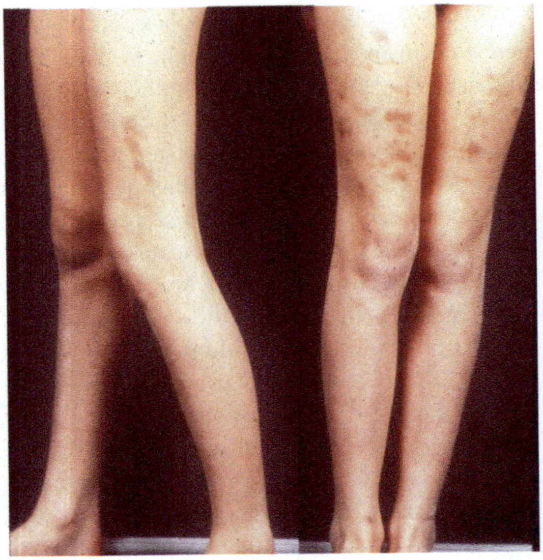

Fig. 5.20 Painful bruising syndrome in a twin

appearance of the bruises. Laboratory testing (coagulation, immunology, serology) was normal. Hagemeier concluded that the diagnosis of Gardner-Diamond syndrome was certain in the 12-year-old girl and should be strongly suspected in the other children. Child abuse (including pediatric condition falsification) and factitious disorder were considered. According to Hagemeier, there was no evidence of child abuse, although a self-inflicted factitious disorder could not be excluded convincingly (Figs. 5.20, 5.21, and 5.22).

It may take years before the diagnosis is made. Lindahl (1977) described a 20-year-old woman who had suffered from the syndrome since the age of 12 years. She claimed to have Von Willebrand disease and was admitted to hospital 14 times in 8 years for a bleeding disorder which was never diagnosed. A consultant psychiatrist was convinced the bruising was self-inflicted. Sawhney et al. (2006) described a 23-year-old woman with recurrent episodes of spontaneous painful bruising over her extremities and trunk for a period of 9 years along with other factitious skin lesions (linear erosion on the accessible areas of the body and a pseudo-ainhum of her left nipple).

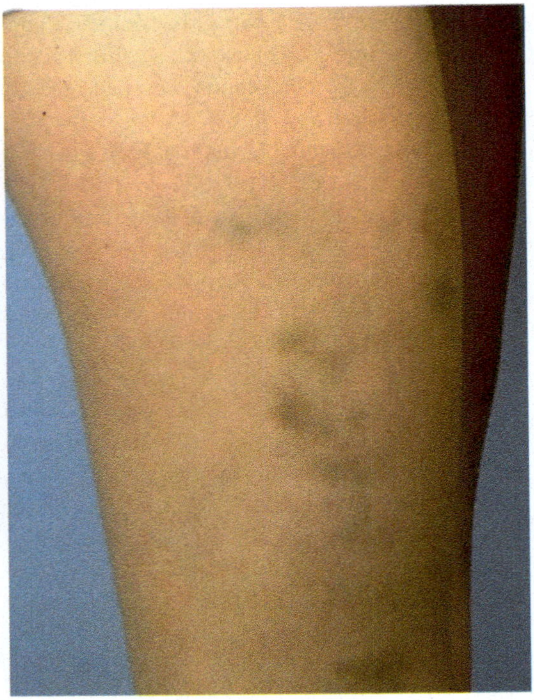

Fig. 5.21 Painful bruising syndrome in a twin: detail of right leg of one of the girls

5.7.4 Intended and Self-Inflicted Bruising and Bleeding: Attempted Suicide

Chua and Friedenberg (1998) described one teenager and one adult with an attempted suicide using superwarfarin. The use of superwarfarin was easily diagnosed in both patients.

5.7.5 Intended Bruising and Bleeding Inflicted by Another Person: Factitious Coagulation Disorder by Proxy – Pediatric Condition Falsification

In Rosenberg (1987), reported that bruising and bleeding were among the most prevalent factitious symptoms in children who were victims of Munchausen syndrome by proxy (now known as fictitious disorder by proxy, pediatric condition falsification, or fabricated/induced illness).

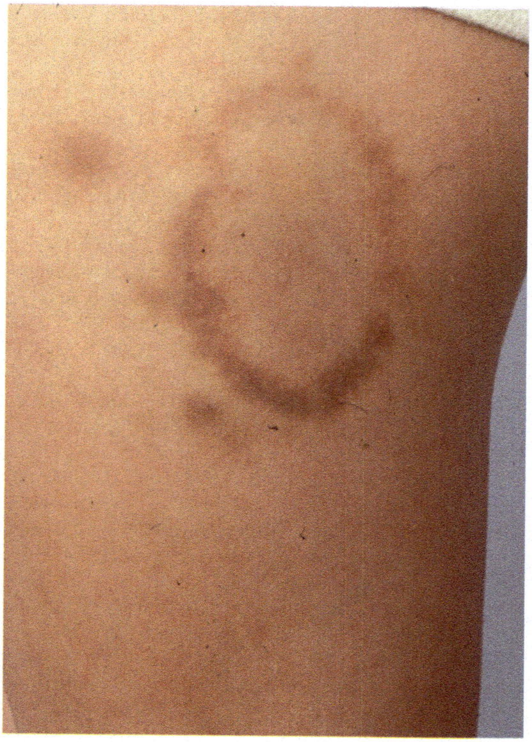

Fig. 5.22 Painful bruising syndrome in a twin: detail of left leg of one of the girls

According to Mehta and Bussing (1993), one should think of a factitious bleeding disorder in a child in the early differential diagnosis of bleeding disorders if the clinical symptoms and laboratory findings do not fit a known bleeding disorder.

As in malingering and factitious disorders in adults, several methods are described in the medical literature to fabricate or induce a factitious coagulation disorder by proxy. Several case reports were published on this issue. The use of warfarin has been described by White et al. (1985) in an 11-month-girl and Souid et al. (1993) in a 13-year-old girl with a mild platelet disorder. Babcock et al. (1993) described a rodenticide-induced coagulopathy (brodifacoum) in a 24-month-old child with bruises. Factitious bleeding ears in children are reported not only by White et al. (1985) as a result of the use of anticoagulants but also by other authors like Griffiths et al. (2001), in which the bleeding ears resulted from trauma inflicted by the mother, and by Bennett et al. (2005), in which the mother spat and placed blood in her child's ear. Kurlandsky et al. (1979) reported an 8-week-old infant with "facial" blood, which presumably resulted from repetitive bleeding episodes, in which the blood originated from the upper respiratory tract. Eventually after extensive investigations, the facial blood turned out to have another Rh subtype (cc) than the child's own blood (Cc). Tüfekçi et al. (2011) reported a 16-year-old girl with complaints of bleeding from multiple sites, including hemoptysis, hematuria, bloody tears, and bloody nipple discharge. The bleeding however was only witnessed by her mother. No organic cause was found and it was concluded that the mother fabricated the symptoms. Gastrointestinal and rectal bleeding has also been reported in children varying in age from several months up to adolescence (Mills and Burke 1990; Guiraldes et al. 1995; Wenk 2003; Ulinski et al. 2004; Sahin et al. 2002). Sometimes complex cases like the before-mentioned cases become even more complicated, for example, if a child with a real illness becomes the victim of a fabricated or induced illness, in which the perpetrator is having a factitious disorder. Ayass et al. (1993) described a boy with hemophilia in which the mother presented the boy to the hospital because of failure to thrive, related to the boy's hemophilia, subsequently for her own self-inflicted mutilating wounds, and finally for bleeding and arthritic complications in the boy, which were simulated by the mother.

References

Almaani WS, Awidi AS (1986) Spontaneous intracranial hemorrhage secondary to Von Willebrand's disease. Surg Neurol 26(5):457–460

Alvin P (1988) Gardner-diamond syndrome and psychogenic purpura. Case report of a 16-year-old adolescent [Article in French]. Ann Pediatr (Paris) 35(5):333–336

American Academy of Pediatrics (2003) Policy statement. Controversies concerning vitamin K and the newborn. Pediatrics 122(1):191–192

American Psychiatric Association (2000) Diagnostic and statistical manual of mental disorders DSM-IV-TR, 4th edn (Text Revision). American Psychiatric Press Inc, Arlington

Anderson JE, DeGoff W, McNamara M (1999) Autoerythrocyte sensitization (psychogenic purpura): a case report and review of the literature. Pediatr Emerg Care 15(1):47–48

Archer-Dubon C, Orozco-Topete R, Reyes-Gutierrez E (1998) Two cases of psychogenic purpura. Rev Invest Clin 50(2):145–148

Ayass M, Bussing R, Mehta P (1993) Munchausen's syndrome presenting as haemophilia: a convenient and economical "steal" of disease and treatment. Paediatr Haematol Oncol 10(3):241–244

Babcock J, Hartman K, Pedersen A et al (1993) Rodenticide-induced coagulopathy in a young child. A case of Munchausen syndrome by proxy. Am J Pediatr Hematol Oncol 15(1):126–130

Bach KP, Schouten-van Meeteren AY, Smit LM, Veenhuizen L, Gemke RJ (2001) Intracranial hemorrhages in infants: child abuse or a congenital coagulation disorder? [Article in Dutch]. Ned Tijdschr Geneeskd 145(17):809–813

Ballas M, Kraut EH (2008) Bleeding and bruising: a diagnostic work-up. Am Fam Physician 77(8): 1117–1124

Bapat K, Zaid Kaylani SHA, Turner C, Regueira O (2011) Bruising in a teenage girl: a manifestation of dermatitis artefacta. Consultant 51(8):573–576. http://www.consultant360.com/content/bruising-teenage-girl-manifestation-dermatitis-artefacta

Bari A, Javaid BK, Rehman S, Naz S (2009) Scurvy: presenting as musculoskeletal pain. J Coll Physicians Surg Pak 19(3):198–200

Beach SR, Stern TA (2011) Malingering involving insurance fraud: when it pays to be ill. Psychosomatics 52(3):280–282

Becker JU (2011) Disseminated intravascular coagulation in emergency medicine. eMedicine Medscape. http://emedicine.medscape.com/article/779097-overview. Accessed on 2010 and 2011

Bennett AM, Bennett SM, Prinsley PR, Wickstead M (2005) Spitting in the ear: a falsified disease using video evidence. J Laryngol Otol 119(11):926–927

Bienenfeld D (2010) Malingering. eMedicine Medscape. http://emedicine.medscape.com/article/293206-overview#a0199 Accessed on 2010 and 2011

Bilo RAC, Robben SGF, van Rijn RR (2010) Section 7.3. Osteogenesis imperfecta. In: Bilo RAC, Robben SGF, van Rijn RR (eds) Forensic aspects of pediatric fractures. Springer, Berlin, Heidelberg, pp 133–140

Bolton-Maggs PHB, Chalmers EA, Collins PW et al (2006) A review of inherited platelet disorders with guidelines for their management on behalf of the UKHCDO. Br J Haematol 135(5):603–633

Boxley JD, Wilkinson DS (1971) Autoerythrocyte sensitization (painful bruising) syndrome. Proc R Soc Med 64(12):1196–1197

Brandrup F (1990) Factitious purpura [Article in Danish. Ugeskr Laeger 152(30):2180–2181

Bray GL, Luban NL (1987) Hemophilia presenting with intracranial hemorrhage. An approach to the infant with intracranial bleeding and coagulopathy. Am J Dis Child 141(11):1215–1217

Brousseau TJ, Kissoon N, McIntosh B (2005) Vitamin K deficiency mimicking child abuse. J Emerg Med 29(3):283–288

Brown J, Melinkovich P (1986) Schönlein-Henoch purpura misdiagnosed as suspected child abuse. JAMA 256(5):617–618

Burk CJ, Molodow R (2007) Infantile scurvy: an old diagnosis revisited with a modern dietary twist. Am J Clin Dermatol 8(2):103–106

Butros LJ, Bussel JB (2003) Intracranial hemorrhage in immune thrombocytopenic purpura: a retrospective analysis. J Pediatr Hematol Oncol 25(8):660–664

Campbell AN, Freedman MH, McClure PD (1983) Autoerythrocyte sensitization. J Pediatr 103(1): 157–160

Canadian Hemophilia Society (2008) Bleeding disorders. http://www.hemophilia.ca/en/bleeding-disorders/

Carpentieri U, Gustavson LP, Haggard ME (1978) Misdiagnosis of neglect in a child with a bleeding disorder and cystic fibrosis. South Med J 71(7):854–855

Chang VY (2011) Thrombasthenia. eMedicine Medscape. http://emedicine.medscape.com/article/955385-overview. Accessed on 2010 and 2011

Chatterjee M, Jaiswal AK (2002) Painful bruising syndrome. Indian J Dermatol Venereol Leprol 68(6):347–348

Chavali KH, Dasari H (2011) Dithranol: an unusual agent to produce artificial (false) bruise: a case report. Am J Forensic Med Pathol. [Epub ahead of print]

Christian CW (2003) Differential diagnosis of inflicted childhood neurotrauma – response. In: Reece RM, Nicholson CE (eds) Inflicted childhood neurotrauma. American Academy of Pediatrics, Elk Grove Village, pp 43–47

Chua JD, Friedenberg WR (1998) Superwarfarin poisoning. Arch Intern Med 158(17):1929–1932

Clark GD, Key JD, Rutherford P, Bithoney WG (1984) Munchausen's syndrome by proxy (child abuse) presenting as apparent autoerythrocyte sensitization syndrome: an unusual presentation of Polle syndrome. Pediatrics 74(6):1100–1102

Clemetson CA (2002) Barlow's disease. Med Hypotheses 59(1):52–56

Clemetson CA (2004) Elevated blood histamine caused by vaccinations and vitamin C deficiency may mimic the shaken baby syndrome. Med Hypotheses 62(4):533–536

Collard MM, Hunter ML, Motley RJ, Lewis MA (2008) Dermatitis artefacta of the lip in an adolescent. Dent Update 35(5):339–340, 343

Cordell WH, Berry G (2004) Faux pox: 2 case reports. JAMA 292(13):1554

Culvert L, Norris T (2006) Coagulation disorders. In Krapp KM, Wilson J (eds) Gale Encyclopedia of Children's Health: volume 1 infancy through adolescence. Gale, Farmingon Hills 1st ed

Daly KC, Siegel RM (1998) Henoch-Schöenlein purpura in a child at risk of abuse. Arch Pediatr Adolesc Med 152(1):96–98

Datta S, Datta H, Kapoor S (2009) A case of psychogenic purpura in a female child. J Indian Med Assoc 107(2):104–106

Davis HW, Carrasco MM (2002) Child abuse and neglect. In: Zitelli BJ, Davis HW (eds) Atlas of pediatric physical diagnosis. Mosby, St Louis, pp 153–222

de Paepe A, Malfait F (2004) Bleeding and bruising in patients with Ehlers-Danlos syndrome and other collagen vascular disorders. Br J Haematol 127(5):491–500

de Tezanos Pinto M, Fernandez J, Perez Bianco PR (1992) Update of 156 episodes of central nervous system bleeding in hemophiliacs. Haemostasis 22(2):259–267

de Waard-van der Spek FB, Oranje AP (1997) Purpura caused by Emla is of toxic origin. Contact Dermatitis 36(1):11–13

Demirören K, Yavuz H, Cam L (2004) Intracranial hemorrhage due to vitamin K deficiency after the newborn period. Pediatr Hematol Oncol 21(7):585–592

Dingle AD (2005) Chapter 13 Disorders with physical symptoms. In: Sexson SB (ed) Child and adolescent psychiatry, 2nd ed. Blackwell Publishing Ltd, Oxford, p 177–189

Duncan CP, Westra SJ, Rosenberg AE (2007) Case records of the Massachusetts General Hospital. Case 23–2007: a 9-year-old boy with bone pain, rash, and gingival hypertrophy. N Engl J Med 357(4):392–400

Early LF, Lifschutz JE (1974) A case of stigmata. Arch Gen Psychiatry 30(2):197–200

Eyster ME, Gill FM, Blatt PM et al (1978) Central nervous system bleeding in hemophiliacs. Blood 51(6):1179–1188

Feldman KW (2009) The bruised premobile infant: should you evaluate further? Pediatr Emerg Care 25(1):37–39

Fenton LZ, Sirotnak AP, Handler MH (2000) Parietal pseudofracture and spontaneous intracranial hemorrhage suggesting nonaccidental trauma: report of 2 cases. Pediatr Neurosurg 33(6):318–322

Fey MF, Beck EA (1986) Psychogenic purpura, idiopathic thrombocytopenic purpura, and platelet dysfunction in the same patient. J Clin Psychiatry 47(7):386–387

Franze I, Forrest TS (1988) Sonographic diagnosis of a subdural hematoma as the initial manifestation of hemophilia in a newborn. J Ultrasound Med 7(3): 149–152

Fung EL, Nelson EA (2004) Could vitamin C deficiency have a role in shaken baby syndrome? Pediatr Int 46(6):753–755

Gahl WA (2010) Hermansky-Pudlak syndrome. Gene Reviews. http://www.ncbi.nlm.nih.gov/bookshelf/br.fcgi?book=gene&part=hps

Ganesh A, Jenny C, Geyer J et al (2004) Retinal hemorrhages in type I osteogenesis imperfecta after minor trauma. Ophthalmology 111(7):1428–1431

Gardner FH, Diamond LK (1955) Autoerythrocyte sensitization; a form of purpura producing painful bruising following autosensitization to red blood cells in certain women. Blood 10(7):675–690

Gedeit RG (2001) Medical management of the shaken infant. In: Lazoritz S, Palusci VJ (eds) The shaken baby syndrome – a multidisciplinary approach. The Haworth Maltreatment & Trauma Press, Binghamton, pp 155–171

Geisler BP, Dezube BJ (2011) Psychogenic purpura (Gardner-Diamond syndrome). UpToDate. http://www.uptodate.com. Accessed on 2010 and 2011

George JN, Caen JP, Nurden AT (1990) Glanzmann's thrombasthenia: the spectrum of clinical disease. Blood 75(7):1383–1395

George JN, Woolf SH, Raskob GE et al (1996) Idiopathic thrombocytopenic purpura: a practice guideline developed by explicit methods for the American Society of Hematology. Blood 88(1):3–40

Gil-Bistes D, Kluger N, Guillot B, Bessis D (2010) Dermatitis artefacta in a young girl [Article in French. Arch Pediatr 17(11):1543–1545

Griffiths H, Cuddihy PJ, Marnane C (2001) Bleeding ears: a case of Munchausen syndrome by proxy. Int J Pediatr Otorhinolaryngol 57(3):245–247

Groninger A, Schaper J, Messing-Juenger M et al (2005) Subdural hematoma as clinical presentation of osteogenesis imperfecta. Pediatr Neurol 32(2):140–142

Guiraldes E, Bènard D, Triviño X, Larraín F (1995) Factitious gastrointestinal hemorrhage in 3 school-age girls [Article in Spanish. Rev Med Chil 123(7):874–879

Hagemeier L, Schyma C, Zillhardt H et al (2011) Gardner-Diamond syndrome: a rare differential diagnosis of child abuse. Br J Dermatol 164(3):672–673

Hampton KK, Preston FE (2003) Chapter 10. Bleeding disorders, thrombosis, and anticoagulation. In: Provan D (ed) ABC of clinical haematology, 2nd edn. BMJ Books, London, pp 43–46

Harley JR (1997) Disorders of coagulation misdiagnosed as nonaccidental bruising. Pediatr Emerg Care 13(5):347–349

Harth W, Gieler U, Kusnir D, Tausk FA (2008) Chapter 1. Primarily psychogenic dermatoses. Section 1.1.4 special forms: Gardner-diamond syndrome. In: Harth W, Gieler U, Kusnir D, Tausk FA (eds) Clinical management in psychodermatology. Springer, Berlin, pp 28–29

Harth W, Taube KM, Gieler U (2010) Facticious disorders in dermatology [Article in English, German]. J Dtsch Dermatol Ges 8(5):361–372

Hazewinkel MH, Hoogerwerf JJ, Hesseling PB et al (2003) Haemophilia patients aged 0–18 years in the Western Cape. S Afr Med J 93(10):793–796

Hennes H, Kini N, Palusci VJ (2001) The epidemiology, clinical characteristics and public health implications of shaken baby syndrome. In: Lazoritz S, Palusci VJ (eds) The shaken baby syndrome – a multidisciplinary approach. The Haworth Maltreatment & Trauma Press, Binghamton, pp 19–40

Hodges RE (1980) Ascorbic acid. In: Goodhart RS, Shils ME (eds) Modern nutrition in health and disease, 6th edn. Lea & Febiger, Philadelphia, pp 259–273

Hymel K, Boos S (2009) Chapter 7. Conditions mistaken for child physical abuse. In: Reece RM, Christian CW (eds) Child abuse: medical diagnosis & management, 3rd edn. American Academy of Pediatrics, Philadelphia, pp 227–255

Hymel KP, Abshire TC, Luckey DW, Jenny C (1997) Coagulopathy in pediatric abusive head trauma. Pediatrics 99(3):371–375

Ingber A, Alcalay J, Feuerman EJ (1985) Autoerythrocyte sensitization (Gardner-Diamond syndrome) in men: a case report and review of the literature. Postgrad Med J 61(719):823–826

International Registry of Rare Bleeding Disorders (2009) http://www.rbdd.org/. Accessed on 2010 and 2011

Izquierdo NJ, Townsend W, Hussels IE (1995) Ocular findings in the Hermansky-Pudlak syndrome. Trans Am Ophthalmol Soc 93:191–200; discussion 200–2

James WD, Berger TG, Elston D et al (2006) Chapter 35. Cutaneous vascular diseases. In: James WD, Berger TG, Elston D (eds) Andrews' Diseases of the skin: clinical dermatology, 10th edn. Saunders, New York

Jenny C, Reece RM (2009) Chapter 1. Cutaneous manifestations of child abuse. In: Reece RM, Christian CW (eds) Child abuse: medical diagnosis & management, 3rd edn. American Academy of Pediatrics, Philadelphia, pp 19–51

Jurk K, Kehrel BE (2007) Inherited and acquired disorders of platelet function. Transfus Med Hemother 34:6–19

Khair K, Liesner R (2006) Bruising and bleeding in infants and children – a practical approach. Br J Haematol 133(3):221–231

Kirschner RH, Stein RJ (1985) The mistaken diagnosis of child abuse. A form of medical abuse? Am J Dis Child 139(9):873–875

Knight DJ, Bennet GC (1990) Nonaccidental injury in osteogenesis imperfecta: a case report. J Pediatr Orthop 10(4):542–544

Kolluri VR, Reddy DR, Reddy PK et al (1986) Subdural hematoma secondary to immune thrombocytopenic purpura: case report. Neurosurgery 19(4):635–636

Kozyreva O (2009) Alpha2-plasmin inhibitor deficiency. eMedicine Medscape. http://emedicine.medscape.com/article/198336-overview. Accessed on 2010 and 2011

Kugler M (2005) Hermansky-Pudlak syndrome. http://rarediseases.about.com/od/rarediseasesh/a/090404.htm. Accessed on 2010 and 2011

Kuhne T, Elinder G, Blanchette VS, Garvey B (1998) Current management issues of childhood and adult immune thrombocytopenic purpura (ITP). Acta Paediatr Suppl 424:75–81

Kumar V, Choudhury P (2009) Scurvy-a forgotten disease with an unusual presentation. Trop Doct 39(3):190–192

Kumar R, Aggarwal A, Faridi MM (2009) Complex regional pain syndrome type 1 and scurvy. Indian Pediatr 46(6):529–531

Kurlandsky L, Lukoff JY, Zinkham WH et al (1979) Munchausen syndrome by proxy: definition of factitious bleeding in an infant by 51Cr labeling of erythrocytes. Pediatrics 63(2):228–231

Labbe J, Caouette G (2001) Recent skin injuries in normal children. Pediatrics 108(2):271–276

Landers MC, Schroeder TL (2004) Bathtub suction-induced purpura. Pediatr Dermatol 21(2):146–149

Lane PA, Hathaway WE, Githens JH et al (1983) Fatal intracranial hemorrhage in a normal infant secondary to vitamin K deficiency. Pediatrics 72(4):562–564

Lee ACW (2008) Bruises, blood coagulation tests and the battered child syndrome. Singapore Med J 49(6):445–450

Leung AKC, Chan KW (2001) Evaluating the child with purpura. Am Fam Physician 64(3):419–428

Levi M, Ten Cate H (1999) Disseminated intravascular coagulation. N Engl J Med 341(8):586–592

Libow JA (2000) Child and adolescent illness falsification. Pediatrics 105(2):336–342

Liesner RJ, Machin SJ (2003) Chapter 7. Platelet disorders. In: Provan D (ed) ABC of clinical haematology, 2nd edn. BMJ Books, London, pp 28–32

Lilleyman JS (1994) Intracranial haemorrhage in idiopathic thrombocytopenic purpura. Paediatric Haematology Forum of the British Society for Haematology. Arch Dis Child 71(3):251–253

Lindahl MW (1977) Psychogenic purpura: report of a case. Psychosom Med 39(5):358–368

Lovejoy FH, Marcuse EK, Landrigan PJ (1971) Two examples of purpura factitia. Clin Pediatr (Phila) 10(3):183–184

Maguire S, Mann MK, Sibert J et al (2005) Are there patterns of bruising in childhood which are diagnostic or suggestive of abuse? a systematic review. Arch Dis Child 90(2):182–186

Mason JD (2010) Munchausen syndrome by proxy in emergency medicine. eMedicine Medscape. http://emedicine.medscape.com/article/806735-overview. Accessed on 2010 and 2011

Matsuda T (1996) Clinical aspects of DIC – disseminated intravascular coagulation. Pol J Pharmacol 48(1):73–75

McClain JL, Clark MA, Sandusky GE (1990) Undiagnosed, untreated acute lymphoblastic leukemia presenting as suspected child abuse. J Forensic Sci 35(3):735–739

Medeiros D (2003) Chapter XI.6. Bleeding disorders. Case based pediatrics for medical students and residents. Department of Pediatrics, University of Hawaii John A. Burns School of Medicine. http://www.hawaii.edu/medicine/pediatrics/pedtext/s11c06.html

Medeiros D, Buchanan GR (1998) Major hemorrhage in children with idiopathic thrombocytopenic purpura: immediate response to therapy and long-term outcome. J Pediatr 133(3):334–339

Medeiros D, Buchanan GR (2000) Idiopathic thrombocytopenic purpura: beyond consensus. Curr Opin Pediatr 12(1):4–9

Meeder R, Bannister S (2006) Gardner-Diamond syndrome: difficulties in the management of patients with unexplained medical symptoms. Paediatr Child Health 11(7):416–419

Mehta P, Bussing R (1993) Factitious coagulopathy due to Munchausen syndrome by proxy. Am J Pediatr Hematol Oncol 15(1):124–125

Menter A (1987) Symmetrical purpura doesn't mirror child abuse. JAMA 257(4):486

Merck Manual Online Medical Library (2007) Vitamin K. http://www.merck.com/mmpe/sec01/ch004/ch004m.html. Accessed on 2010 and 2011

Mills RW, Burke S (1990) Gastrointestinal bleeding in a 15 month old male. A presentation of Munchausen's syndrome by proxy. Clin Pediatr (Phila) 29(8):474–477

Mimasaka S, Funayama M, Adachi N et al (2000) A fatal case of infantile scurvy. Int J Legal Med 114(1–2):122–124

Minford AMB, Richards EM (2010) Excluding medical and haematological conditions as a cause of bruising in suspected non-accidental injury. Arch Dis Child Educ Pract Ed 95(1):2–8

Mishra P, Naithani R, Dolai T et al (2008) Intracranial haemorrhage in patients with congenital haemostatic defects. Haemophilia 14(5):952–955

Montgomery RR, Scott JP (2003) Part 20: diseases of the blood; section 7: hemorrhagic and thrombotic diseases. In: Behrman RE, Kliegman RM, Jenson HB (eds) Nelson textbook of pediatrics, 17th edn. Saunders, Philadelphia, pp 1650–1674

Myles LM, Massicotte P, Drake J (2001) Intracranial hemorrhage in neonates with unrecognized hemophilia A: a persisting problem. Pediatr Neurosurg 34(2):94–97

Nadjem H, Sutor AH (1991) Hematoma in acute leukemia – suspected diagnosis of child abuse [Article in German. Beitr Gerichtl Med 49:227–231

National Hemophilia Foundation (2006) Learning about coagulation disorders. http://www.hemophilia.org/NHFWeb/MainPgs/MainNHF.aspx?menuid=2&contentid=577&rptname=bleeding

Nelson MD, Maeder MA, Usner D et al (1999) Prevalence and incidence of intracranial haemorrhage in a population of children with haemophilia. The Hemophilia Growth and Development Study. Haemophilia 5(5):306–312

Newland AC, Evans TGJR (2003) Haematological disorders at the extremes of life. In: Provan D (ed) ABC of clinical haematology, 2nd edn. BMJ Books, London, pp 57–60

Newman RS, Jalili M, Kolls BJ et al (2002) Factor XIII deficiency mistaken for battered child syndrome: case of "correct" test ordering negated by a commonly accepted qualitative test with limited negative predictive value. Am J Hematol 71(4):328–330

Nimavat DJ (2009) Hemorrhagic disease of newborn. eMedicine Medscape. http://emedicine.medscape.com/article/974489-overview. Accessed on 2010 and 2011

Nosek-Cenkowska B, Cheang MS, Pizzi NJ et al (1991) Bleeding/bruising symptomatology in children with and without bleeding disorders. Thromb Haemost 65(3):237–241

O'Hare AE, Eden OB (1984) Bleeding disorders and non-accidental injury. Arch Dis Child 59(9):860–864

Olivieri M, Kurnik K, Bidlingmaier C (2009) Coagulation testing in the evaluation of suspected child abuse. Hamostaseologie 29(2):190–192

Owen SM, Durst RD (1984) Ehlers-Danlos syndrome simulating child abuse. Arch Dermatol 120(1):97–101

Patel P (2008) Vitamin K deficiency. eMedicine Medscape. http://emedicine.medscape.com/article/126354-overview. Accessed on 2010 and 2011

Pinto FC, Porro FF, Suganuma L et al (2003) Hemophilia and child abuse as possible causes of epidural hematoma: case report. Arq Neuropsiquiatr 61(4):1023–1025

Popovich D, McAlhany A, Adewumi AO, Barnes MM (2009) Scurvy: forgotten but definitely not gone. J Pediatr Health Care 23(6):405–415

Pridmore S (2009) Chapter 23. Factitious disorder and malingering. Download of Psychiatry. http://eprints.utas.edu.au/287/28/Chapter_23._Factitious_disorder_and_malingering.pdf. Accessed on 2010 and 2011

Puckett RM, Offringa M. Prophylactic vitamin K for vitamin K deficiency bleeding in neonates. Cochrane database of systematic reviews 2000, Issue 4. Art. No.: CD002776. DOI: 10.1002/14651858.CD002776 published on line 2009

Ratanachu-Ek S, Sukswai P, Jeerathanyasakun Y, Wongtapradit L (2003) Scurvy in pediatric patients: a review of 28 cases. J Med Assoc Thai 86(Suppl 3): S734–S740

Ratnoff OD (1989) Psychogenic purpura (autoerythrocyte sensitization): an unsolved dilemma. Am J Med 87(3N):16N–21N

Ries M, Klinge J, Rauch R et al (1998) Spontaneous subdural hematoma in a 18-day-old male newborn infant with severe hemophilia A. Klin Padiatr 210(3):120–124

Roberts DL, Pope FM, Nicholls AC, Narcisi P (1984) Ehlers-Danlos syndrome type IV mimicking non-accidental injury in a child. Br J Dermatol 111(3):341–345

Rogers M, Fairley M, Santhanam R (2001) Artefactual skin disease in children and adolescents. Australas J Dermatol 42(4):264–270

Rooms L, Fitzgerald N, McClain KL (2003) Hemophagocytic lymphohistiocytosis masquerading as child abuse: presentation of three cases and review of central nervous system findings in hemophagocytic lymphohistiocytosis. Pediatrics 111(5 Pt 1):e636–e640

Rosenberg DA (1987) Web of deceit: a literature review of Munchausen syndrome by proxy. Child Abuse Negl 11(4):547–563

Royal College of Paediatrics and Child Health (2006) Child Protection Companion. Royal College of Paediatrics and Child Health, London, pp 20–21

Russell-Eggitt IM, Thompson DA, Khair K et al (2000) Hermansky-Pudlak syndrome presenting with subdural haematoma and retinal haemorrhages in infancy. J R Soc Med 93(11):591–592

Rutty GN, Smith CM, Malia RG (1999) Late-form hemorrhagic disease of the newborn: a fatal case report with illustration of investigations that may assist in avoiding the mistaken diagnosis of child abuse. Am J Forensic Med Pathol 20(1):48–51

Sahin F, Kuruoğlu A, Işik AF et al (2002) Munchausen syndrome by proxy: a case report. Turk J Pediatr 44(4):334–338

Sawhney M, Arora G, Arora S, Prakash J (2006) Undiagnosed purpura: a case of autoerythrocyte sensitization syndrome associated with dermatitis artefacta and pseudo-ainhum. Indian J Dermatol Venereol Leprol 72(5):379–381

Schmitt BD (1987) The child with nonaccidental trauma. In: Helfer RE, Kempe RS (eds) The battered child, 4th edn. The University of Chicago Press, Chicago, pp 178–196

Schulman S (2006) Drugs that can cause bleeding. World Federation of Hemophilia. http://www.wfh.org/index.asp?lang=EN. Accessed on 2010 and 2011

Schwer W, Brueschke EE, Dent T (1982) Family practice grand rounds: hemophilia. J Fam Pract 14:661–674

Seçkin H, Kazanci A, Yigitkanli K et al (2006) Chronic subdural hematoma in patients with idiopathic thrombocytopenic purpura: a case report and review of the literature. Surg Neurol 66(4):411–414; discussion 414

Sham RL, Francis CW (1994) Evaluation of mild bleeding disorders and easy bruising. Blood Rev 8(2):98–104

Sharathkumar AA, Shapiro A (2008) Platelet function disorders, 2nd edn. World Federation of Hemophilia, Montreal

Shearer MJ (2009) Vitamin K deficiency bleeding (VKDB) in early infancy. Blood Rev 23(2):49–59

Shih SL, Lin JC, Liang DC et al (1993) Computed tomography of spontaneous intracranial haemorrhage due to haemostatic disorders in children. Neuroradiology 35(8):619–621

Sibert J (2004) Bruising, coagulation disorder, and physical child abuse. Blood Coagul Fibrinolysis 15(Suppl 1):S33–S39

Silverman MA (2011) Idiopathic thrombocytopenic purpura. eMedicine Medscape. http://emedicine.medscape.com/article/779545-overview. Accessed on 2010 and 2011

Sirotnak AP (2006) Medical disorders that mimic abusive head trauma. In: Frasier L, Rauth-Farley K, Alexander R et al (eds) Abusive head trauma in infants and children – a medical, legal, and forensic reference. GW Medical, St. Louis, p 191–226

Smith OP, White B (1999) Infectious purpura fulminans: diagnosis and treatment. Br J Haematol 104(2):202–207

Sorensen RU, Newman AJ, Gordon EM (1985) Psychogenic purpura in adolescent patients. Clin Pediatr (Phila) 24(12):700–704

Souid A, Sadowitz PD (1995) Acute childhood immune thrombocytopenic purpura. Diagnosis and treatment. Clin Pediatr 34(9):487–494

Souid AK, Korins K, Keith D et al (1993) Unexplained menorrhagia and hematuria: a case report of Munchausen's syndrome by proxy. Pediatr Hematol Oncol 10(3):245–248

Stanziale SF, Christopher JC, Fisher RB (1997) Brodifacoum rodenticide ingestion in a patient with shigellosis. South Med J 90(8):833–835

Stray-Pedersen A, Omland S, Nedregaard B et al (2011) An infant with subdural hematoma and retinal hemorrhages: does Von Willebrand disease explain the findings? Forensic Sci Med Pathol 7(1):37–41

Strijks E, Poort SR, Renier WO et al (1999) Hereditary prothrombin deficiency presenting as intracranial haematoma in infancy. Neuropediatrics 30(6):320–324

Swedish Information Centre for Rare Diseases (2011) Osteogenesis imperfecta. The Sahlgrenska Academy at the University of Gothenburg. http://www.socialstyrelsen.se/rarediseases/osteogenesisimperfecta. Accessed on 2010 and 2011

Swerdlin A, Berkowitz C, Craft N (2007) Cutaneous signs of child abuse. J Am Acad Dermatol 57(3):371–392

Tamura Y, Welch DC, Zic JA et al (2000) Scurvy presenting as painful gait with bruising in a young boy. Arch Pediatr Adolesc Med 154(7):732–735

Taylor GP (1982) Severe bleeding disorders in children with normal coagulation screening tests. Br Med J (Clin Res Ed) 284(6332):1851–1852

Thomas AE (2004) The bleeding child: is it NAI? Arch Dis Child 89(12):1163–1167

Thomas A (2009) Chapter 4. Haematological abnormalities that can simulate abuse. In: Busuttil A, Keeling JW (eds) Paediatric forensic medicine & pathology. Hodder Arnold, London, pp 76–105

Tüfekçi Ö, Gözmen S, Yılmaz Ş et al (2011) A case with unexplained bleeding from multiple sites: Munchausen syndrome by proxy. Pediatr Hematol Oncol 28(5):439–443

Tunnessen WW, Chessar IJ (1984) Factitious cutaneous bleeding: a case of pseudostigmata. Am J Dis Child 138(4):354–355

Ulinski T, Lhopital C, Cloppet H et al (2004) Munchausen syndrome by proxy with massive proteinuria and gastrointestinal hemorrhage. Pediatr Nephrol 19(7):798–800

Vaillant L, Le Marchand D, Alison Y, Lorette G (1986) Gardner-Diamond syndrome in a 14-year-old girl. Discussion on the diagnostic value of skin tests [Article in French]. Ann Pediatr (Paris) 33(5):429–431

van Oostrom CG, Werkman HP, Fiselier TJ (1984) Bruising: a coagulation disorder, abuse or abnormality of the vessel wall? [Article in Dutch]. Tijdschr Kindergeneeskd 52(4):152–155

Venkateswaran L, Wilimas JA, Jones DJ et al (1998) Mild hemophilia in children: prevalence, complications, and treatment. J Pediatr Hematol Oncol 20(1):32–35

Vitale A, La Torre F, Martini G et al (2009) Arthritis and gum bleeding in two children. J Paediatr Child Health 45(3):158–160

Vora A, Makris M (2001) Personal practice: an approach to investigation of easy bruising. Arch Dis Child 84(6):488–491

Vorstman EB, Anslow P, Keeling DM et al (2003) Brain haemorrhage in five infants with coagulopathy. Arch Dis Child 88(12):1119–1121

Vun YY, Muir J (2004) Periodic painful purpura: fact or factitious? Australas J Dermatol 45(1):58–63

Walker JS (2011) Malingering in children: fibs and faking. Child Adolesc Psychiatr Clin N Am 20(3):547–556

Walker M, Payne J, Wagner B, Vora A (2007) Hermansky-Pudlak syndrome. Br J Haematol 138(6):671

Wardinsky TD, Vizcarrondo FE, Cruz BK (1995) The mistaken diagnosis of child abuse: a three-year USAF Medical Center analysis and literature review. Mil Med 160(1):15–20

Weinstein M, Babyn P, Zlotkin S (2001) An orange a day keeps the doctor away: scurvy in the year 2000. Pediatrics 108(3):E55

Wenk RE (2003) Molecular evidence of Munchausen syndrome by proxy. Arch Pathol Lab Med 127(1):e36–e37

Werner EJ, Broxson EH, Broxson EH, Tucker EL et al (1993) Prevalence of Von Willebrand disease in children: a multiethnic study. J Pediatr 123(6):893–898

Wetzel RC, Slater AJ, Dover GJ (1995) Fatal intramuscular bleeding misdiagnosed as suspected nonaccidental injury. Pediatrics 95(5):771–773

Wetzstein V, Budde U, Oyen F et al (2006) Intracranial hemorrhage in a term newborn with severe Von Willebrand disease type 3 associated with sinus venous thrombosis. Haematologica 91(12 Suppl):ECR60

Wheeler DM, Hobbs CJ (1988) Mistakes in diagnosing non-accidental injury: 10 years' experience. Br Med J (Clin Res Ed) 296(6631):1233–1236

White JG, Pearson HA, Coddington RD (1966) Purpura factitia Attracting attention by self-inflicted lesions. Clin Pediatr (Phila) 5(3):157–160

White ST, Voter K, Perry J (1985) Surreptitious warfarin ingestion. Child Abuse Negl 9(3):349–352

Willmott NS, Bryan RA (2008) Case report: scurvy in an epileptic child on a ketogenic diet with oral complications. Eur Arch Paediatr Dent 9(3):148–152

Wood J, Rubin DM, Nance ML, Christian CW (2005) Distinguishing inflicted versus accidental abdominal injuries in young children. J Trauma 59(5):1203–1208

Wynne J (2003) Chapter 30. The physical and emotional abuse of children. In: Payne-James J, Busuttil A, Smock W (eds) Forensic medicine, clinical and pathological aspects, 1st edn. Greenwich Medical Media Ltd, London, pp 469–485

Yamada K, Sakurai Y, Shibata M et al (2009) Factitious purpura in a 10-year-old girl. Pediatr Dermatol 26(5):597–600

Yates VM (1992) Factitious purpura. Clin Exp Dermatol 17(4):238–239

Yoshida M, Hayashi T, Kuramoto S et al (1979) Traumatic intracranial hematomas in hemophiliac children. Surg Neurol 12(2):115–118

Dermatological Disorders and Artifacts

6

6.1 Introduction

In the medical literature, many case histories and review articles have been written about the misinterpretation of skin findings as child abuse; these may concern normal variants, typical dermatological disorders, or artifacts (traditional medicine, pediatric condition falsification, or postmortem changes) (Nong The Anh 1976; Yeatman et al. 1976; Waskerwitz et al. 1981; Oates 1984; Kirschner and Stein 1985; Wheeler and Hobbs 1988; Oranje and Bilo 2011).

The study by Wheeler and Hobbs (1988) showed that over diagnosing child abuse may happen with a variety of different skin findings. They evaluated the data of 2,578 children who were reported because of suspected child abuse. In 50 cases, the initial suspicion was incorrect: "bruising" was present in 23 of these cases (Table 6.1).

In the differential diagnosis of bruising in child abuse, many of these findings are not rare, as is shown in the medical literature. Moreover, the manifestation of the findings is not always atypical but suspicion may have been aroused because of background risk factors in the family. Sometimes the diagnosis is considerably more difficult where the finding follows an atypical clinical course or has an atypical location. Disorders, which are extremely rare, are often described only once in the medical literature as a single case report, for example, hepatoerythropoietic porphyria by Cantatore-Francis et al. (2010).

If in doubt, the practitioner is advised to photograph the findings systematically or to let the skin findings be documented by a professional photographer (Chap. 9). In addition, it is extremely important to review the physical findings periodically after a suitable length of time. Consultation with a specialized pediatrician, dermatologist, or pediatric dermatologist is advised. If the suspicion of child abuse continues, the child should be seen by a specialized pediatrician who can call on the services of a pediatric dermatologist. Confusion may be avoided by a detailed registration of the physical examination and repeated examination (Hobbs et al. 1999).

Table 6.1 Skin findings misinterpreted as abusive bruising

Bleeding disorders	Idiopathic thrombocytopenic purpura
	Hemophilia
	Hemorrhagic disease of newborn (vitamin K-deficient bleeding disorder)
Dermatological abnormalities	Blue spots – Mongolian spots
	Hemangioma of infancy
	Atopic dermatitis
	Erythema nodosum
	Allergic periorbital swelling
	Prominent facial veins
Artifacts	Ink, paint, or dye on face
	Vietnamese folk medicine (cao gio)
	Dental treatment (bruised face)

Wheeler and Hobbs (1988)

R.A.C. Bilo et al., *Cutaneous Manifestations of Child Abuse and Their Differential Diagnosis*,
DOI 10.1007/978-3-642-29287-3_6, © Springer-Verlag Berlin Heidelberg 2013

6.2 Pigment Abnormalities

6.2.1 Mongolian Spots

In young children, Mongolian spots occur frequently and should not be confused with child abuse-related bruising. It involves a uniform bluish hyperpigmentation (blue-green, greenish-blue, blue-gray, blue-black, or sometimes brown) with a diffuse border. The spot is already present at birth, but sometimes becomes visible only after several days once the edema after delivery has disappeared. The spots are more frequently seen in individuals of Asian background and darker skin color than in those with a lighter skin color (Table 6.2). The spots are usually located on the back, particularly in the lower lumbar region, sacral region, and on the buttocks. Sometimes, extensive lesions are seen on the shoulders and the extremities (almost always on the extensor surfaces) or smaller lesions in the face (Cordova 1981) (Figs. 6.1, 6.2, 6.3, 6.4, 6.5, 6.6, 6.7, 6.8, 6.9, and 6.10). Mongolian spots will usually fade within the first 2 or 3 years of life, but may persist into the school-age years and beyond (Kos and Shwayder 2006).

Due to the very typical location and the characteristics of Mongolian spots, they are rarely mistaken for bruises. Moreover, there is never any swelling that may accompany bruises. However, they may cause confusion when the location is atypical (Oates 1984; Asnes 1984; Leung and Kao 1999; AlJasser and Al-Khenaizan 2008; Leung and Robson 2008).

Table 6.2 Incidence of Mongolian spots

Population group	Incidence (%)
Negroid children	95–96
Asian and red-skinned children	65–81
Children of Southern European and South American descent	46–70
Caucasian children	3–10

Jacobs and Walton (1976), Cordova (1981), Osburn et al. (1987)

6.2.2 Café Au Lait Spots

Café au lait spots (maculae) (Figs. 6.11, 6.12, and 6.13) are light-brown patches, which occur in about 3% of all newborns. This percentage increases to about 25% in all children up to the age of 5 years. These macules may be confused with healing bruises. Sekula et al. (1986) describes a child with an epidermal nevus and multiple café au lait spots who was erroneously thought to be a victim of abuse.

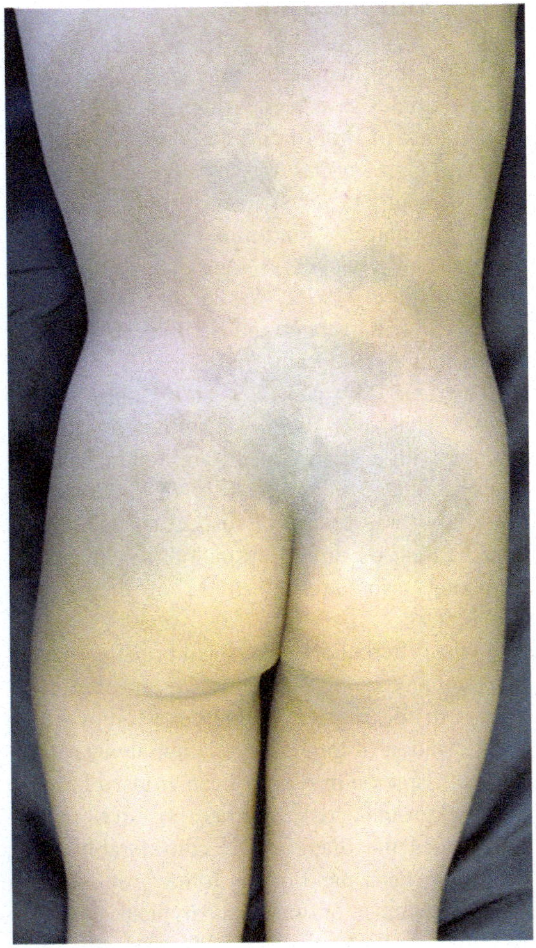

Fig. 6.1 Mongolian spots

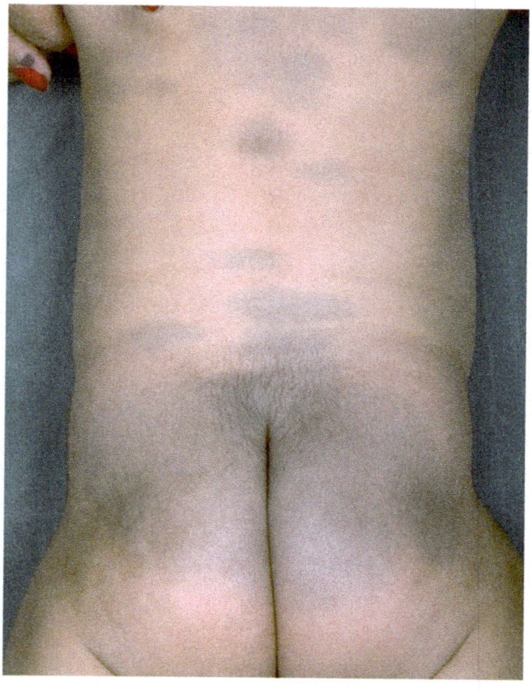

Fig. 6.2 Mongolian spots

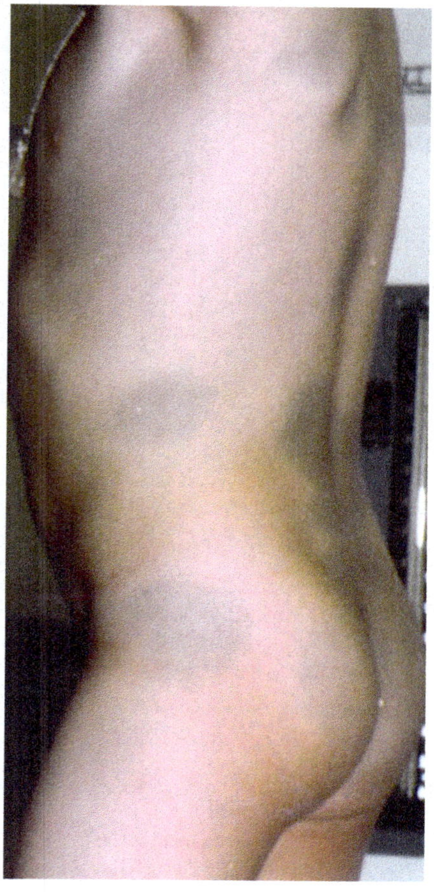

Fig. 6.4 Same child as in Fig. 6.3

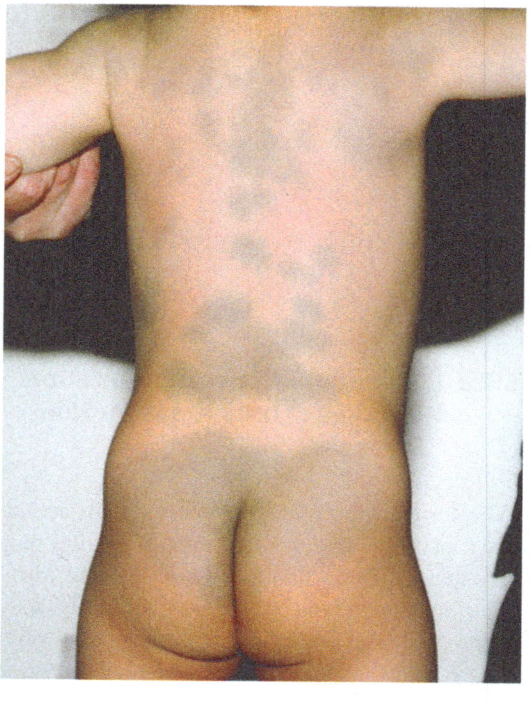

Fig. 6.3 Mongolian spots

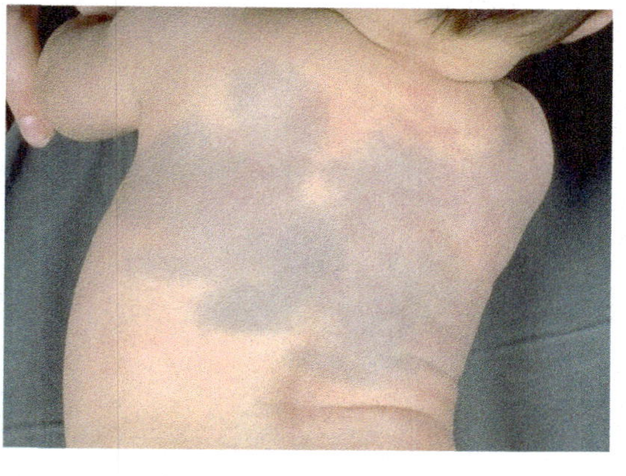

Fig. 6.5 Mongolian spots

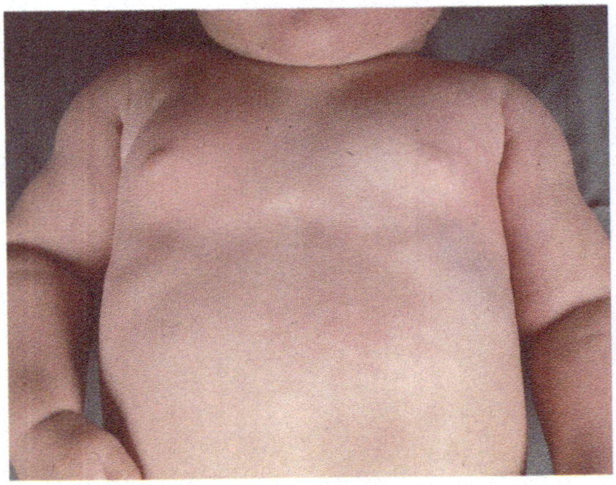

Fig. 6.6 Mongolian spots

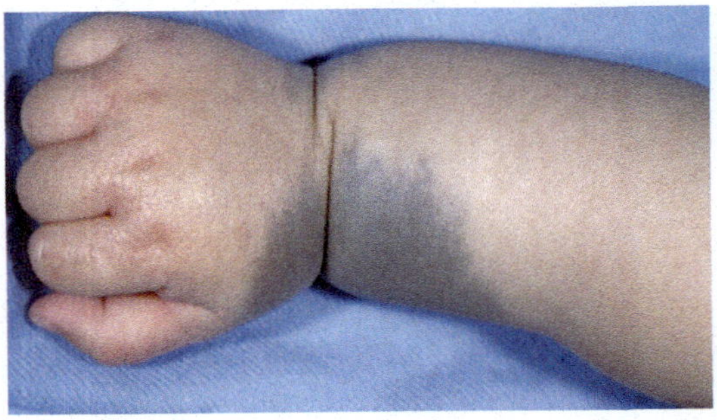

Fig. 6.7 Mongolian spots on less typical locations

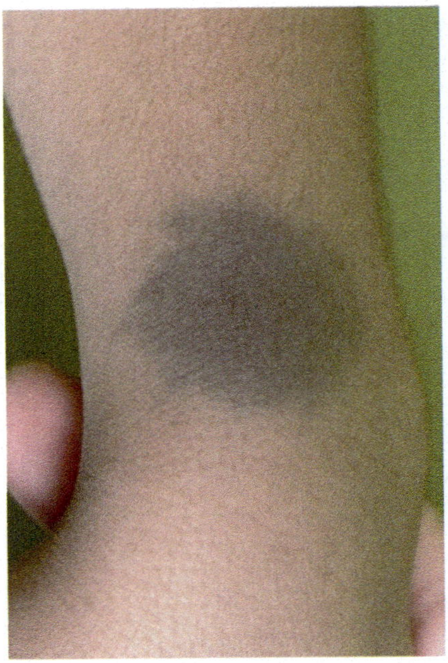

Fig. 6.8 Mongolian spots on less typical locations (= Fig. 3.5)

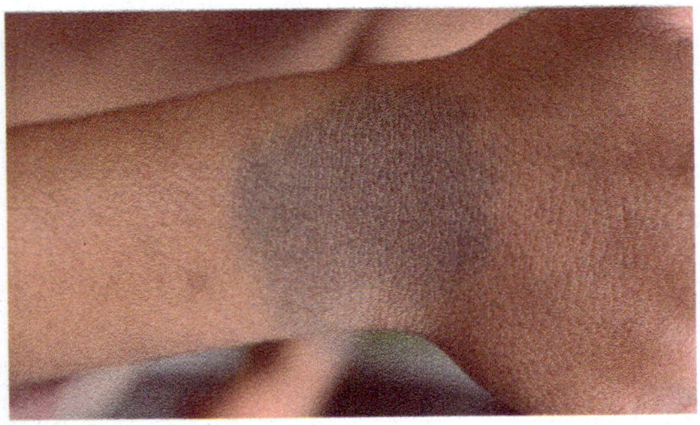

Fig. 6.9 Mongolian spots on less typical locations

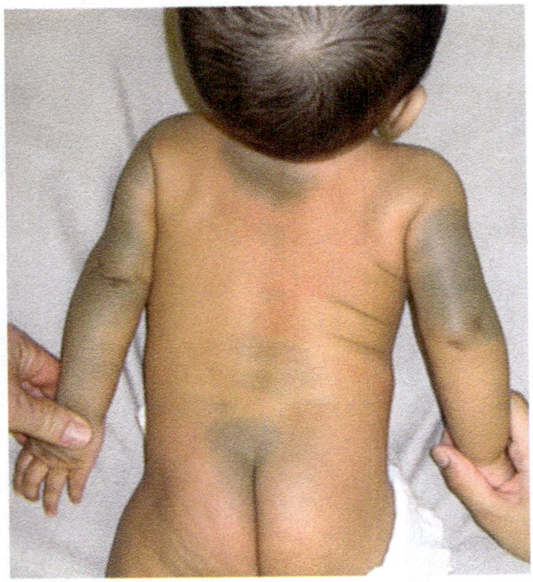

Fig. 6.10 Mongolian spots on typical and less typical locations

6.2.3 Secondary Hyperpigmentation Because of Inflammatory Skin Diseases

Wheeler and Hobbs (1988) reported that secondary (post inflammatory) hyperpigmentation may lead to confusion with assault injuries. The "dirty neck" phenomenon in atopic dermatitis may eventually lead to suspected child neglect by physicians, especially those who have no experience with this phenomenon. The same phenomenon is found in other anatomical locations, like the armpits and the feet (Figs. 6.14, 6.15, and 6.16).

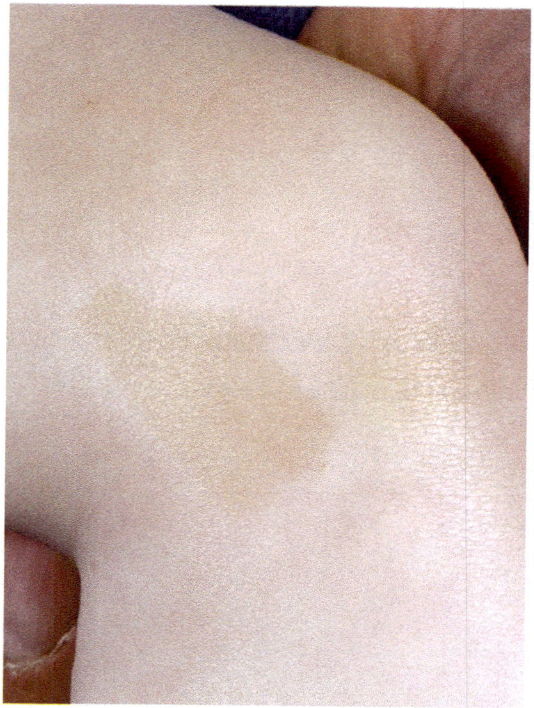

Fig. 6.11 Café au lait spot

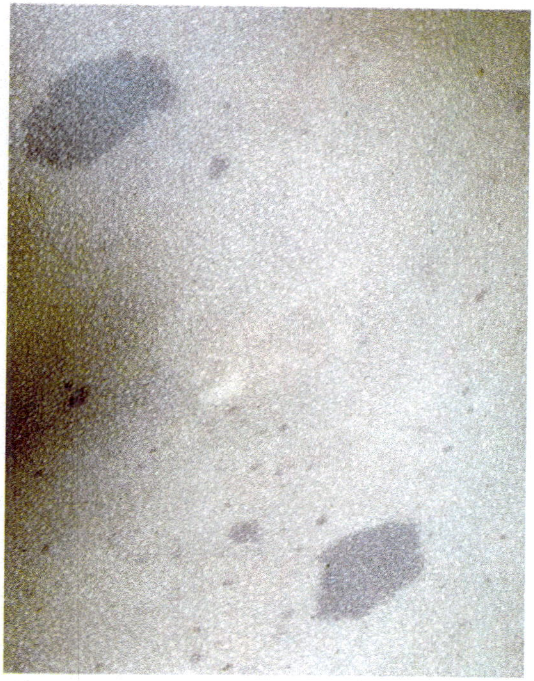

Fig. 6.13 Café au lait spots with freckling in a child with neurofibromatosis I

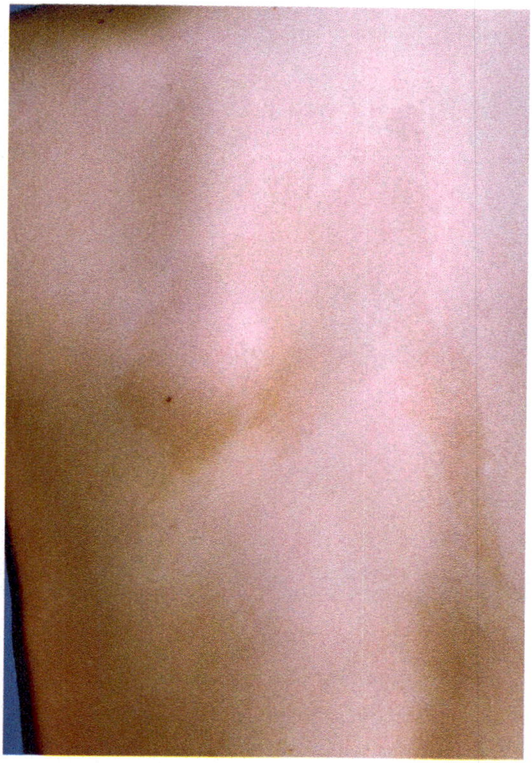

Fig. 6.12 Café au lait spot

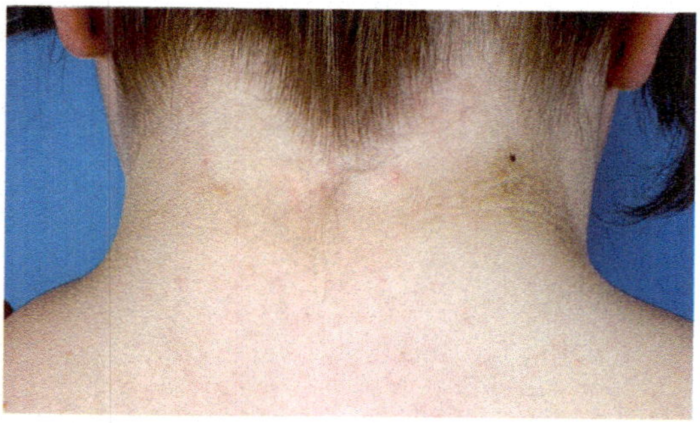

Fig. 6.14 "Dirty neck" in atopic dermatitis

6.2.4 Congenital Nevi

Mayes and MacLeod reported three male infants aged 3 months with a 1-week history of bruising to both parietal areas of the scalp (Mayes and Macleod 1999). The mother of the infant was initially reassured by the physician. Based on the abnormalities, child abuse was suspected. The infant was reexamined, and a consulting dermatologist confirmed the diagnosis of congenital melanocytic nevi (Fig. 6.17).

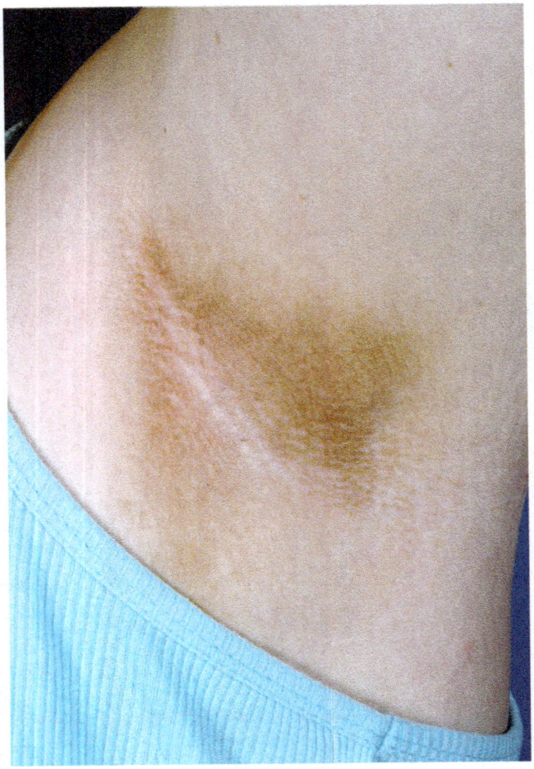

Fig. 6.15 "Dirty lesions" in armpit in atopic dermatitis

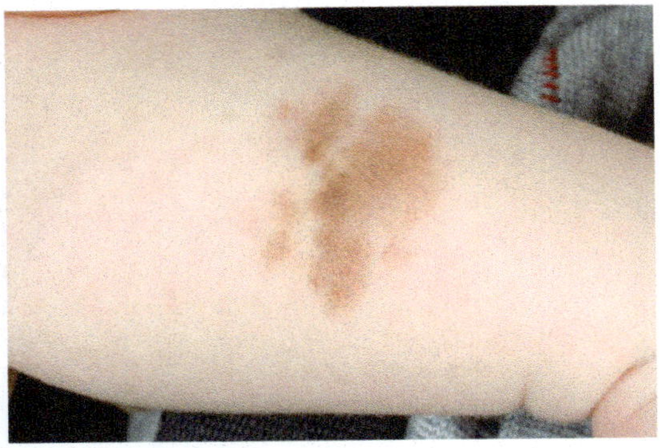

Fig. 6.17 Atypical congenital melanocytic nevus

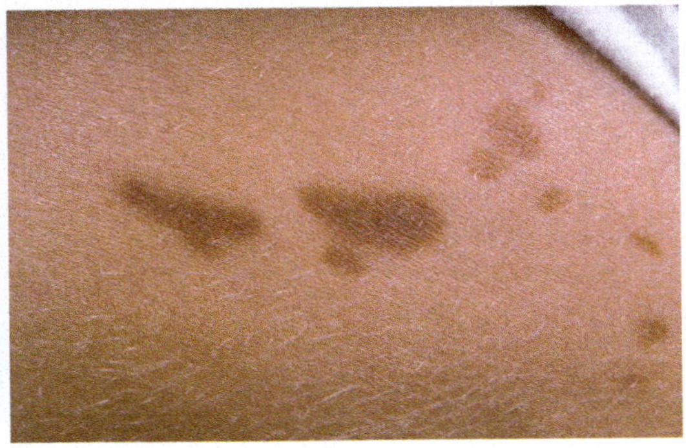

Fig. 6.18 Pigmented lesions in pseudoporphyria

Fig. 6.16 "Dirty lesions" on feet in atopic dermatitis

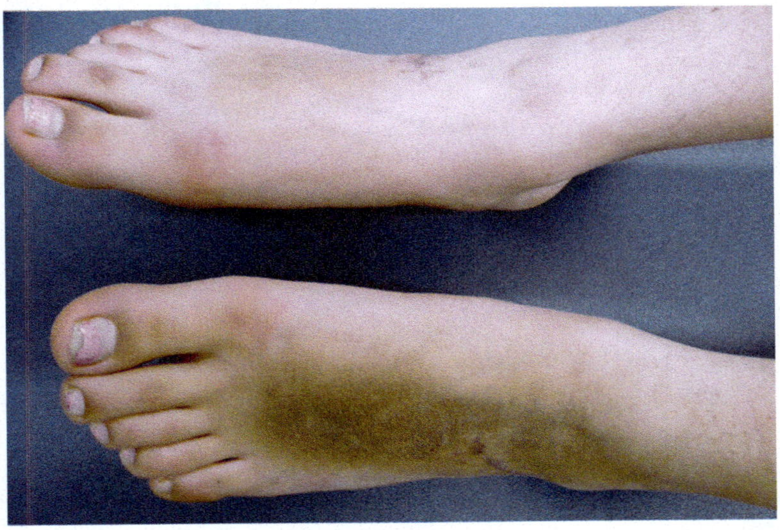

6.2.5 Other Pigmented Skin Findings

In the medical literature, some case descriptions are found of children with other pigmented skin findings which are erroneously thought to have been caused by child abuse, for example, in children with pseudoporphyria (Fig. 6.18), urticaria pigmentosa (mastocytosis) (Gordon et al. 1998)

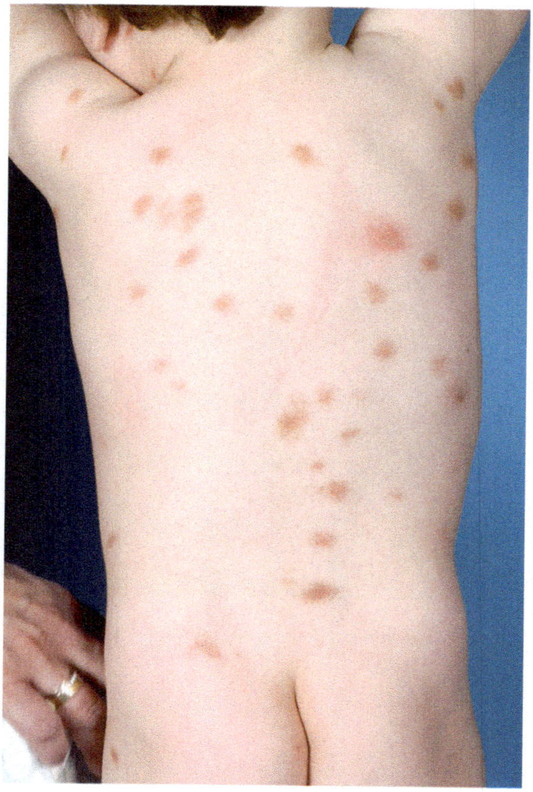

Fig. 6.19 Cutaneous maculopapular mastocytosis

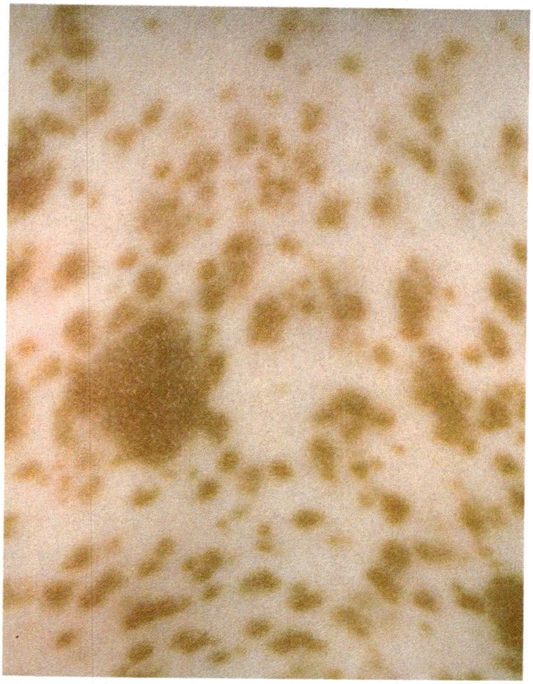

Fig. 6.20 Cutaneous maculopapular mastocytosis

Fig. 6.21 Incontinentia pigmenti

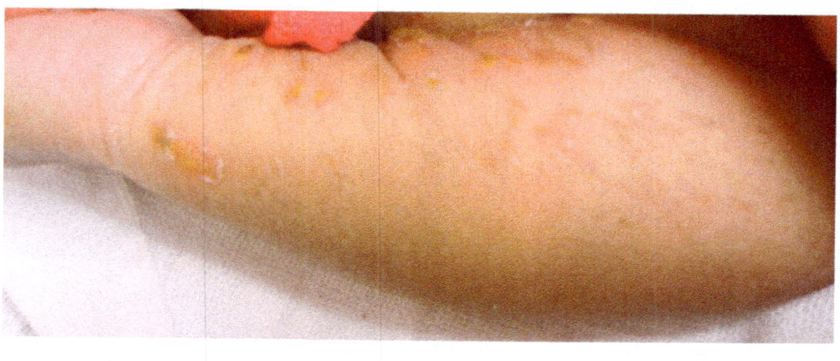

(Figs. 6.19 and 6.20), and incontinentia pigmenti (Ciarallo and Paller 1997) (Figs. 6.21 and 6.22).

Another skin finding with hyperpigmentation which may lead to confusion is erythema ab igne ("redness from fire"): a reticulated, erythematous, or hyperpigmented dermatosis that results from chronic and repeated exposure to low levels of infrared radiation (Miller et al. 2011). Multiple heat sources have been reported to cause this condition, which include heated reclining chairs, heating pads, hot water bottles, car heaters, electric space heaters, and laptop computers (Miller et al. 2011). The condition is also known as fire stains, hot water bottle rash, laptop leg, and toasted skin syndrome (Figs. 6.23, 6.24, and 6.25).

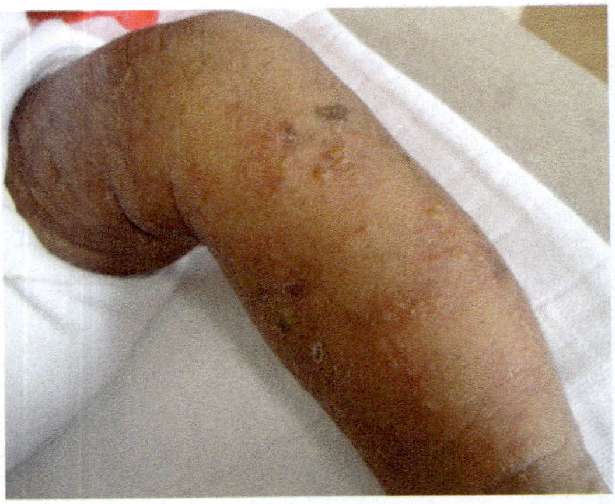

Fig. 6.22 Incontinentia pigmenti

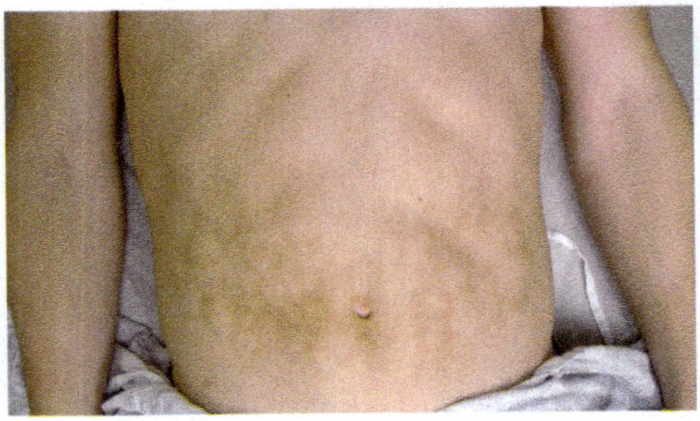

Fig. 6.23 Erythema ab igne on trunk (= Fig. 2.41)

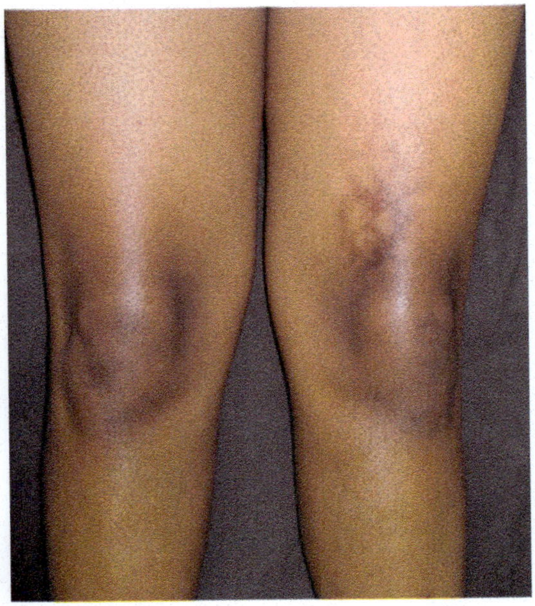

Fig. 6.24 Erythema ab igne on left thigh – laptop leg

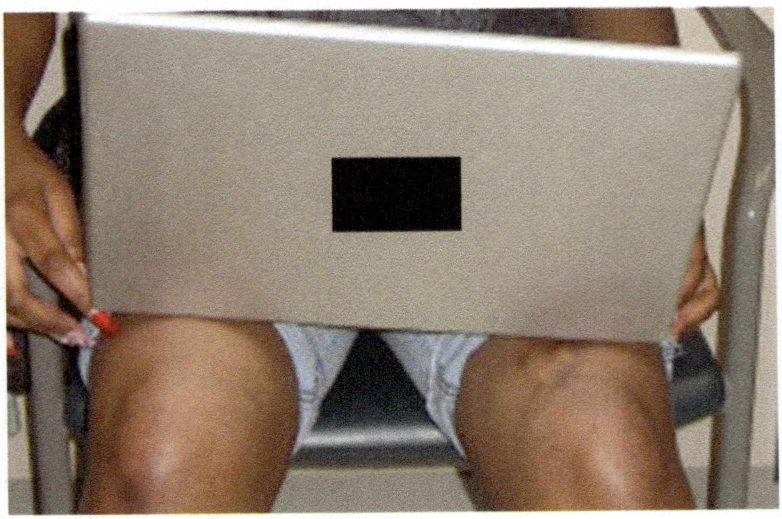

Fig. 6.25 Erythema ab igne – laptop leg (same person as in Fig. 6.24)

6.3 Various Allergic or Toxic Reactions Due to Inflammatory Skin Diseases

Child abuse may be erroneously suspected in children with various allergic or toxic reactions, such as in periorbital swellings, phyto-photodermatitis, or vasculitis allergica. Two other disorders belonging to this category, which are often mentioned in the differential diagnosis of non-accidental bruising, are erythema nodosum (Figs. 6.26, 6.27, and 6.28) and erythema multiforme (Kos and Shwayder 2006; Swerdlin et al. 2007; AlJasser and Al-Khenaizan 2008; Jenny and Reece 2009). Both conditions are reported only sporadically as wrongly diagnosed non-accidental bruising (Adler and Kane-Nussen 1983; Rose 1985; Labbe et al. 1996).

6.3.1 Periorbital Swellings and Bruising

Child abuse can be suspected erroneously in children with periorbital swelling and bruising. The swelling and bruising may suggest a traumatic origin.

Swelling may be due to an allergic reaction or an insect bite. Allergic swellings result from prolonged venous congestion in allergic rhinitis or allergic eye reactions. In general, the color will more often be brownish than blue. Allergic swelling is seen more frequently in the lower eyelid.

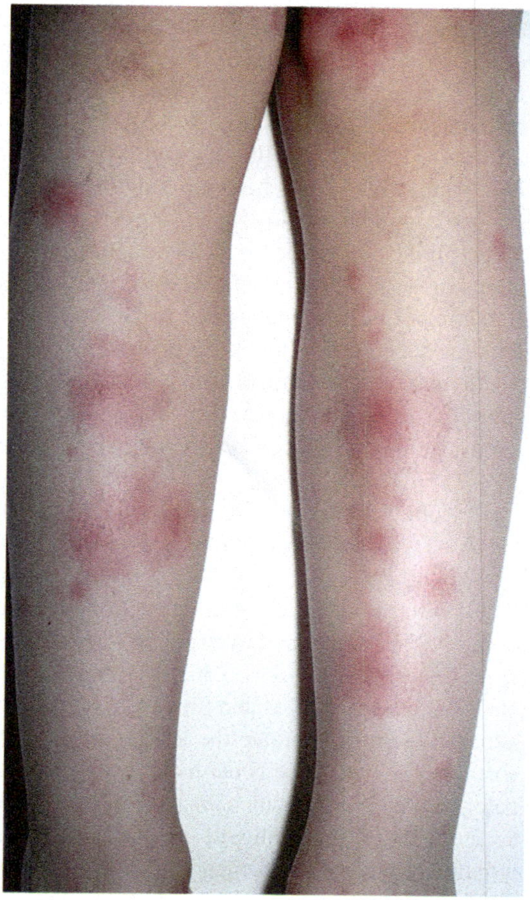

Fig. 6.26 Erythema nodosum

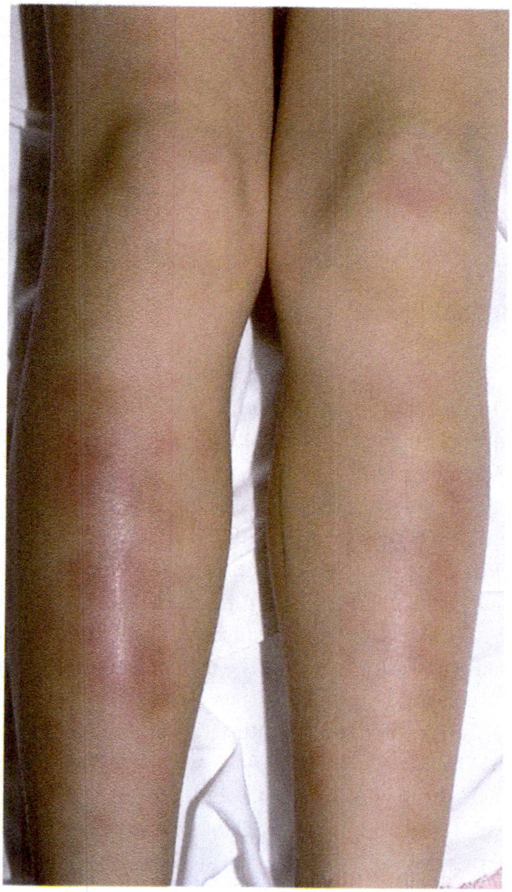

Fig. 6.27 Erythema nodosum

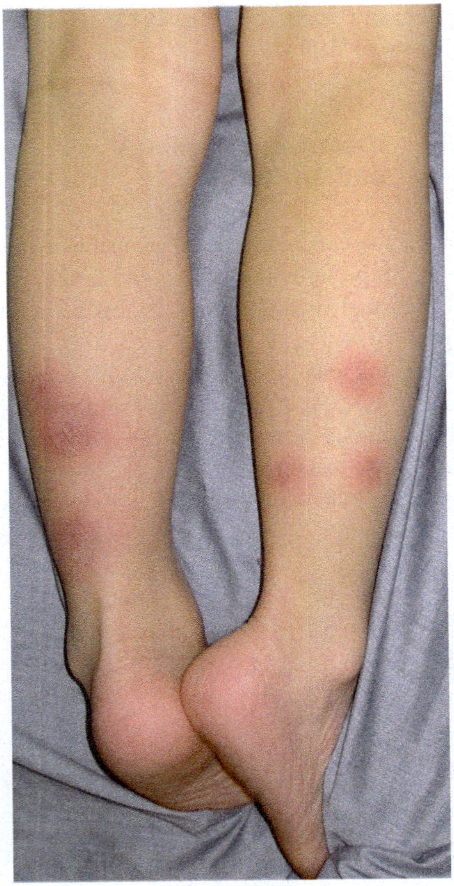

Fig. 6.28 Erythema nodosum

Differentiation is facilitated by the presence of an allergy and the typical location (Schmitt 1987; Wheeler and Hobbs 1988).

Thakur and Kaplan (1996) report a young child who presented with atypical angioedema (noninflammatory scalp or facial swelling without recurrence on other parts of the body and without urticaria). Because of the unexplained scalp swelling, initially non-accidental blunt force trauma to the head was suspected.

In the medical literature, several descriptions are found of children with neuroblastoma who had periorbital swelling and bruising (raccoon eyes) resulting from osseous metastasis to the orbits and skull (Dober et al. 2007; Bohdiewicz et al. 1995). This periorbital bruising may initially be misinterpreted as child abuse.

6.3.2 Phytophotodermatitis

Phytophotodermatitis is an acute cutaneous reaction that may develop after skin contact with the sap of various plants and the subsequent immediate exposure to sunlight. However, according to Barradell et al. (1993), one may even find the reaction on a more or less sunless day.

It has been described among others to result from limes, lemon juice, and umbellifers, such as hogweed, parsley, celery, parsnip, wild rhubarb, common rue, and other garden weeds (Coffman et al. 1985; Dannaker et al. 1988; Barradell et al. 1993; Lagey et al. 1995; Hill et al. 1997; Furniss and Adams 2007). Contact with figs has also been implicated (Watemberg et al. 1991).

The sap contains toxic substances that cause a phototoxic reaction in the skin through the influence of ultraviolet A (UVA) irradiation. The abnormality initially consists of linearly arranged erythema and blisters, sometimes resembling a hand imprint. At a later stage, the lesions may resemble recently developed bruising (redness with some swelling), somewhat older hematomas (brown patches with a sharp border), or partial-thickness hot water burns (bullae). Hyperpigmented lesions typically appear on the hands or around the mouth (Kung et al. 2009). Sometimes one may find lesions on a less specific location such as the buttocks (Hill et al. 1997).

Phytophotodermatitis is usually mild and self-limiting, although the hyperpigmentation may persist for weeks, or even years (Watemberg et al. 1991).

Phytophotodermatitis is easily (and often) confused with bruising or burning as seen in child abuse (Coffman et al. 1985; Dannaker et al. 1988; Watemberg et al. 1991; Barradell et al. 1993; Hill et al. 1997; Carlsen and Weismann 2007; Kung et al. 2009) (Figs. 6.29, 6.30, 6.31, 6.32, and 6.33). According to Kos and Shwayder (2006), it is possible to differentiate the lesions from abusive lesions since there is hardly any variation in color, as is expected in a healing bruise, and because the history should reveal an earlier inflammatory and/or vesicular eruption.

Gruson and Chang (2002) reported a 9-year-old girl with Berloque dermatitis, result-

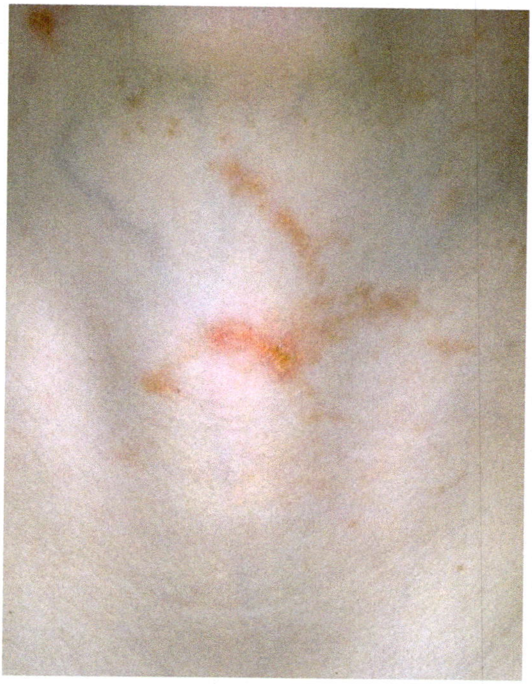

Fig. 6.29 Phytophotodermatitis, resembling grip marks in the neck

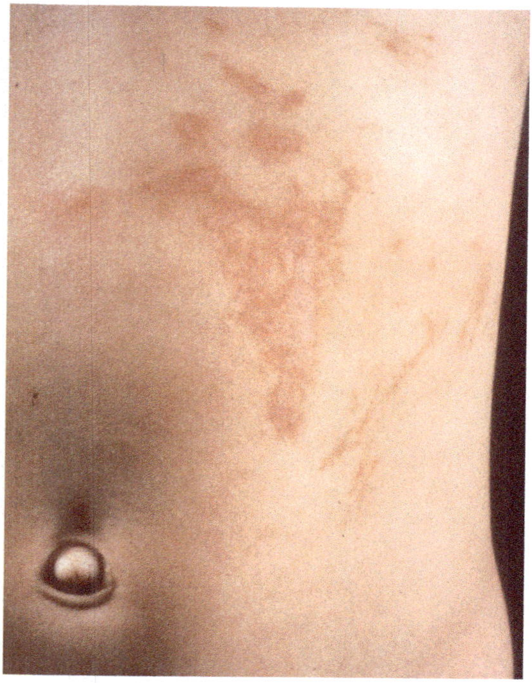

Fig. 6.31 Phytophotodermatitis, resembling healing bruises

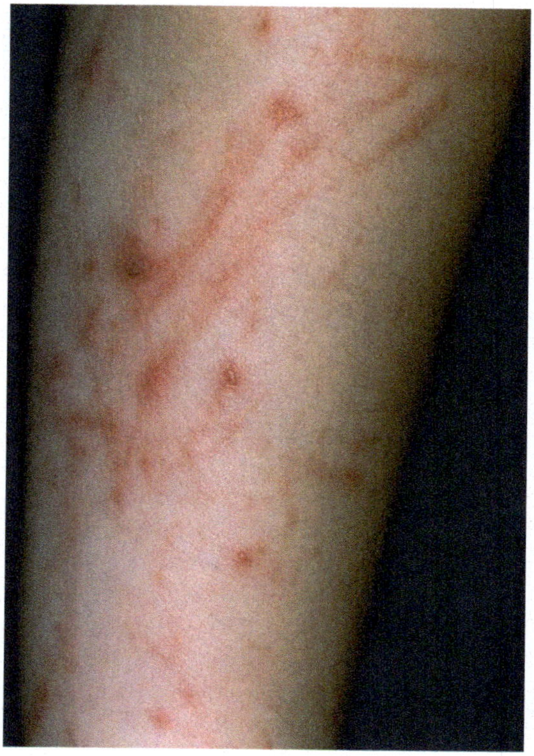

Fig. 6.30 Phytophotodermatitis mimicking strap marks or loop-shaped bruising (Chap. 3)

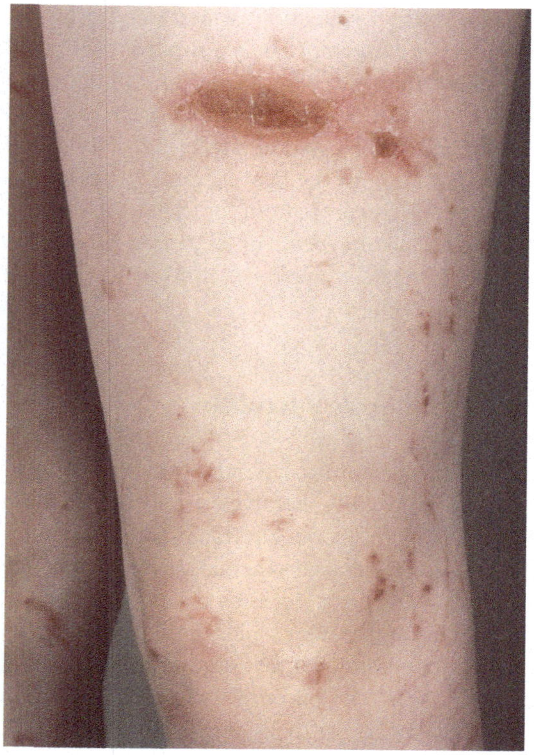

Fig. 6.32 Phytophotodermatitis

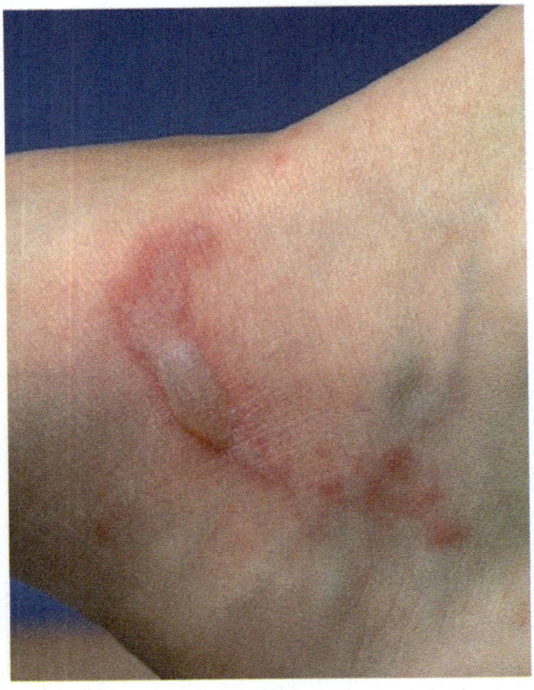

Fig. 6.33 Phytophotodermatitis, resembling a burn

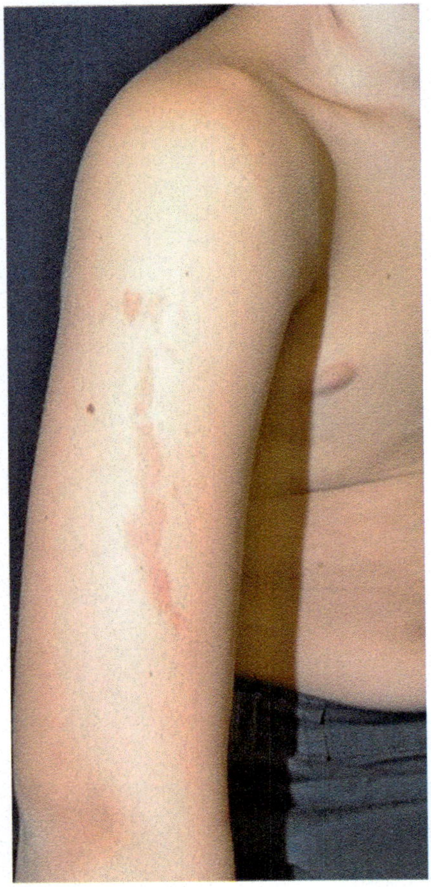

Fig. 6.34 Berloque dermatitis

ing from the application of perfumed products containing bergamot (or a psoralen), followed by exposure of the skin to sunlight. In the acute phase of Berloque dermatitis, one may find patterned redness and/or blistering. Due to the typical pattern of the healing dermatitis (hyperpigmented linear pattern or handprint marks localized on the neck or any area where the product has been applied), child abuse may be suspected (Fig. 6.34).

6.3.3 Allergic Vasculitis

Allergic vasculitis depends on various processes. It usually involves Henoch-Schönlein purpura in childhood, but it may also be a manifestation of lupus erythematosus. On the one hand, its diagnosis depends on the clinical picture and, on the other hand, in case of doubt on the histopathological investigation (Legrain and Taieb 2006). The purpura is especially seen on the legs and the buttocks (Figs. 6.35, 6.36, 6.37, and 6.38), often as symmetrical bruising on extensor surfaces (Menter 1987; Daly and Siegel 1998). There may have been a recent infection or associated symptoms such as joint complaints or a stomachache (intussusception), blood in the feces, and renal (proteinuria, hematuria) complaints. A biopsy for histopathological investigation is indicated in case of doubt or in an atypical course. In the early stages of the disease, lesions may impress as multiple bruises and confusion with child abuse may arise, especially in case of an atypical course or an atypical location (Brown and Melinkovich 1986; Menter 1987; Daly and Siegel 1998;). Tender swollen joints, as seen in children with hemophilia, acute leukemia, and neuroblastoma, have also been described in children with Henoch-Schönlein purpura (Thomas 2004).

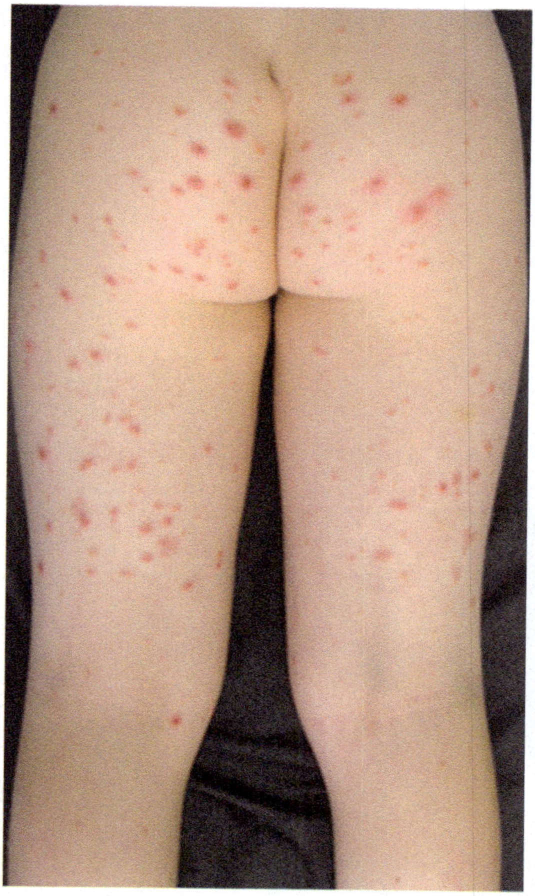

Fig. 6.35 Henoch-Schönlein purpura

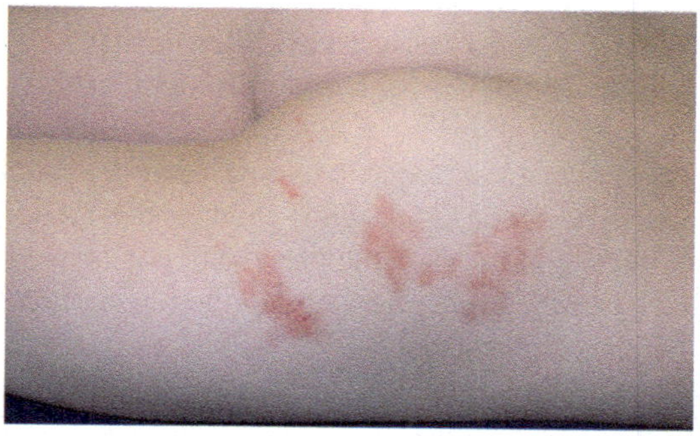

Fig. 6.36 Unilateral Henoch-Schönlein purpura

Fig. 6.38 Same child as in Fig. 6.37

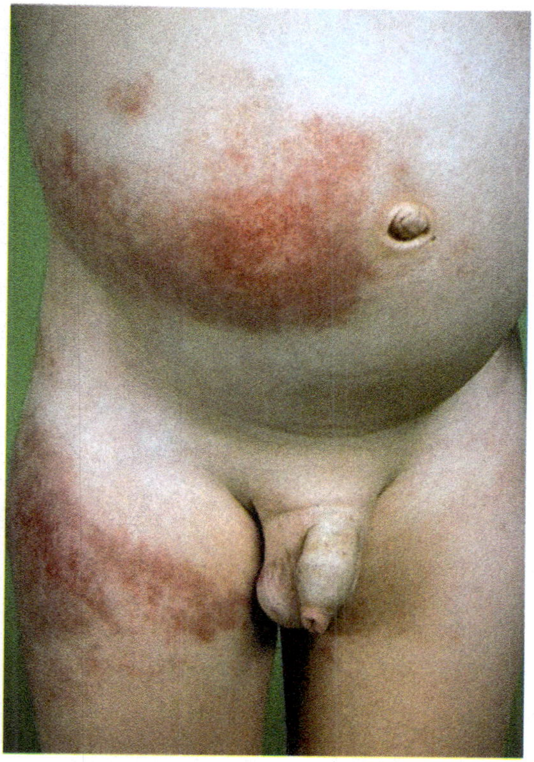

Fig. 6.37 Atypical Henoch-Schönlein purpura

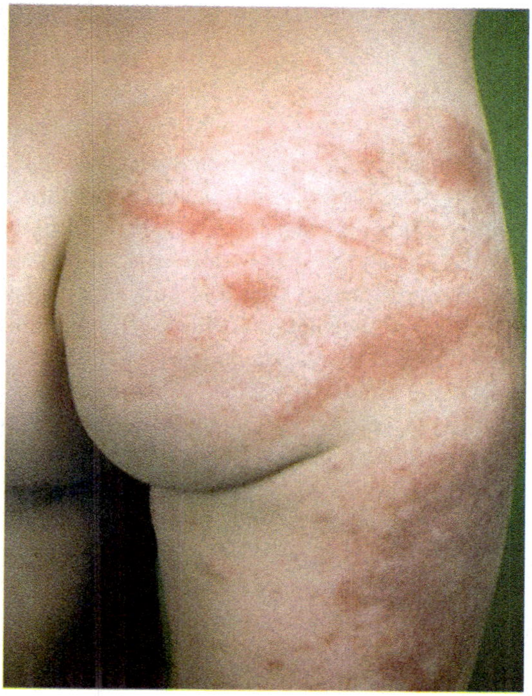

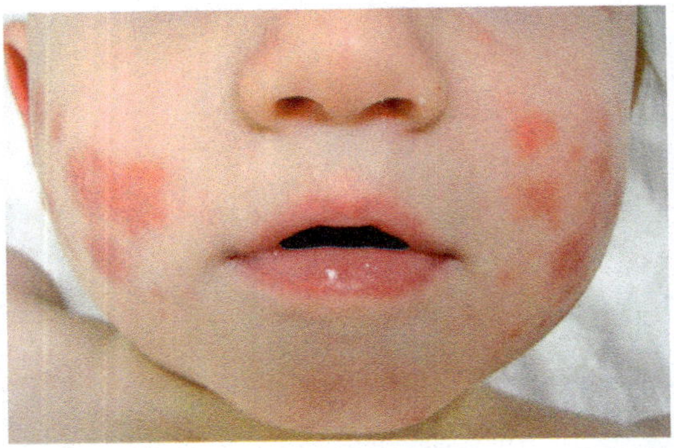

Fig. 6.39 Acute hemorrhagic edema of infancy resembling grip marks

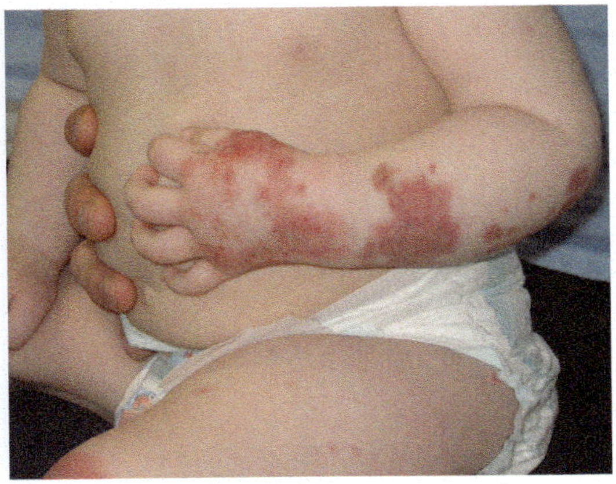

Fig. 6.40 Acute hemorrhagic edema of infancy

Fig. 6.41 Acute hemorrhagic edema of infancy

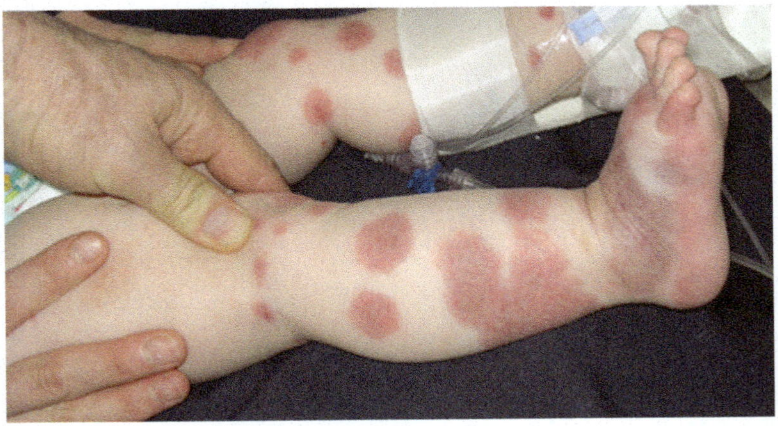

Children with Henoch-Schönlein purpura (HSP) or children with acute hemorrhagic edema of infancy (AHEI) (Figs. 6.39, 6.40, 6.41, and 6.42) may present with edema, erythema, and purpura on the face and ears before any other sites become affected (Brown and Melinkovich 1986; Scaramuzza et al. 1997). These symptoms in a young child may easily lead to suspected abuse. Infants with AHEI also show lesions on the extremities, as well as on the face and ears. Occasionally, lesions can be seen on the scrotum, another area suspect for abuse (Calişkan et al. 1995). The patients are febrile although otherwise they appear to be well (Scaramuzza et al. 1997).

In addition to HSP and AHEI, the purpuric lesions of any of the forms of vasculitis may be confused with abuse (Waskerwitz et al. 1981).

6.4 Disease-Related "Bruising" and "Petechiae": Other Causes

A number of infrequent findings and disorders are rarely confused with child abuse-related bruises, except when the presentation is atypical or when the evaluation is performed by an inexperienced physician.

6.4.1 Hemangioma of Infancy and Other Vascular Malformations in Infancy

Hemangioma of infancy (HOI) is the most frequently occurring benign neoplasm in children (Drolet et al. 1999). It occurs in 10% of all infants. About 60% are found on the head and neck.

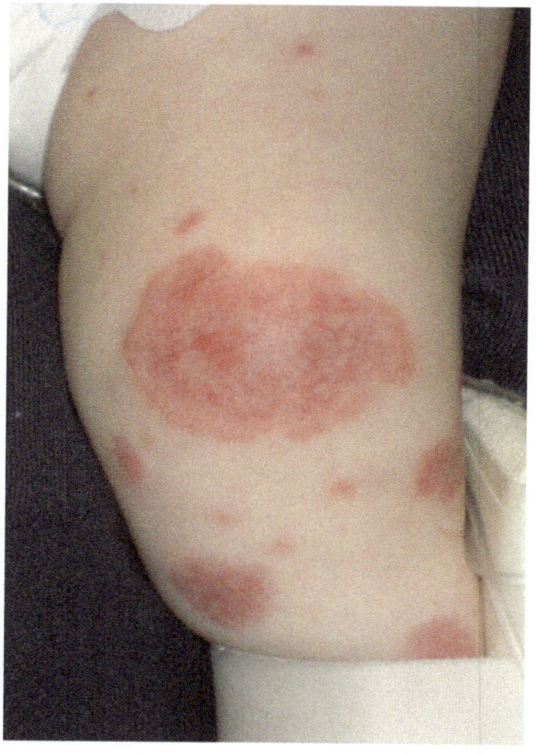

Fig. 6.42 Acute hemorrhagic edema of infancy

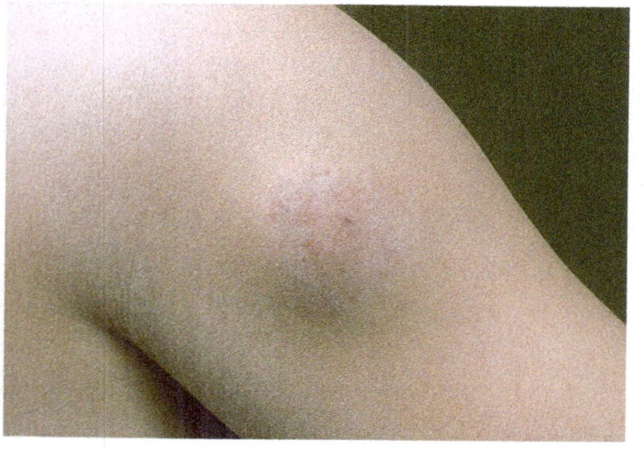

Fig. 6.43 Deep hemangioma of infancy

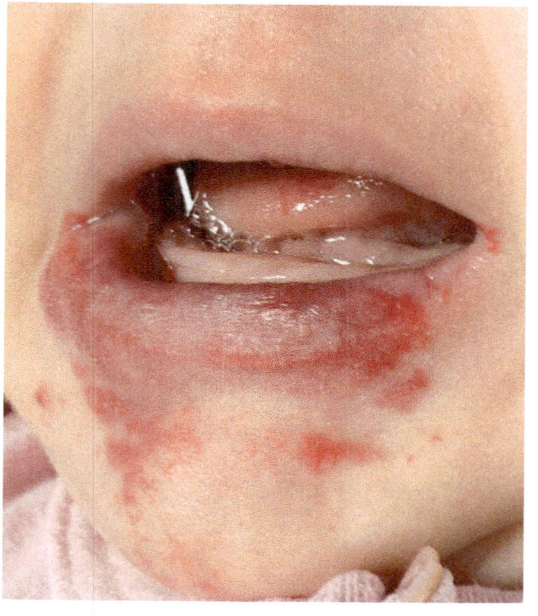

Fig. 6.44 Superficial hemangioma of infancy

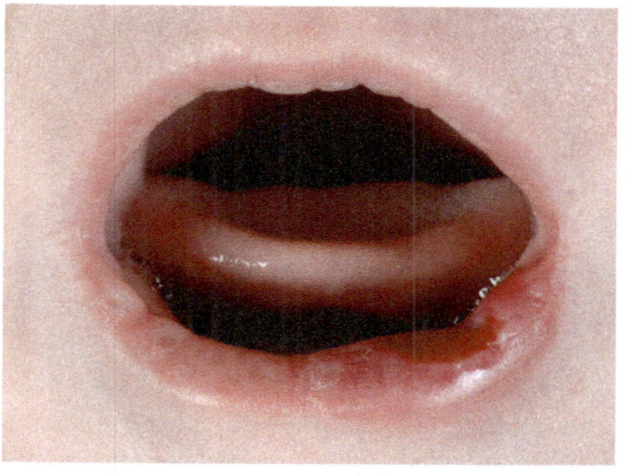

Fig. 6.45 Ulcerating hemangioma of infancy

About 20% of the children with HOI have more than one lesion (Drolet et al. 1999).

When the true nature of the finding is not recognized, HOI may be misdiagnosed as bruising by child abuse (Drolet et al. 1999; AlJasser and Al-Khenaizan 2008); there are cases in which parents have been falsely accused of child abuse by strangers (Tanner et al. 1998; Drolet et al. 1999; Greig and Harris 2003) (Figs. 6.43, 6.44, 6.45, 6.46, 6.47, 6.48, 6.49, 6.50, and 6.51). Also other vascular malformations can be misdiagnosed as bruising due to child abuse (Figs. 6.52, 6.53, 6.54, 6.55, 6.56, 6.57, 6.58, 6.59, 6.60, 6.61, 6.62, 6.63, 6.64, and 6.65).

Greig and Harris (2003) evaluated the perceptions of facial hemangiomas in two professional groups (health visitors and primary school teachers) involved in child-abuse surveillance. Only one health visitor (5%) and one teacher (5%) thought that the lesion was a non-accidental injury. Based on these findings, one may assume that the risk of an incorrect diagnosis by a professional appears to be low.

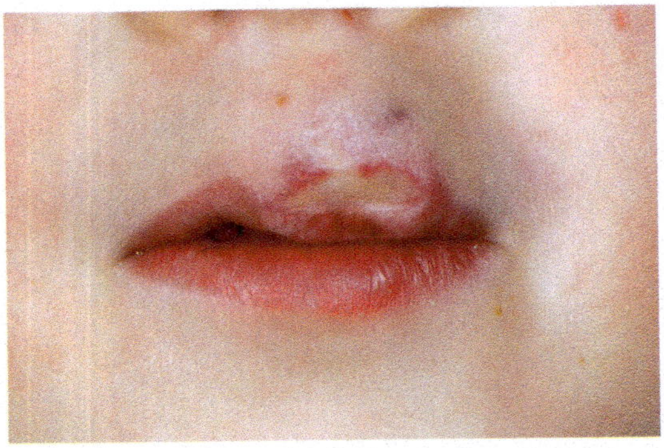

Fig. 6.46 Hemangioma of infancy in regression with scarring

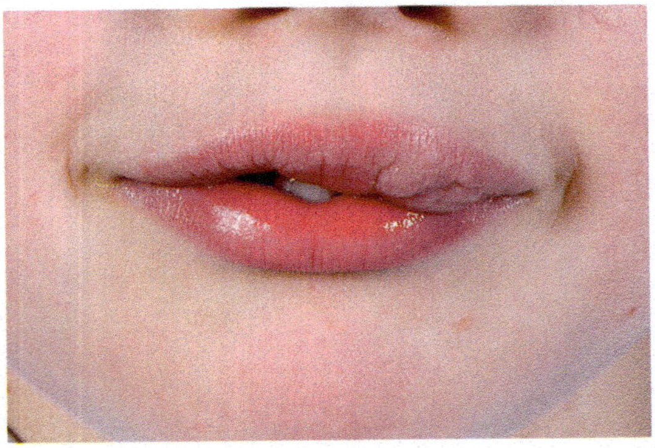

Fig. 6.47 Scarring after regressing of hemangioma of infancy

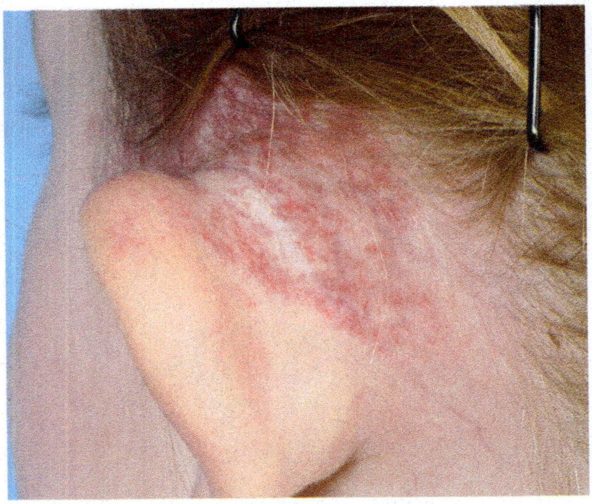

Fig. 6.48 Hemangioma of infancy in regression

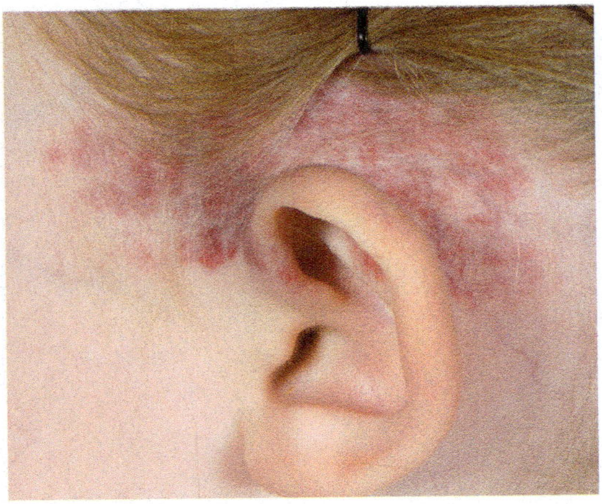

Fig. 6.49 Same child as in Fig. 6.48

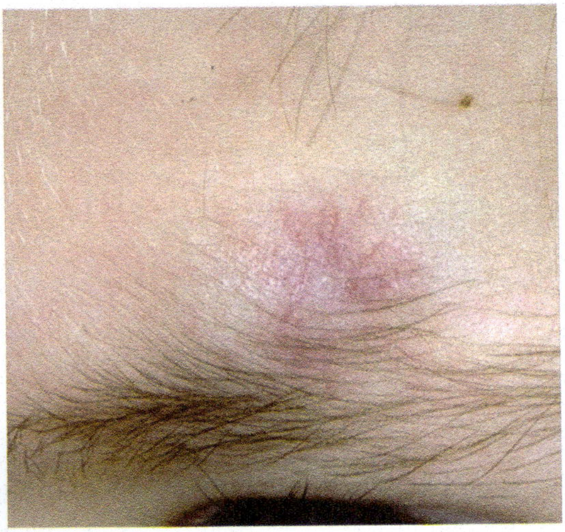

Fig. 6.50 Hemangioma of infancy in regression

However, in case of complications like ulceration, even medical professionals are at risk. Levin and Selbst (1988) reported an infant with a vulvar hemangioma that had undergone extensive ulcerative changes which were initially diagnosed as a perineal burn secondary to child abuse.

6.4.2 *Haemophilus influenzae*

Haemophilus influenzae may lead to a bluish transparent cellulitis on the cheek. Differentiation from child abuse is based on the fact that these children are sick and have a fever and that the involved area is sensitive and swollen. Laboratory investigations indicate increased sedimentation rate and leukocytosis (Speight 1992).

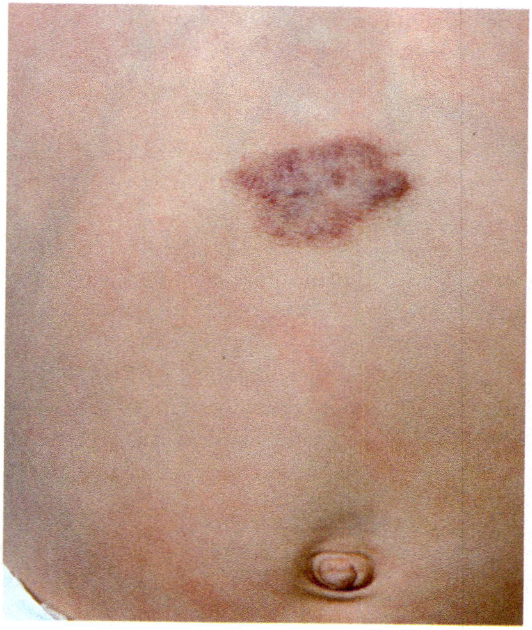

Fig. 6.51 Hemangioma of infancy in regression

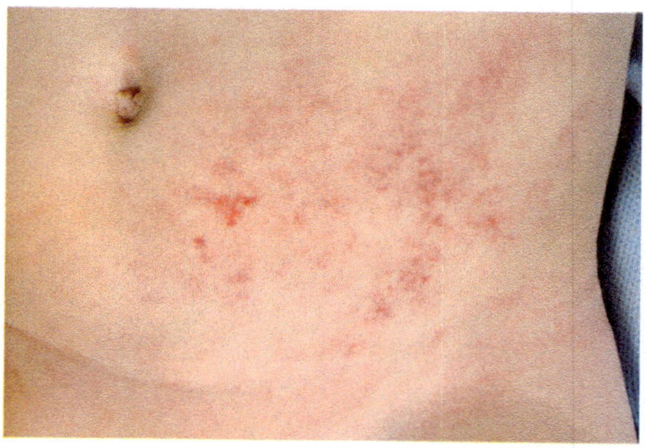

Fig. 6.52 Capillary vascular malformation

6.4.3 Maculae Ceruleae

Maculae ceruleae are blue linear skin lesions (linear bruises) which occur simultaneously with a head or pubic lice infection. Whether this is due to lice bites or an accompanying phenomenon is not clear. The maculae ceruleae disappear when the infection is adequately treated (Schmitt 1987; Ragosta 1989). In most parts of the world, pubic

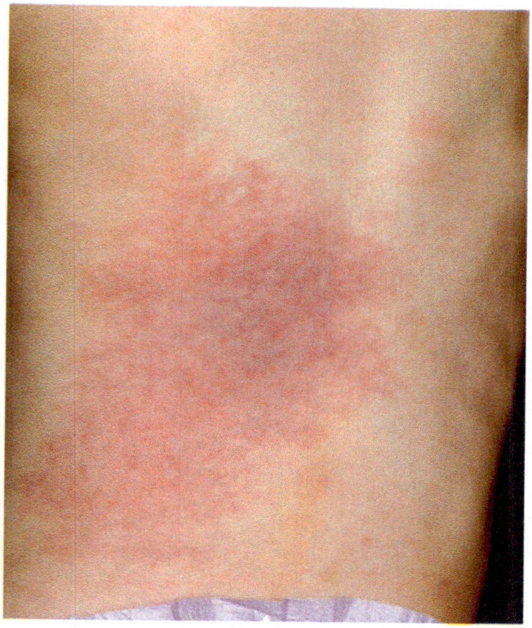

Fig. 6.53 Cutis marmorata telangiectatica congenita on the back of an infant (CMTC)

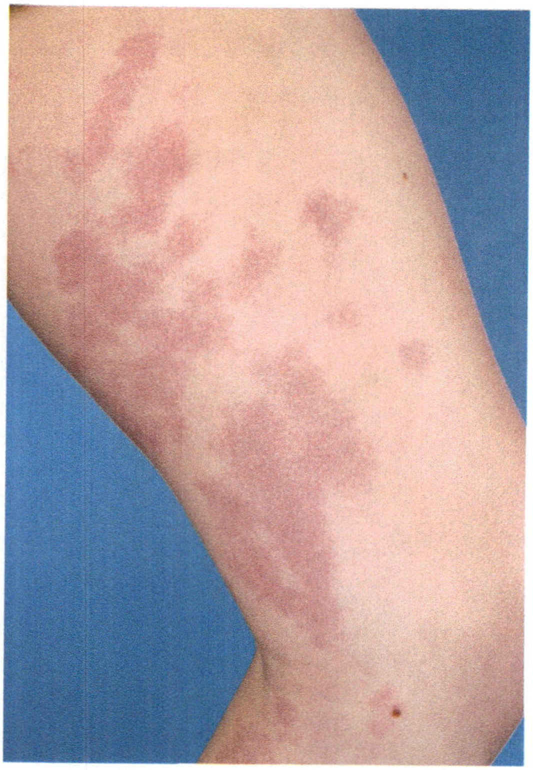

Fig. 6.54 Capillary vascular malformation

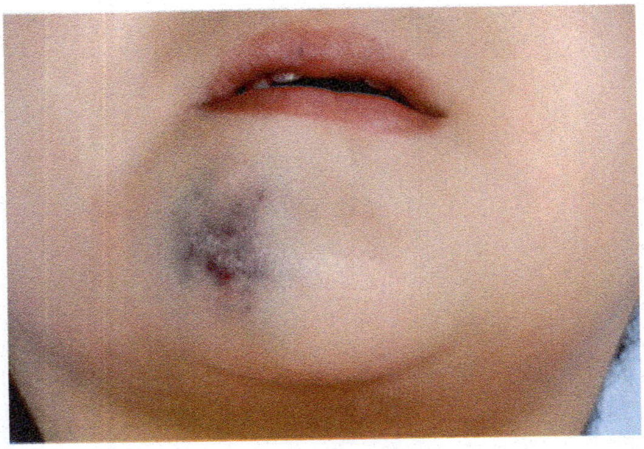

Fig. 6.55 Vascular malformation

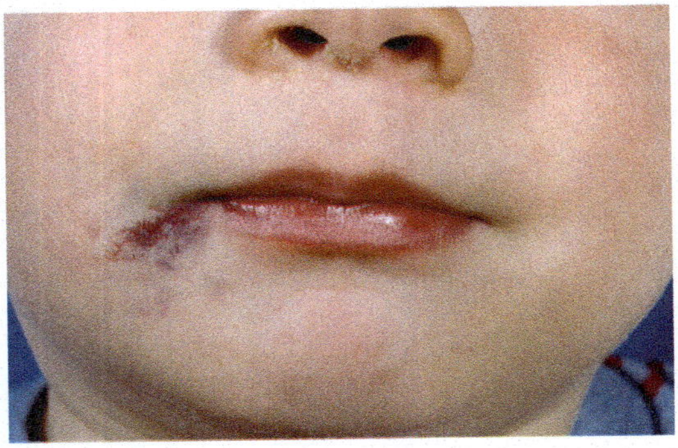

Fig. 6.56 Vascular malformation

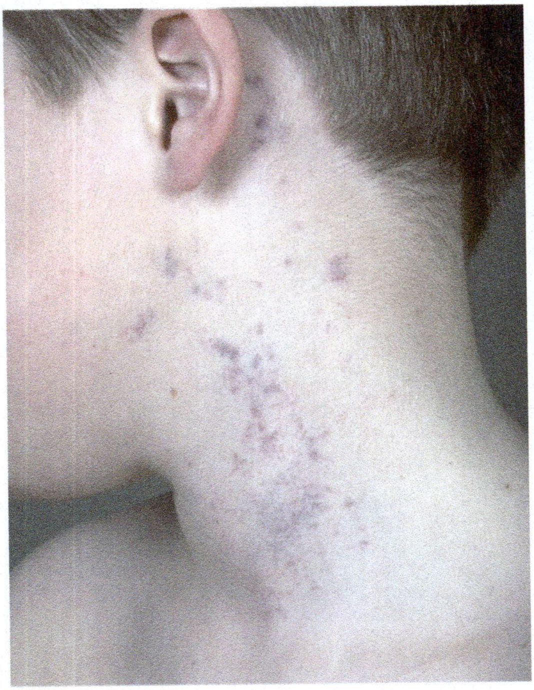

Fig. 6.57 Vascular malformation

lice infection only rarely occurs in children but if found, sexual abuse may need to be considered.

6.4.4 Dermographism and Factitious Urticaria

Dermographism, dermatographism, or "skin writing" is a skin disorder seen in 1.5–4.5% of the population. Dermographism is one of the most common types of urticaria in which the skin becomes raised and inflamed when stroked, scratched, or rubbed. In older patients, it has been observed in association with atopic dermatitis,

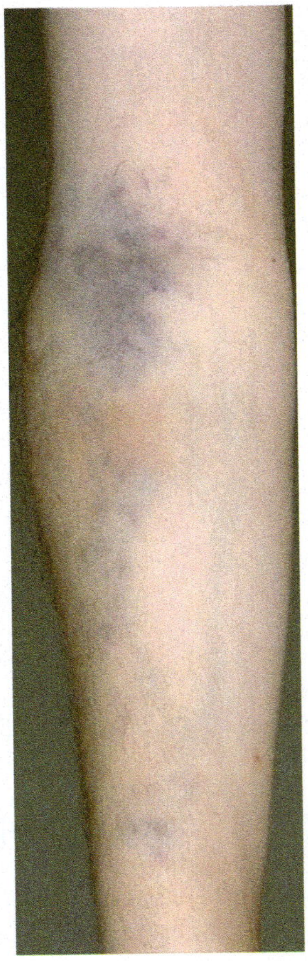

Fig. 6.58 Vascular malformation

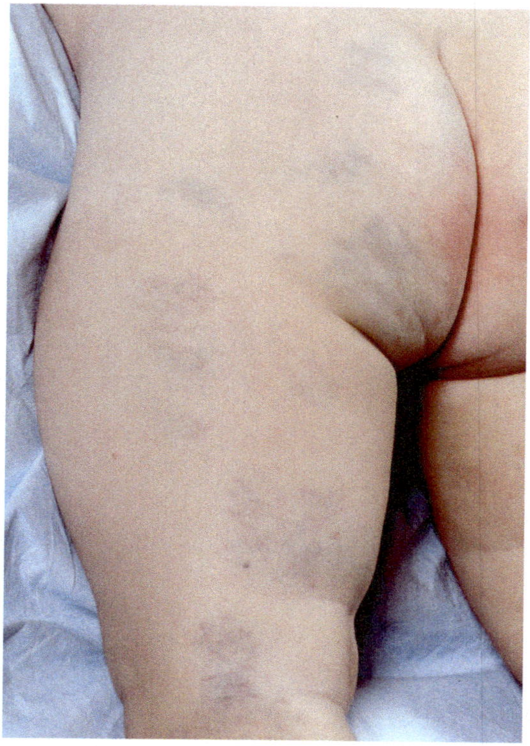

Fig. 6.59 Vascular malformation

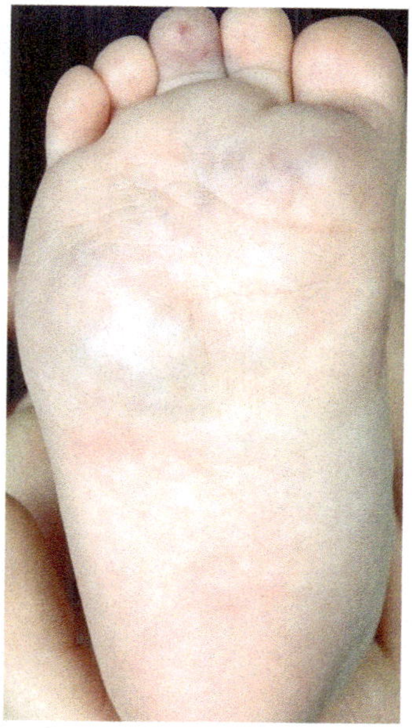

Fig. 6.61 Vascular malformation

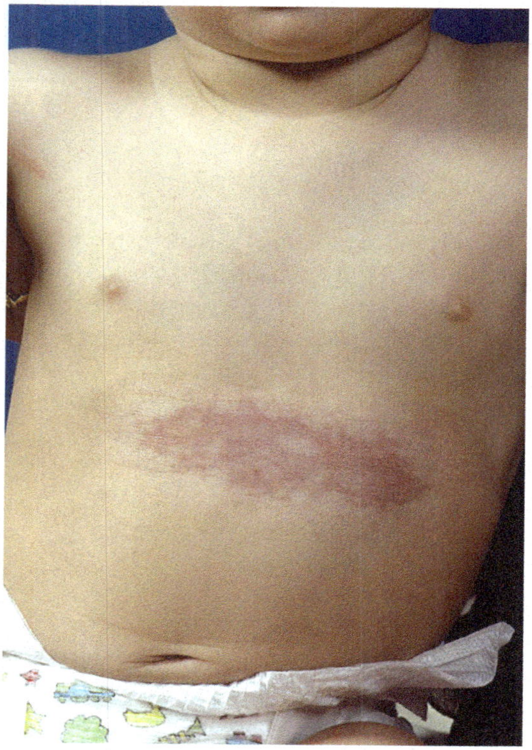

Fig. 6.62 Kaposiform hemangio-endothelioma in regression

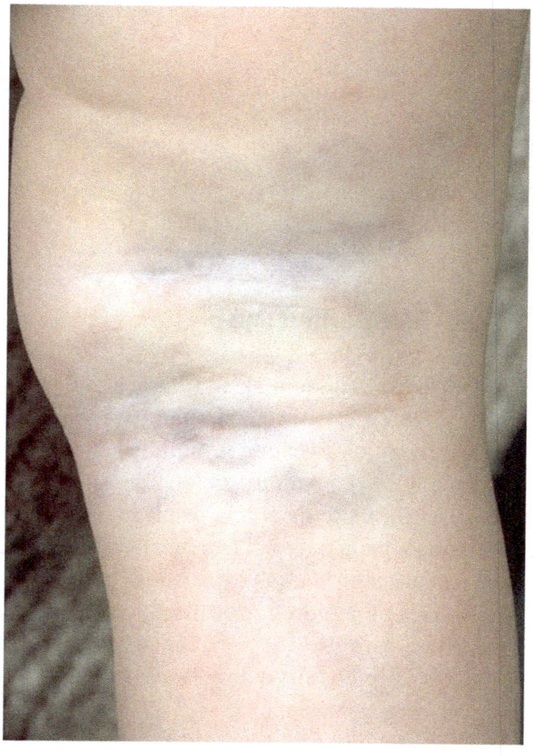

Fig. 6.60 Vascular malformation

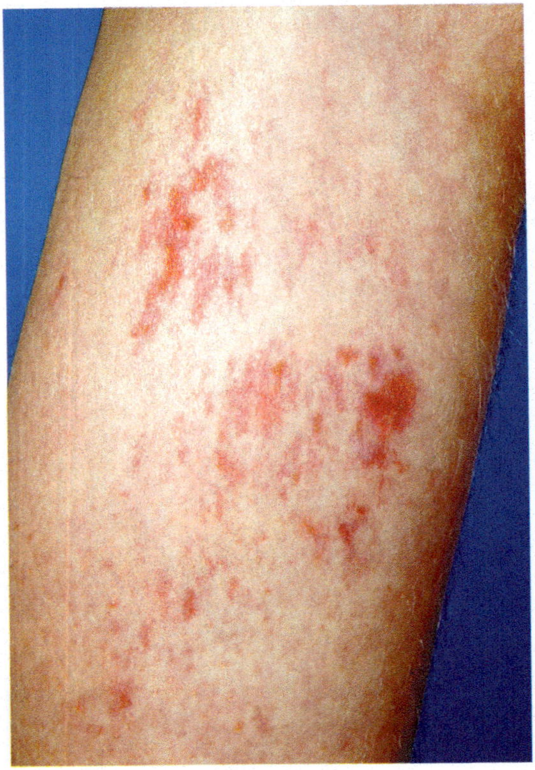

Fig. 6.63 Linear telangiectasia

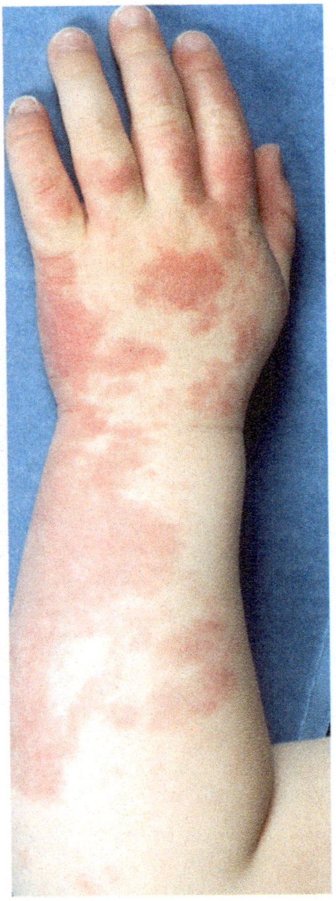

Fig. 6.64 Nevus flammeus

urticaria, and mastocytosis (Leaute-Labreze 2006; Oranje 2010) (Figs. 6.66, 6.67, 6.68, and 6.69).

In infants, one may observe reactive redness after touching the skin. This phenomenon is physiological and disappears within 1–2 years. It is also known as factitious urticaria (Figs. 6.70 and 6.71).

6.4.5 Ehlers-Danlos Syndrome (Classical Type)

Ehlers-Danlos syndrome (EDS) is a group of inherited connective tissue disorders caused by a defect in the synthesis of collagen. In earlier publications, 11 different subtypes were recognized, but nowadays, only four subtypes are described: classical type (types I and II), type III of benign hypermobility type, or type IV (vascular type) (Lawrence 2005) (Figs. 6.72, 6.73, and 6.74). In particular, the classical type can be misdiagnosed as child abuse (see also Sect. 5.4.1.1).

6.4.6 Ectodermal Dysplasia

Hypohidrotic ectodermal dysplasia is one of about 150 types of ectodermal dysplasia in humans in which sweating is diminished, leading to temperature regulation problems (Irvine 2006). Before birth, these disorders result in the abnormal development of structures including the skin, hair, nails, teeth, and sweat glands. The symptomatology of anhidrotic ectodermal dysplasia is even more serious. These patients however are more easily recognized than those with hypohidrotic ectodysplasia.

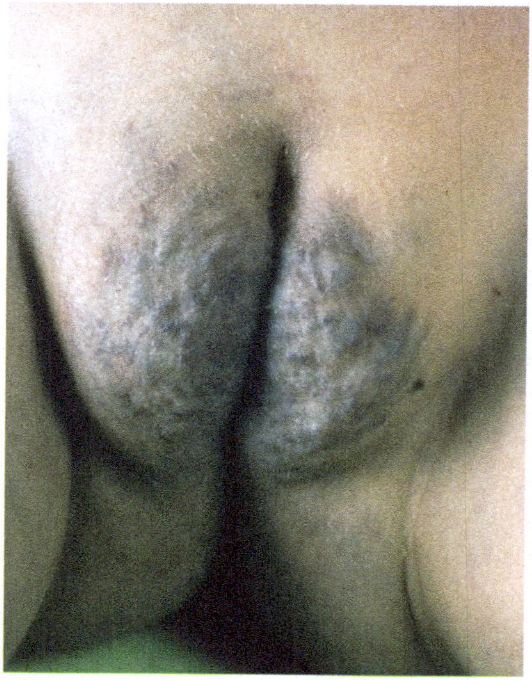

Fig. 6.65 Vascular malformation as part of blue rubber bleb nevus syndrome

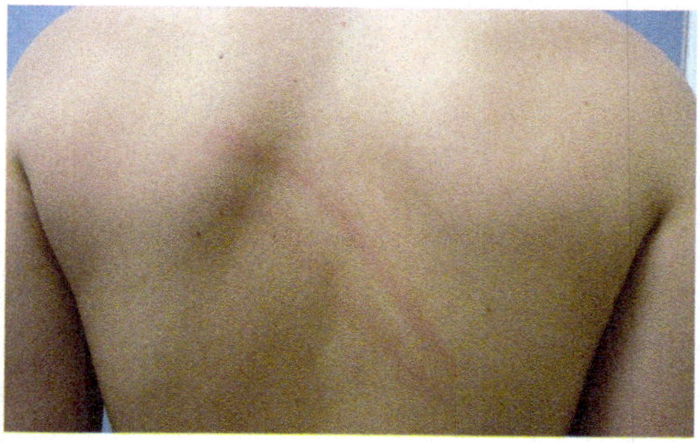

Fig. 6.66 Dermographism mimicking strap mark – tram-line bruising

If the symptomatology of these diseases is misinterpreted, parents may show "medical shopping" behavior to find proper treatment for their child. This behavior may be labeled incorrectly as child abuse, especially pediatric condition falsification (Oranje, own observation).

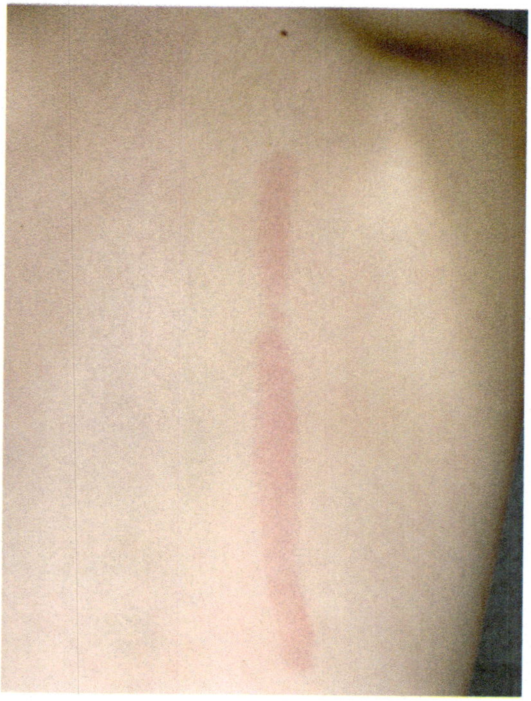

Fig. 6.67 Dermographism mimicking strap mark

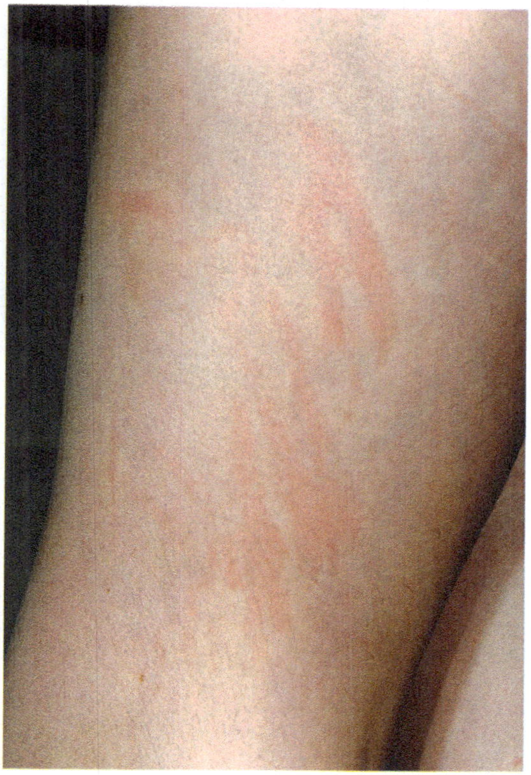

Fig. 6.68 Dermographism mimicking strap mark

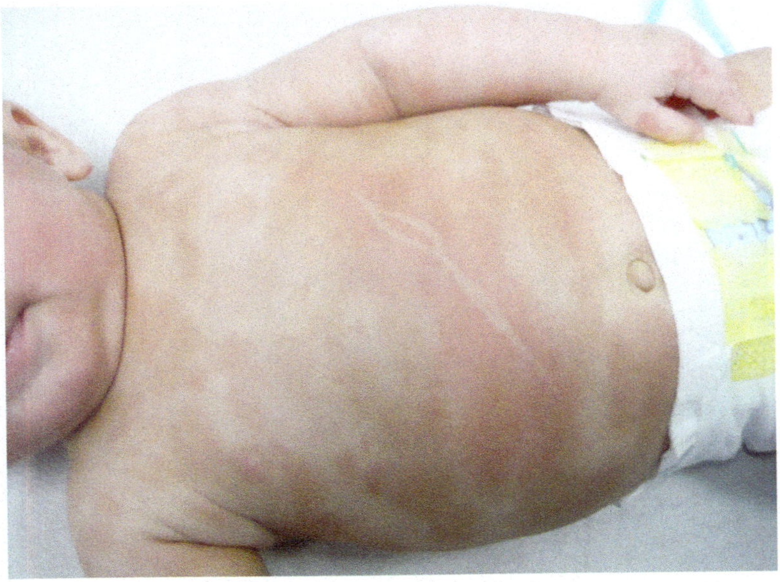

Fig. 6.69 Dermographism in a child with mastocytosis

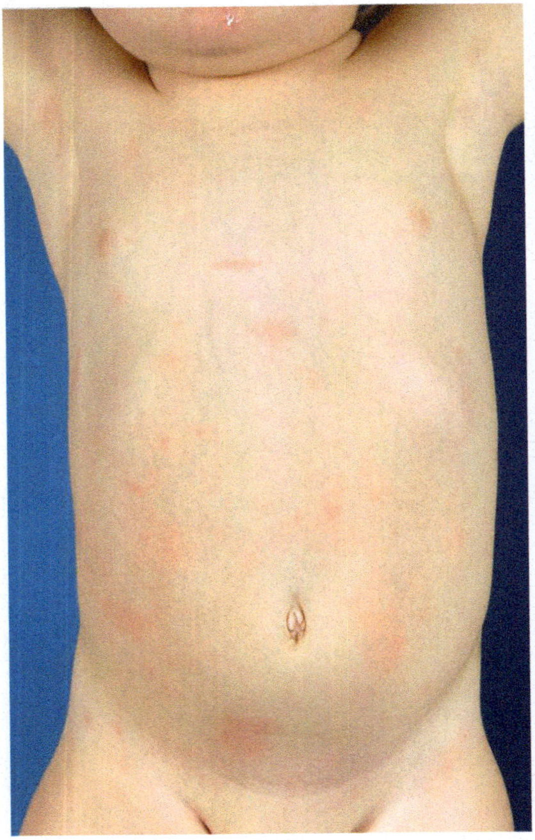

Fig. 6.70 Factitious urticaria

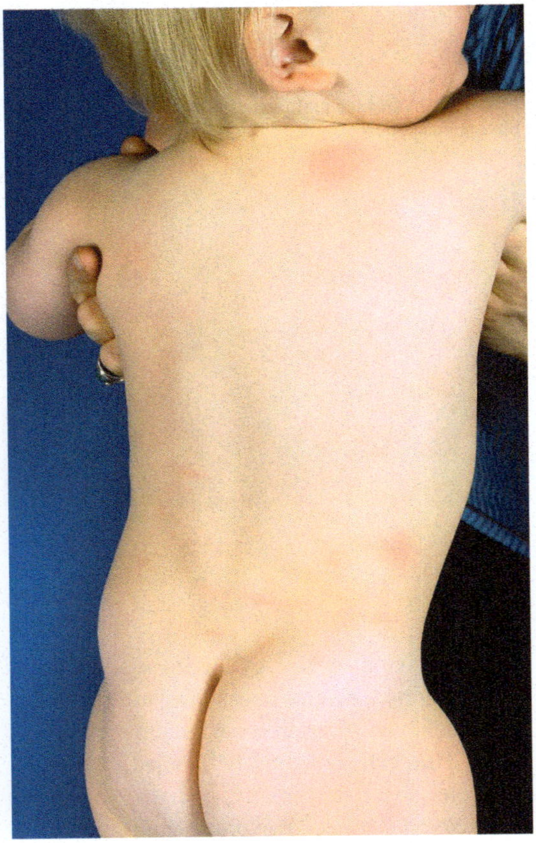

Fig. 6.71 Same child as in Fig. 6.70

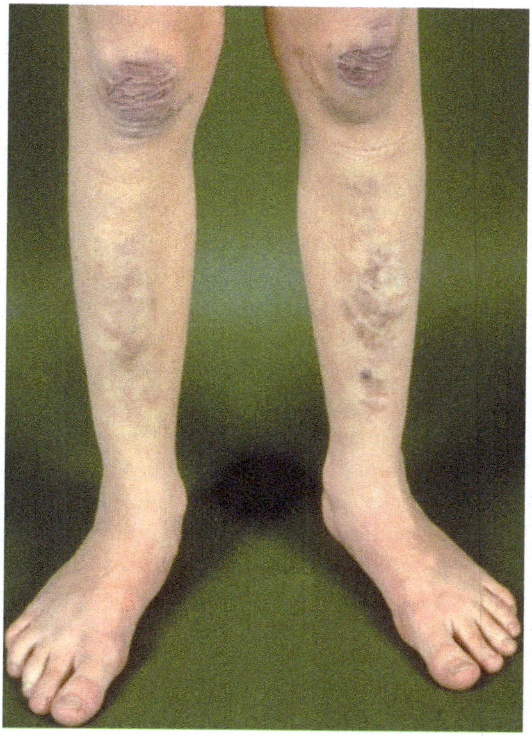

Fig. 6.72 Characteristic findings in classical type Ehlers-Danlos syndrome (types I and II): extensive bruising and cigarette paper tissue scars (= Fig. 5.5)

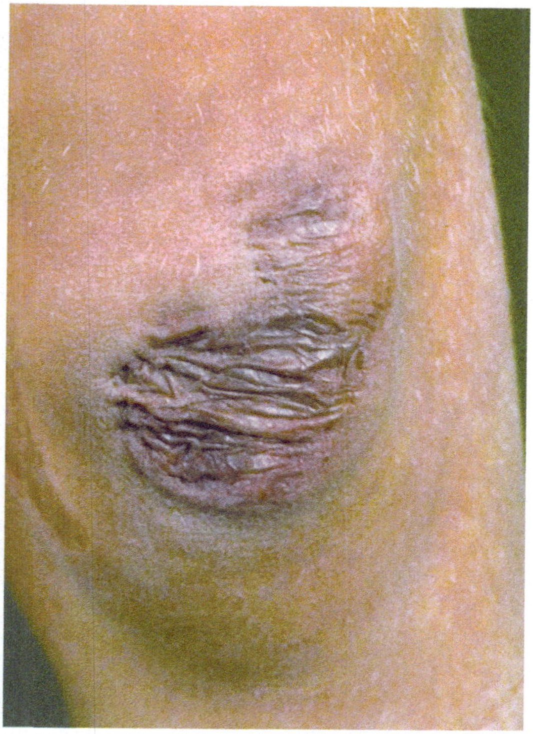

Fig. 6.73 Characteristic findings in classical type Ehlers-Danlos Syndrome (types I and II): cigarette paper tissue scar (= Fig. 5.6)

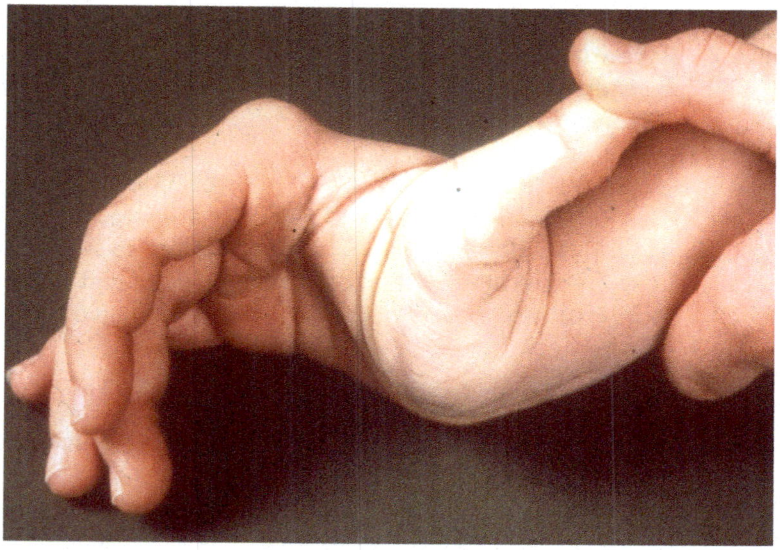

Fig. 6.74 Characteristic findings in classical type Ehlers-Danlos Syndrome (types I and II): joint hypermobility (= Fig. 5.7)

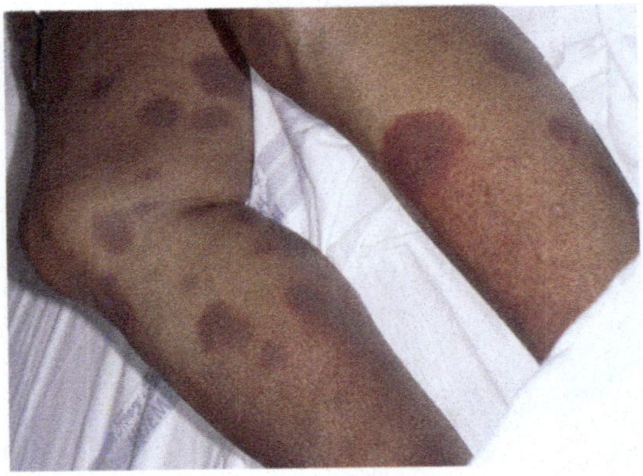

Fig. 6.75 Fixed drug eruption

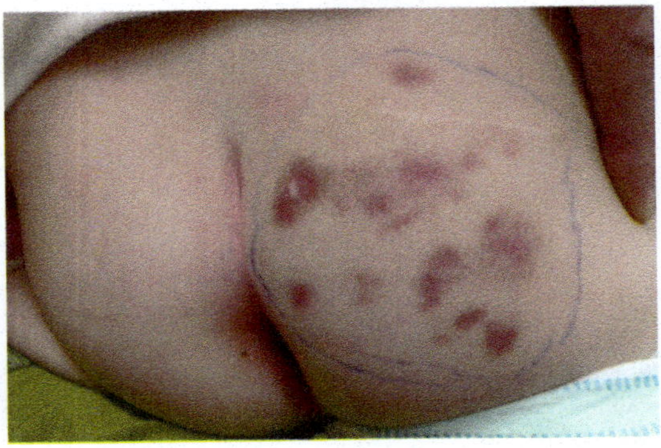

Fig. 6.76 Dermatofibrosarcoma protuberans (DFSP) (extent marked with ink)

6.4.7 Potentially Confusing Disease-Related Skin Lesions in the Differential Diagnosis

See Figs. 6.75 and 6.76.

6.5 Low Temperature-Related Skin Findings

6.5.1 Introduction

Exposure of the child to low temperatures may lead to (Long et al. 2005):

- Systemic hypothermia as a result of heat loss by radiation, evaporation, conduction, and convection.
- Changes to the skin and subcutaneous tissues as a result of localized cold injuries.

Young children are at greater risk because they have a less adaptive behavioral reaction to cold stress, especially during outdoor activities in low temperatures, for example, skating, skiing, and playing in the snow. In addition, they have a larger body surface area-to-weight (volume) ratio than adults and are more prone to lose body heat at low temperatures, leading to hypothermia. Abusive induction of hypothermia can follow prolonged placement of an inadequately clothed child in a cold environment or may be due to immersion in cold water (Gustavson and Levitt 1996). Victoria Climbié was left in a cold bathroom inadequately clothed and wetted by her own urine for a long period of time. Malnutrition may also have contributed to her death (Laming 2003). Hypothermia with serious morbidity and a high mortality may also be found in abandoned children, mostly neonates and young infants (Mehta 1982).

Frostbite and hypothermia (core body temperature below 35°C) may occur simultaneously. In this context, hypothermia in children will not be addressed any further.

Peripheral cold injuries can be categorized in:

- Swollen red hands and feet, also known as "deprivation hands and feet," but in reality resulting from hypothermia. The nose and cheeks may also be affected.
- Chilblains arising in low nonfreezing temperatures.
- Frostbite resulting from freezing temperatures.

Low temperature-related injuries in children are usually the result of accidental causes or occur secondary to disorders. Non-accidental causes, such as child abuse and neglect and self-inflicted injuries, such as in drug abuse, are only reported rarely in medical literature (Sect. 6.5.4).

6.5.2 Chilblains

Chilblain (pernio, erythema pernio, or perniones) is an inflammatory reaction of the skin, which occurs after exposure to low nonfreezing temperatures, especially in combination with humid conditions. Chilblains are most often seen in the

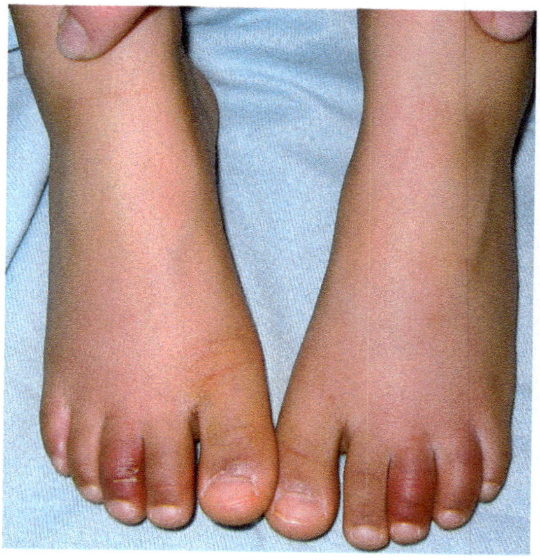

Fig. 6.77 Chilblains of the toes

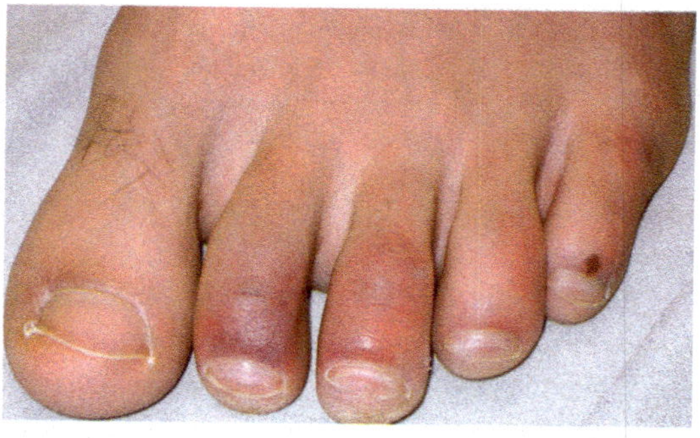

Fig. 6.78 Chilblains of the toes

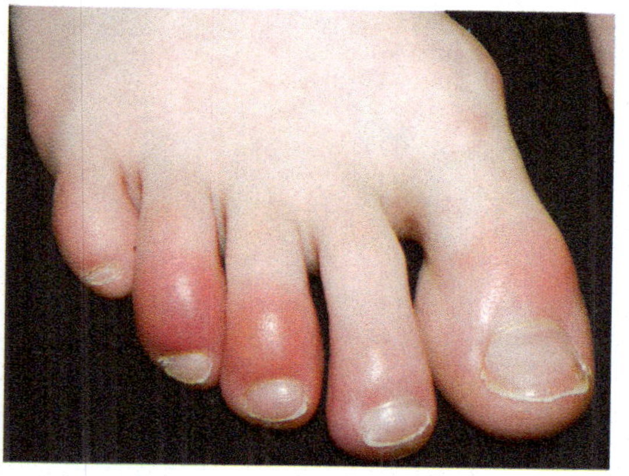

Fig. 6.79 Chilblains of the toes (Sapp 2007 from Wikimedia Commons 2011: Wintertenen.jpg) (= Fig. 2.43)

autumn or winter and will disappear in the spring or early summer (Simon et al. 2005). Symptoms occur within 12–24 h after exposure to cold (Simon et al. 2005; Cheng et al. 2008) and will disappear within 1–3 weeks, usually without treatment (Edlich 2008).

Chilblains are characterized by local itching and/or painful burning lesions, which are erythematous and edematous. Sometimes one may find cyanosis, particularly of the hands, feet (Figs. 6.77, 6.78, and 6.79), and face (nose and ears). A minor trauma can provoke the development of symptoms, even in otherwise normal weather conditions.

Chilblains may occur as an idiopathic primary disorder but also secondary to an underlying disease (Goette 1990; Giusti and Tunnessen 1997; Simon et al. 2005; Maroon 2009). According to Weston and Morelli (2000), it is rare in childhood. According to Simon et al. (2005), it is most frequently seen in young women, although it may occur in children and the elderly.

The symptoms of chilblains may give rise to erroneously suspected child abuse (Kos and Shwayder 2006; Jenny and Reece 2009).

6.5.3 Frostbite

Frostbite or congelatio is defined as the freezing and crystallizing of fluids in the interstitial and cellular spaces due to prolonged exposure to freezing temperatures (Cheng et al. 2008). Frostbite leads to tissue destruction due to the direct damage to the cells and indirect damage secondary to vasospasm and arterial thromboses (Golant et al. 2008).

The risk of frostbite occurs when the temperature drops to 0°C or below. In temperatures below zero, the intradermal blood flow is reduced to such an extent that the skin is at risk for freezing (Cheng et al. 2008). The skin temperature drops about 0.5°C per minute after the blood flow has stopped (Cheng et al. 2008).

The body's extremities, such as fingers, hands, toes, feet, ears, nose, and cheeks, are most susceptible to frostbite (Figs. 6.80 and 6.81). The vasoconstriction in the skin enhances this effect and will

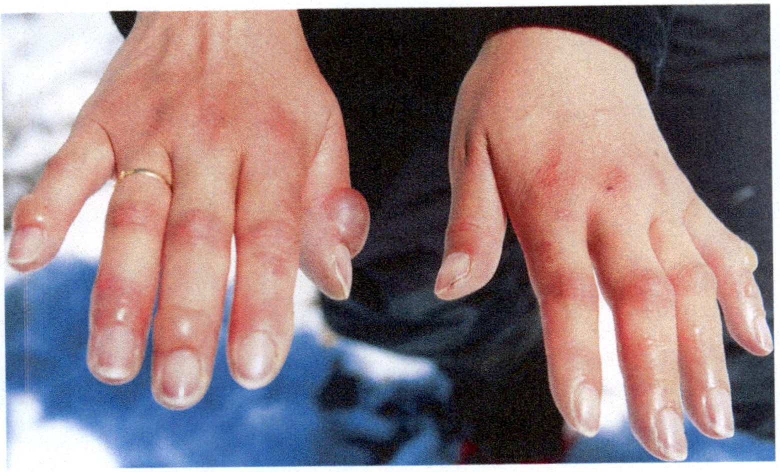

Fig. 6.80 Frostbite in an adult (Winky 2005 from Wikimedia Commons 2011: Frostbite.jpg)

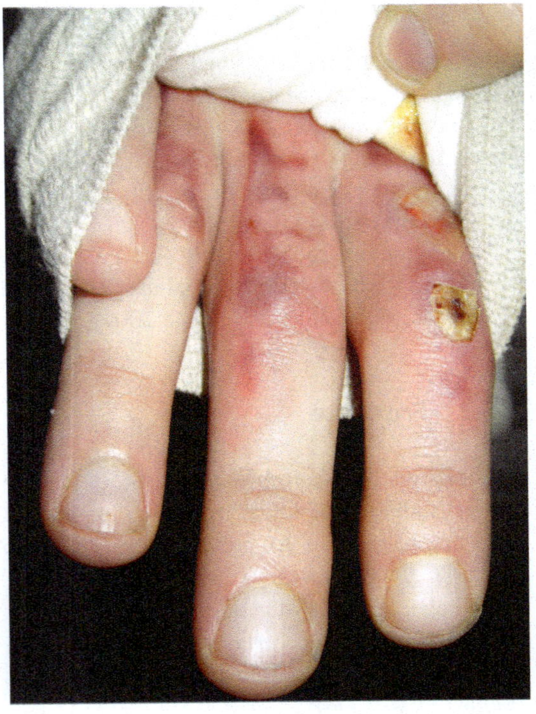

Fig. 6.81 Frostbite (Eli Duke 2010 from Wikimedia Commons 2011: Injuries at Antarctica – ouch!.jpg) (= Fig. 2.44)

lead to an increased risk of frostbite in temperatures below 0°C. In less severe frostbite, only the most peripheral body parts are affected, including the tips of the fingers and toes or the most exposed body parts, such as cheeks, nose, and ears. Indicative dating of lesions in frostbite is shown in Table 6.3.

Table 6.3 Dating of frostbite

Time course	Findings
First hour	Endothelial leakage
First 6 h	Erythrocyte extravasation
Within 6–24 h	Leukocyte migration and vasculitis
Within 1–2 weeks	Medial degeneration, loss of intracellular attachments, and vacuolization of keratinocytes

Cheng et al. (2008)

The severity of frostbite depends, besides the temperature, on factors such as length of exposure, windchill factor/wind speed, altitude, dampness, and the type of clothing worn (Golant et al. 2008).

Frostbite injury to the hands and feet of a child can have long-term sequelae, namely, premature fusion, destruction, and abnormal growth in the epiphyseal cartilage (Reed 1988; Crouch and Smith 1990; Golant et al. 2008).

6.5.4 Accidental Versus Non-accidental Cold Injuries

6.5.4.1 Child Abuse and Neglect

Although usually resulting from an accidental cause, cold injuries in children is basically a completely preventable injury. For this reason, in children with cold injuries, one should always investigate the possibility of serious physical neglect, for example, inadequate protection against cold (abandonment, lack of shelter, inadequate clothing, and/or wet clothing, possibly combined with malnutrition or exhaustion) or less frequently, physical abuse (Mehta 1982; Gustavson and Levitt 1996; Laming 2003; Green 2009).

6.5.4.2 Self-Inflicted Cold Injuries

Lacour and Le Coultre (1991) describe a boy of 8.5 years with a deep frostbite. The freezing was caused by improper use of a toilet air refreshener, which the boy sprayed directly on his skin. The temperature of the aerosol during spraying turned out to be minus 40°C. The propellants in the spray were propane and butane.

Several authors draw attention to the risk of oral and orofacial frostbite caused by inhalant abuse, often containing fluorinated hydrocarbon propellants (Elliott 1991; Anderson and Loomis 2003).

6.5.4.3 Other Skin Reactions Due to Low Temperatures

Popsicle panniculitis is predominantly seen in summer and characterized by a local inflammatory response to cold exposure, secondary to holding popsicles in the corner of the mouth (Jenny and Reece 2009). This type of panniculitis is characterized by non-painful bruising, swelling, and induration, especially in the corner of the mouth, spreading to the cheeks (Day and Klein 1992; van Wie 2008). Popsicle panniculitis may be confused with bruising and swelling due to child abuse (slapping or gagging).

Jaddoe and Oranje (2008) reported a young boy with "blue ears," which initially were not diagnosed. The cause was found to be a chronic persistent Mycoplasma infection (Figs. 6.82, 6.83, and 6.84).

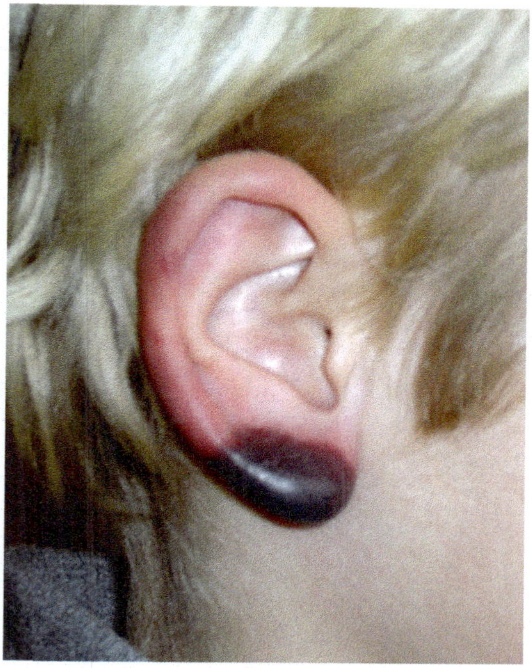

Fig. 6.82 "Blue ears" (purpura) due to a chronic persistent Mycoplasma infection

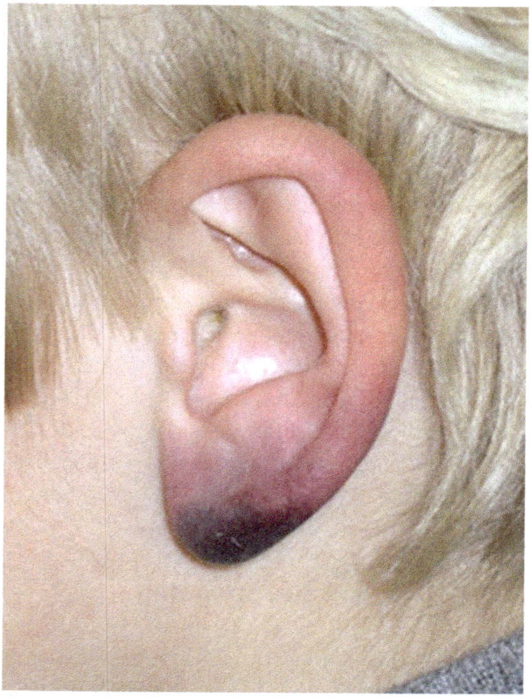

Fig. 6.83 "Blue ears" (purpura) due to a chronic persistent Mycoplasma infection

6.6 Artifacts Caused by Traditional Medicine and Cultural Practices

Traditional medicine and cultural practices do often present in the pediatric population with cutaneous manifestations (Ravanfar and Dinulos

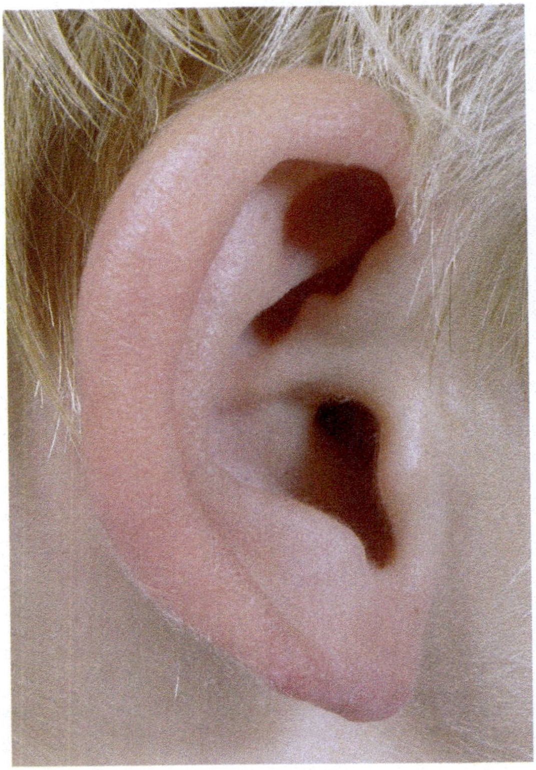

Fig. 6.84 Same child as in Fig. 6.82: as a result, the child lost the tips of both ears

2010). If not recognized, the skin findings may be misinterpreted as injuries caused by child abuse. The suspicion may even increase if these manifestations are patterned, which is usual in skin manifestations of cultural practices.

Generally, cultural practices are not considered to be abusive, although they can result in bruising and burns. Parents do not intend to harm their children but to treat them according to their traditional methods. The differential diagnosis of abusive burns and scalds from burns resulting from traditional medicine will not be discussed here.

6.6.1 Coining and Spooning

Coining (coin rubbing or cao gio) and spooning (spoon rubbing or quat sha/gua sha) are traditional medical habits practiced by the Vietnamese and the Chinese. It is used in the treatment of fever, com-

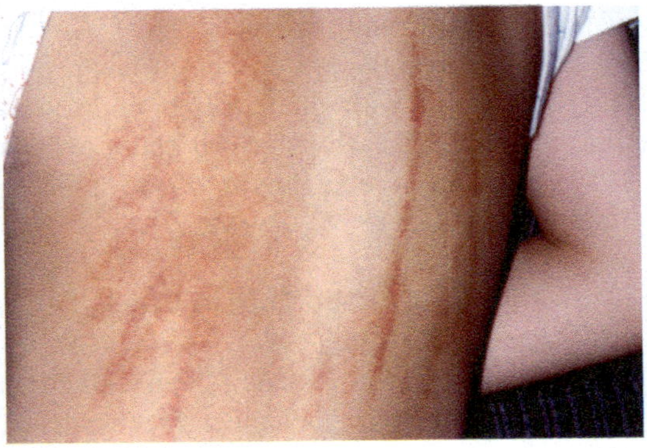

Fig. 6.85 Coining

mon cold, and headaches. The chest and the back are lubricated with warm oil and are forcefully massaged downward and sideways with the edge of a worn coin, a spoon, or other objects with a rounded edge, for example, an animal bone, a water buffalo bone, a piece of jade (Ravanfar and Dinulos 2010). This leads to the development of bilateral, symmetrical linear hematomas or multiple petechiae or purpura that show a sharp border with the normal skin (Figs. 6.85, 6.86, and 6.87) (Nong The Anh 1976; Yeatman et al. 1976; Yeatman and Dang 1980; Feldman 1984; Rosenblat and Hong 1989; Stewart and Rosenberg 1996). Coining or spooning probably causes no pain or inconvenience to the patient and leaves no scars, or at least pain and inconvenience from the procedure is denied (Ravanfar and Dinulos 2010). Scars are found when deep burn wounds develop, which have never been described in children (Amshel and Caruso 2000).

Quat sha is another traditional medical habit comparable with cao gio. Instead of a coin, a spoon is used (Stewart and Rosenberg 1996). The resulting appearance will be the same as in coin rubbing (Figs. 6.88, 6.89, and 6.90).

The cutaneous manifestations of coining and spooning have been misinterpreted as bruising caused by child abuse (Primosch and Young 1980; David et al. 1986; Davis 2000).

6.6.2 Cupping

Cupping is a traditional medical habit, particularly in Russia and other Eastern European

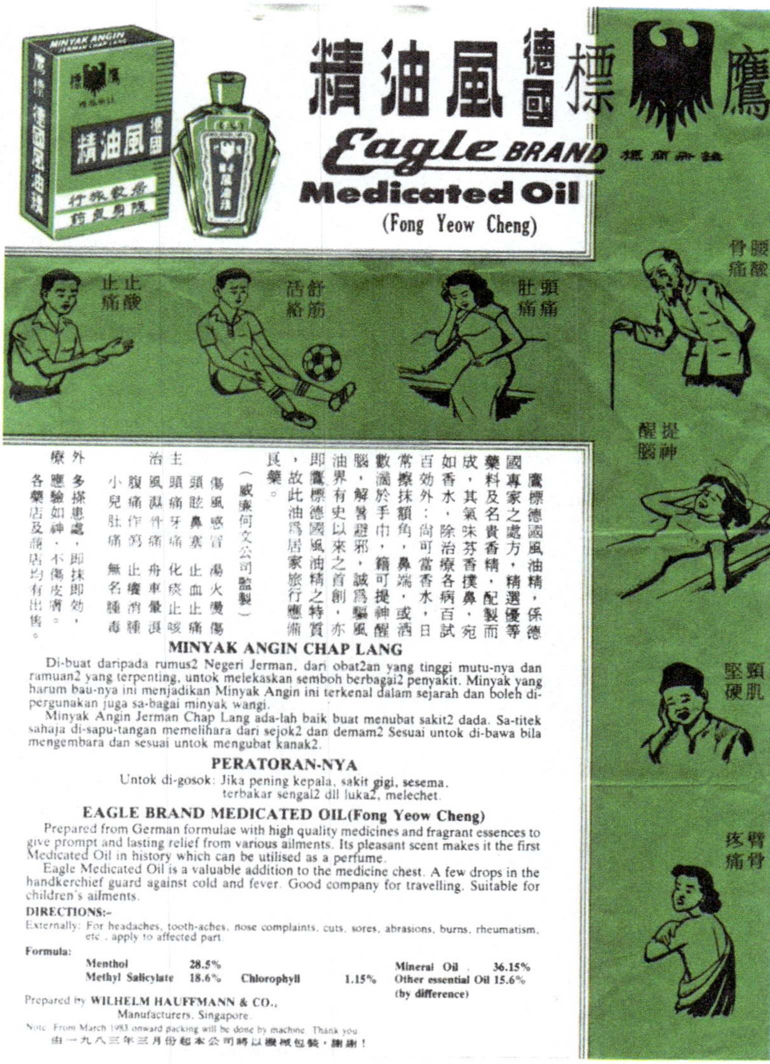

Fig. 6.86 Leaflet of an oil brand used in coining

countries, but recently seems to be adopted by the celebrity. It is also used in Latin America and Asia. It is used to alleviate pain. A cup or a glass is warmed and placed onto the skin, usually on the trunk. A vacuum develops as soon as the cup or the glass cools down. Erythematous patches with defined borders develop as a result of the vacuum (Sandler and Haynes 1978; Asnes and Wisotsky 1981; Feldman 1984; Stewart and Rosenberg 1996). Eventually a circular purpura factitia may develop. Similar to cao gio, cupping should cause no pain and inconvenience to the child and leaves no scars. However, a circular burn may result if the cup or the glass is too hot. A blister may eventually arise in the middle of the burn (Sandler and Haynes 1978; Asnes and Wisotsky 1981; Look and Look 1997). In a variation called "wet cupping," the skin is abraded first (Look and Look 1997) (Figs. 6.91, 6.92, 6.93, 6.94, 6.95, 6.96, and 6.97).

6.6.3 Tui na

Tui na (translated: push and grasp) is a form of Chinese massage often used together with other

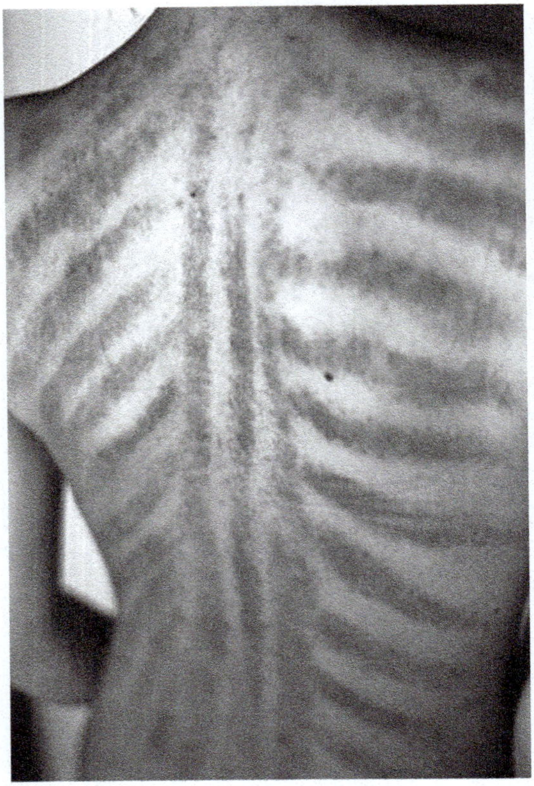

Fig. 6.87 Coining

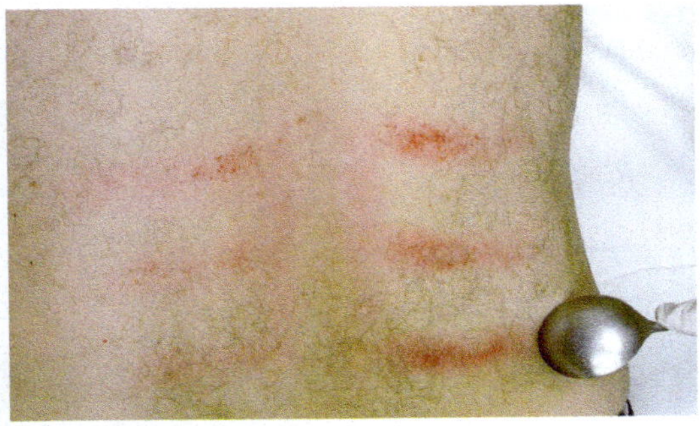

Fig. 6.88 Vietnamese spooning

types of traditional medicine and cultural practices, for example, acupuncture, moxibustion, cupping, and herbalism (Wikipedia 2011) (Figs. 6.98 and 6.99). Ribeiro et al. (2010) presented a Chinese boy of 10 years who was evaluated because of the presence of suspicious bruises on his body, which eventually could be explained to result from Tui na.

6.7 Artifacts: Other Causes

6.7.1 Purpura Factitia and Other Artificial Causes of Bruising and Petechiae

Purpura factitia may develop by a vacuum created by placing a cup, cap of a pen, or something similar on the skin or through a hickey (Lovejoy

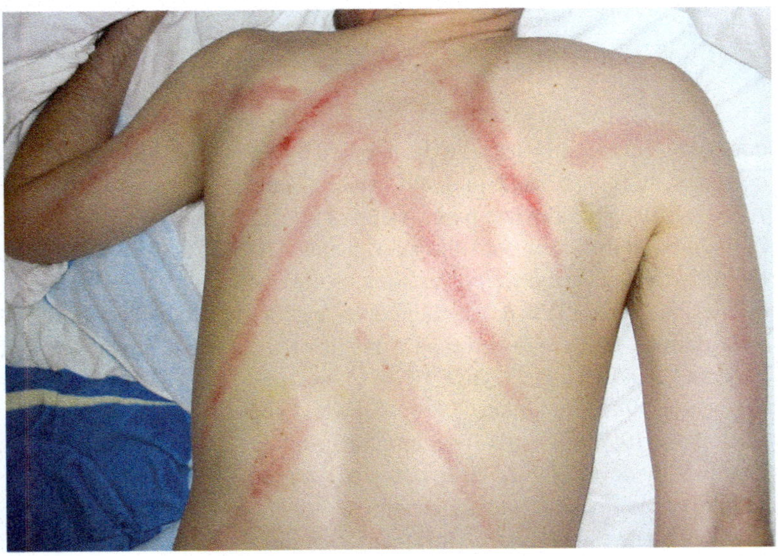

Fig. 6.89 Spooning (Gua sha) in an adult, as practiced in Indonesia: not only on the back but also on the arms (Loder 2008 from Wikimedia Commons 2011: Gua Sha.jpg)

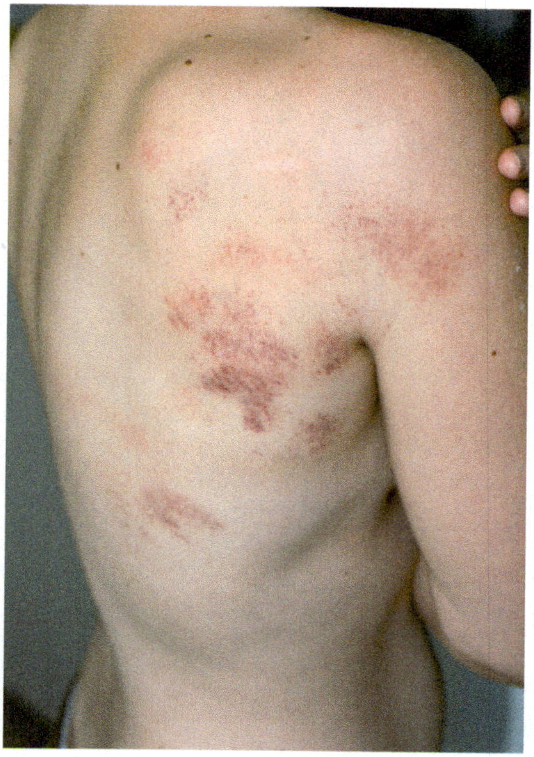

Fig. 6.90 Spooning (Gua sha) in an adult (Amy Selleck 2007, Flickr.com)

et al. 1971) (Sec. 5.7). The presence of a hickey (a suction mark) and a bitemark may indicate sexual abuse (Sec. 3.3.3).

Multiple petechiae on the face and the neck result from a severe rise in intravascular pressure as can occur in severe vomiting or coughing (as in whooping cough) or mechanical asphyxiation (Sect. 3.3). This is probably related due to a sudden increase in pressure in the vena cava superior. Petechiae and purpura may eventually also develop in the mouth and on the conjunctivae.

Purpura on the soft palate may also follow forceful sucking on sweets, fellatio in sexual abuse, and glandular fever (Schmitt 1987).

Petechiae may also be observed following use of a tourniquet or sphygmomanometer cuff, particularly in children who already have an erythematous disorder or a bleeding disorder with thrombocytopenia (Schmitt 1987; Lee 2008; Chap. 5). Occasional petechiae may be seen in normal children (Downes et al. 2002; Sect. 3.3.2) and can be a feature of many disorders (Sect. 3.3).

6.7.2 Hair-Thread Tourniquet Syndrome

The hair-thread tourniquet syndrome is a relatively common and well-described phenomenon in infants and children. It is characterized by the tight wrapping of a hair or hairlike fiber around an end-perfusion appendage, leading to a sharp circumferential demarcation (Barton et al. 1988; Alverson 2007). The wrapping of the hair or hairlike fiber around an appendage is thought to result from repetitive movement of the appendage in a confined area, for example, in a mitten, pajamas, diaper, or underpants (Bothner 2003).

The hair-thread tourniquet syndrome involves toes (Barton et al. 1988; Vázquez Rueda et al. 1996; Strahlman 2003; Haene and Loeffler 2007), sometimes multiple toes and bilateral (Mackey et al. 2005), fingers (Hack and Brish 1972; Wang and Schott 2001; Kumaravel 2008), wrist (Cardriche 2009), tongue (Cardriche 2009), uvula (Krishna and Paul 2003), ear lobe (Cardriche 2009), umbilicus (Cardriche 2009), nipple (Cardriche 2009), penis (Toguri et al. 1979; Garty et al. 1983; Vázquez Rueda et al. 1996; Hussain 2008; Okeke 2008), scrotum (Cardriche 2009), clitoris (Rich and Keating 1999; Alverson 2007; Serour et al. 2007), and labia majora (Golshevsky et al. 2005) and minora (Bacon and Burgis 2005; Pomeranz et al. 2009) (Figs. 6.100, 6.101, and 6.102).

Excessive crying, redness and swelling of the appendage distal to the tourniquet, pain, and sometimes necrosis and auto-amputation may be found. Amputation has been found in toes, fingers, penis (shaft or glans) (Thomas et al. 1977; Sheinfeld et al. 1985), and clitoris (Kuo et al. 2002).

Most cases are found in infants and young children. Toe and finger tourniquets are mainly seen from as early as shortly after birth up to almost 2 years (Barton et al. 1988). Penis tourniquets

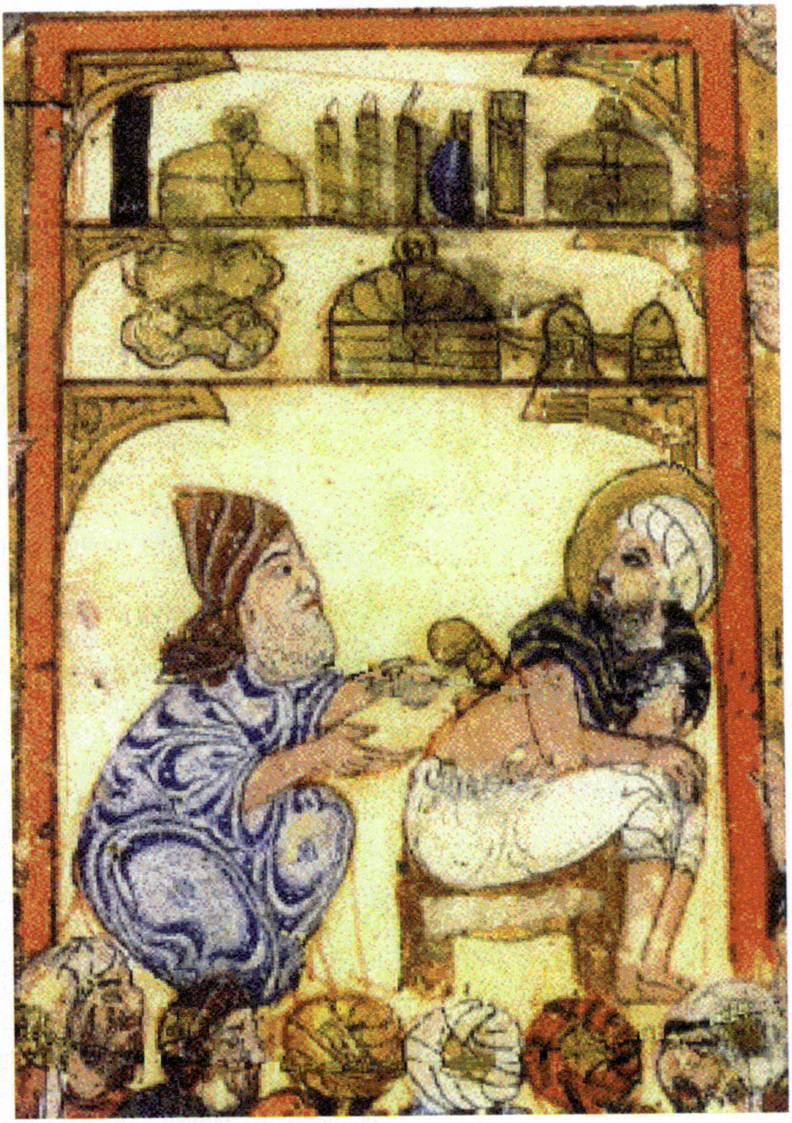

Fig. 6.91 Cupping

are most prevalent in young boys between 4 months and 6 years (Barton et al. 1988), although it has also been seen in an adolescent (Pantuck et al. 1997). Labial and clitoral wrapping have been described in girls between 4 years and 14 years (Rich and Keating 1999; Bacon and Burgis 2005; Alverson 2007; Serour et al. 2007).

Tourniquet syndrome has been described both in non-abused and abused children (Biehler et al. 1994). Most cases of hair-thread tourniquet syndrome are considered to be non-inflicted (accidental). However, the findings may be misinterpreted as an intentionally inflicted injury by nonmedical personnel or inexperienced medical personnel (Oates 1984; Biehler et al.

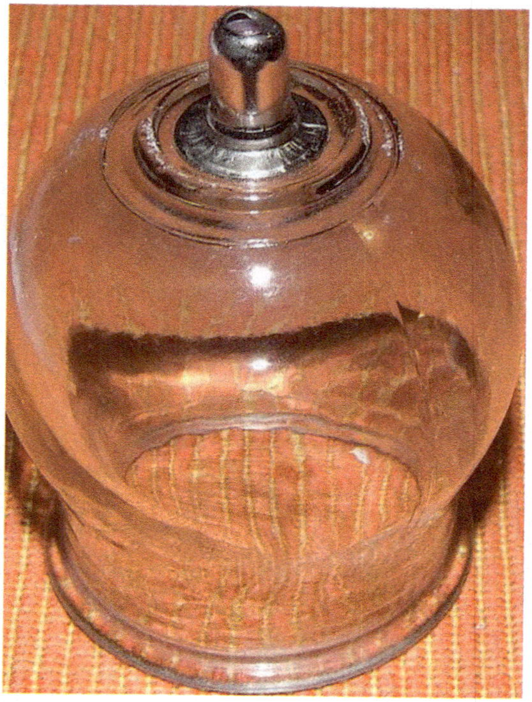

Fig. 6.92 Cupping: a vacuum cup (Śmietanka 2006 from Wikimedia Commons 2011: Vacuum suction close up.jpg)

1994; Lohana et al. 2006). Children with inflicted tourniquet syndrome have been described in the medical literature; so, child abuse can and should not be excluded without further investigation (Johnson 1988; Kornberg 1992). Mhiri et al. (1987) states that hair-thread tourniquet is more frequently seen in socially disadvantaged children, suggesting that perhaps some kind of neglect or lack of hygiene could play a role. Failure to seek prompt medical care should attract concern.

Because of the lack of any reasonable explanation and the meticulous wrapping, Klusmann and Lenard (2004) suggest that hair-thread tourniquet syndrome is often the result of child abuse. They conclude that child abuse should be included in the differential diagnosis of the cause of the hair-thread tourniquet syndrome until another etiology can be proven convincingly. According to Sudhan et al. (2000), most cases of toe or finger wrapping tend to be non-inflicted, whereas when wrapping in the genital area is found, it could indicate inflicted injuries. According to Hobbs et al. (1993), involvement of the penis may indicate sexual abuse.

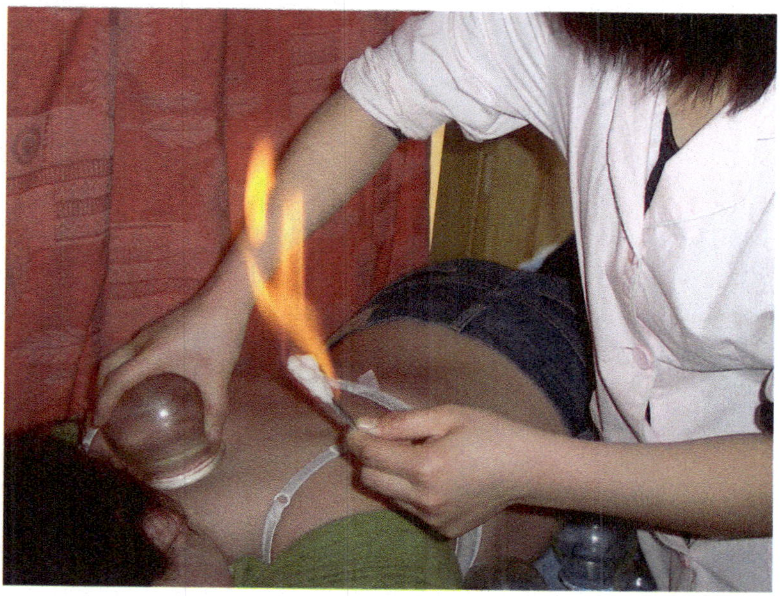

Fig. 6.93 Fire cupping (Ralph 2004 from WikiMedia Commons 2011: Fire Cupping.jpg)

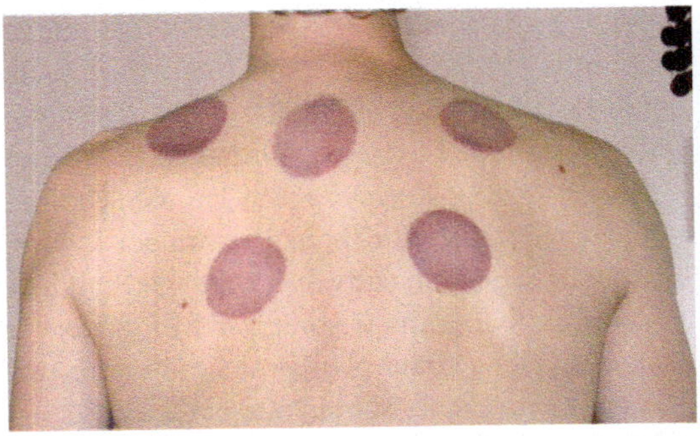

Fig. 6.94 Fire cupping: the result (Bentevb 2007 from Wikimedia Commons 2011: Cupping results.jpg)

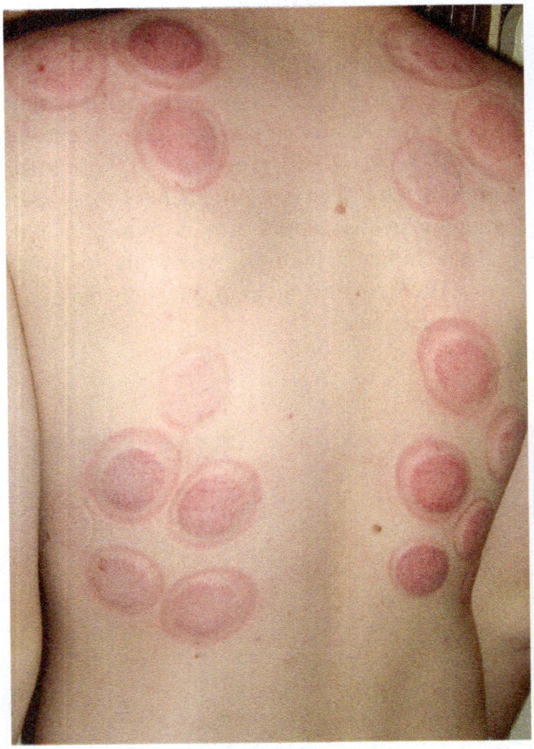

Fig. 6.95 Fire cupping (Piotrus 2010 from Wikimedia Commons 2011: Ślady po bańkach.JPG)

A case of a physical abuse-related tourniquet syndrome, which could be proven beyond reasonable doubt, is reported by Tournel et al. (2006). The authors describe a 3-year-old boy who had been abused by his mother's boyfriend. The boyfriend wrapped the boy's penis and perforated the boy's eyes with a knife, masquerading

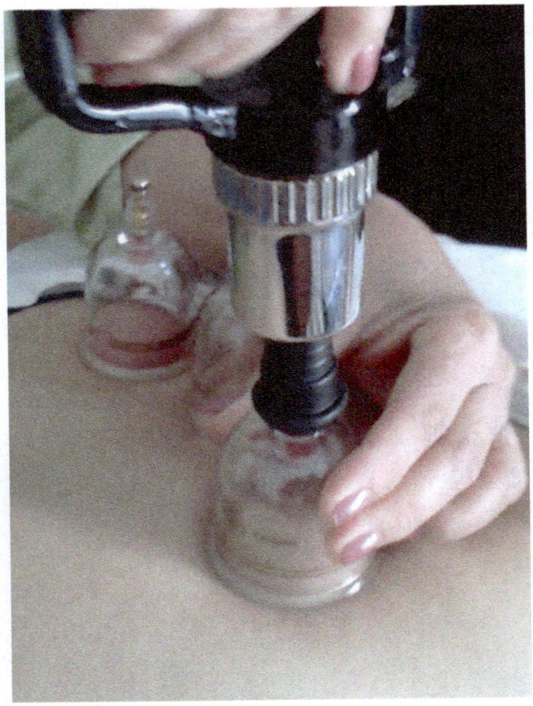

Fig. 6.96 Vietnamese cupping: vacuum cupping

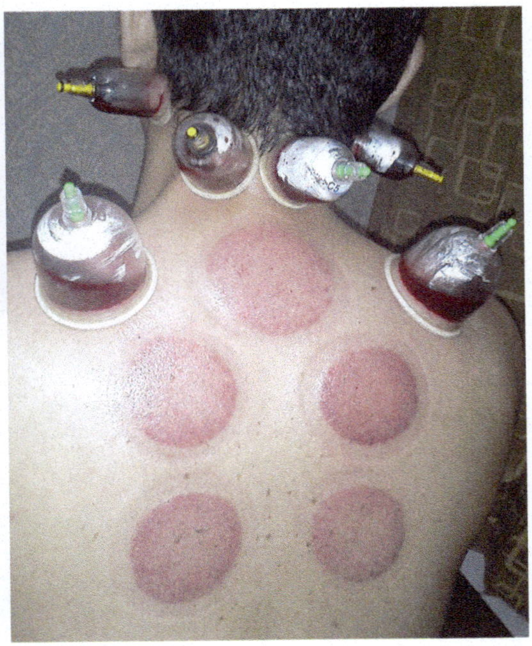

Fig. 6.97 Wet cupping (Hijama) (Iwansw 2011 from Wikimedia Commons 2011: Hijama therapy1.jpg)

the perforation by using previous surgical and infectious lesions.

6.7.2.1 Ink, Crayon, Paint, or Dyes

Wheeler and Hobbs (1988) reported that dyes on the face may erroneously lead to suspected child abuse. Also clothing dyes, especially the dyes in often new and unwashed jeans (blue, gray, or black), may lead to a bluish-blue gray discoloration/rash of the skin, which may be confused with abuse-related bruising. The discoloration will be found on places with the closest contact between the clothing and the skin, for example, the hands, the thighs and abdomen, and the legs and hips (Harris et al. 1984; Lantner and Ros 1991; Leiferman and Gleich 1991; Predescu 2004). It is seen in children as young as 18 months (Lantner and Ros 1991) up to adolescence (Predescu 2004). Removing the dye with soap and water is often not possible, so the discoloration will persist after bathing (Predescu 2004). In general, alcohol will be effective to remove the dye.

6.8 Rarely Reported Non-Disease-Related Skin Findings

An overview of skin lesions in the differential diagnosis, which are not disease-related and are only rarely reported in the medical literature is given in Table 6.4.

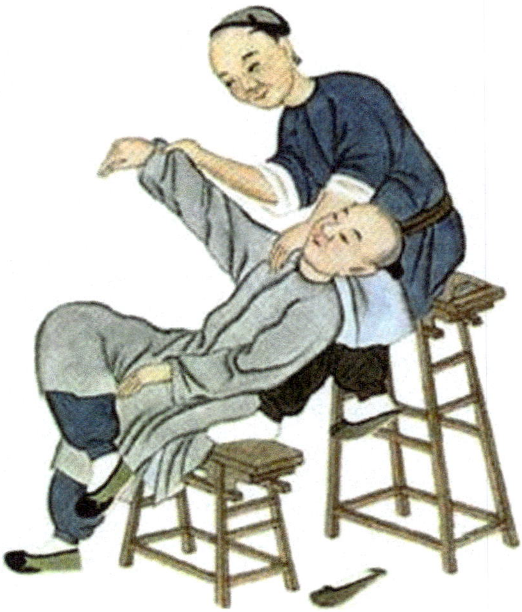

Fig. 6.98 Tui na

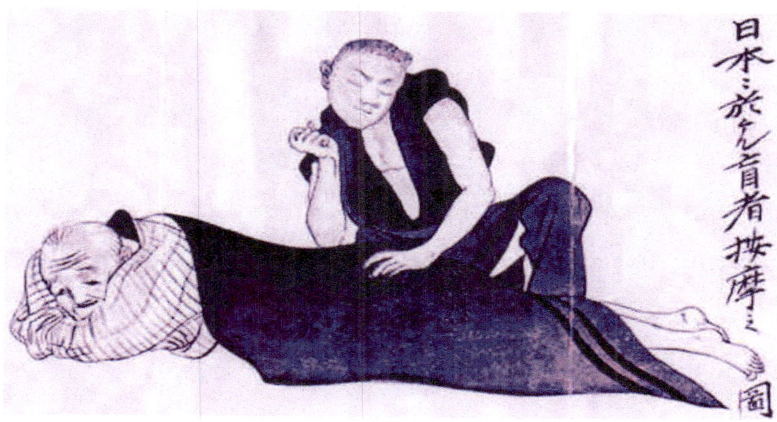

Fig. 6.99 Tui na

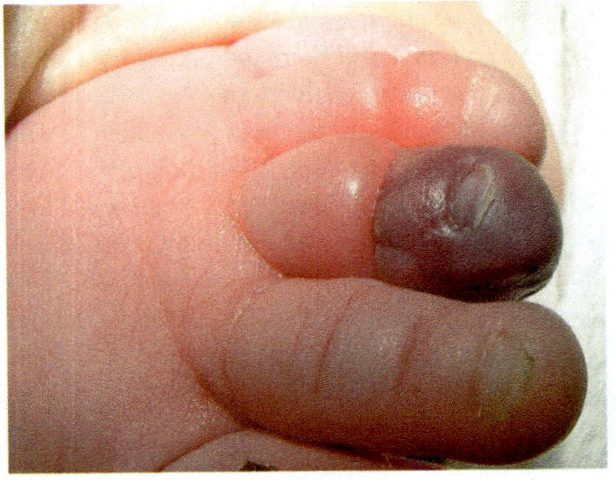

Fig. 6.100 Hair tourniquet syndrome of two toes

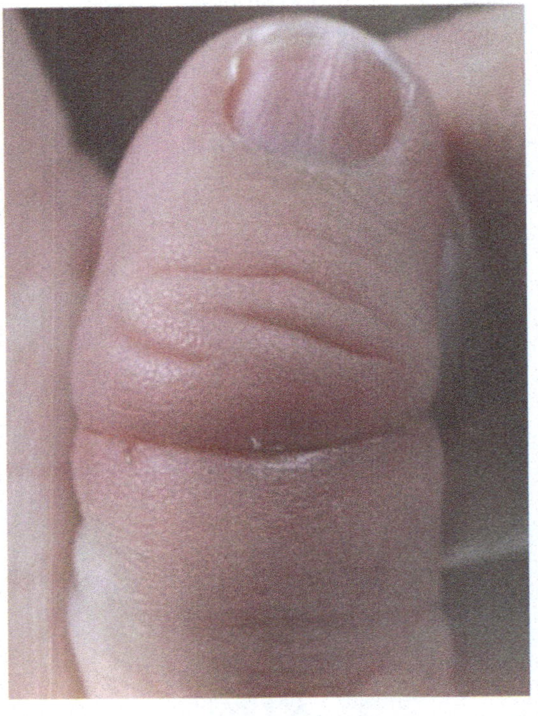

Fig. 6.101 Hair tourniquet syndrome of a thumb

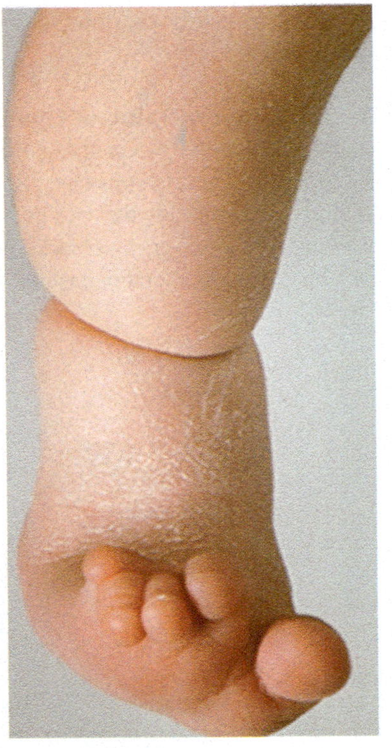

Fig. 6.102 Intrauterine ligature

Table 6.4 Rarely reported non-disease-related skin findings

Cause	Symptoms	Author
Prominent facial veins	Bruising	Wheeler and Hobbs (1988)
Dental treatment	Facial bruising	Wheeler and Hobbs (1988)
EMLA cream application	Petechial eruption	Calobrisi et al. (1998); de Waard-van der Spek and Oranje (1997)
Calcium chloride necrosis	Bruising with deep dermal thigh necrosis caused by percutaneous penetration of calcium chloride (an industrial defrosting calcium salt, also an ingredient of many commercially available deicers)	Zurbuchen et al. (1996)
Brown recluse spider bite	Bruising with ulcerating	Newcomer and Young (1993)
Postmortem cockroach bites	Strangulation-like "bruising" in the neck and burn-like findings	Denic (1997)

References

Adler R, Kane-Nussen B (1983) Erythema multiforme: confusion with child battering syndrome. Pediatrics 72(5):718–720

AlJasser M, Al-Khenaizan S (2008) Cutaneous mimickers of child abuse: a primer for pediatricians. Eur J Pediatr 167(11):1221–1230

Alverson B (2007) A genital hair tourniquet in a 9-year-old girl. Pediatr Emerg Care 23(3):169–170

Amshel CE, Caruso DM (2000) Vietnamese "coining": a burn case report and literature review. J Burn Care Rehabil 21(2):112–114

Anderson CE, Loomis GA (2003) Recognition and prevention of inhalant abuse. Am Fam Physician 68(5):869–874

Asnes RS (1984) Buttock bruises – Mongolian spot. Pediatrics 74(2):321

Asnes RS, Wisotsky DH (1981) Cupping lesions simulating child abuse. J Pediatr 99(2):267–268

Bacon JL, Burgis JT (2005) Hair thread tourniquet syndrome in adolescents: a presentation and review of the literature. J Pediatr Adolesc Gynecol 18(3): 155–156

Barradell R, Addo A, McDonagh AJG et al (1993) Phytophotodermatitis mimicking child abuse. Eur J Pediatr 152(4):291–292

Barton DJ, Sloan GM, Nichter LS et al (1988) Hair-thread tourniquet syndrome. Pediatrics 82(6):925–928

Biehler JL, Sieck C, Bonner B et al (1994) A survey of health care and child protective services provider knowledge regarding the Toe Tourniquet syndrome. Child Abuse Negl 18(11):987–993

Bohdiewicz PJ, Gallegos E, Fink-Bennett D (1995) Raccoon eyes and the MIBG super scan: scintigraphic signs of neuroblastoma in a case of suspected child abuse. Pediatr Radiol 25(Suppl 1):S90–S92

Bothner J (2003) Hair entrapment removal techniques. Accessed on 2010

Brown J, Melinkovich P (1986) Schönlein-Henoch purpura misdiagnosed as suspected child abuse. JAMA 256(5):617–618

Calişkan S, Taşdan Y, Kasapçopur O et al (1995) Picture of the month. Acute hemorrhagic edema of infancy. Arch Pediatr Adolesc Med 149(11):1267–1268

Calobrisi SD, Drolet BA, Esterly NB (1998) Petechial eruption after the application of EMLA cream. Pediatrics 101(3 Pt 1):471–473

Cantatore-Francis JL, Cohen-Pfeffer J, Balwani M et al (2010) Hepatoerythropoietic porphyria misdiagnosed as child abuse: cutaneous, arthritic, and hematologic manifestations in siblings with a novel UROD mutation. Arch Dermatol 146(5):529–533

Cardriche D, Doty CI (2009) Hair tourniquet removal. eMedicine http://emedicine.medscape.com/article/1348969-overview. Accessed on 2011

Carlsen K, Weismann K (2007) Phytophotodermatitis in 19 children admitted to hospital and their differential diagnoses: child abuse and herpes simplex virus infection. J Am Acad Dermatol 57(5 Suppl):S88–S91

Cheng D, Thompson TM, Yakobi R (2008) Frostbite. eMedicine http://emedicine.medscape.com/article/926249-overview. Accessed on 2010

Ciarallo L, Paller AS (1997) Two cases of incontinentia pigmenti simulating child abuse. Pediatrics 100(4):E6

Coffman K, Boyce T, Hansen RC (1985) Phytophotodermatitis simulating child abuse. Am J Dis Child 139(3):239–240

Cordova A (1981) The Mongolian spot: a study of ethnic differences and a literature review. Clin Pediatr (Phila) 20(11):714–719

Crouch C, Smith WL (1990) Long term sequelae of frostbite. Pediatr Radiol 20(5):365–366

Daly KC, Siegel RM (1998) Henoch-Schöenlein purpura in a child at risk of abuse. Arch Pediatr Adolesc Med 152(1):96–98

Dannaker CJ, Glover RA, Goltz RW (1988) Phytophotodermatitis. A mystery case report. Clin Pediatr (Phila) 27(6):289–290

David A, Mechinaud F, Roze JC, Stalder JF (1986) A case of Cao-Gio. Possible confusion with abuse. [Article in French]. Arch Fr Pediatr 43(2):147

Davis RE (2000) Cultural health care or child abuse? The Southeast Asian practice of cao gio. J Am Acad Nurse Pract 12(3):89–95

Day S, Klein BL (1992) Popsicle panniculitis. Pediatr Emerg Care 8(2):91–93

de Waard-van der Spek FB, Oranje AP (1997) Purpura caused by Emla is of toxic origin. Contact Dermatitis 36(1):11–13

Denic N, Huyer DW, Sinal SH et al (1997) Cockroach: the omnivorous scavenger. Potential misinterpretation of postmortem injuries. Am J Forensic Med Pathol 18(2):177–180

Dober I, Stranzinger E, Kellenberger CJ et al (2007) [Periorbital ecchymosis–trauma or tumor?] [Article in German]. Praxis (Bern 1994) 96(20):811–814

Downes AJ, Crossland DS, Mellon AF (2002) Prevalence and distribution of petechiae in well babies. Arch Dis Child 86(4):291–292

Drolet BA, Esterly NB, Frieden IJ (1999) *Hemangiomas* in Children. N Engl J Med 341(3):173–181

Edlich RF, Long WB (2008) Cold injuries. eMedicine http://emedicine.medscape.com/article/1278523-overview. Accessed on 2010

Elliott DC (1991) Frostbite of the mouth: a case report. Mil Med 156(1):18–19

Feldman KW (1984) Pseudoabusive burns in Asian refugees. Am J Dis Child 138(8):768–769

Furniss D, Adams T (2007) Herb of grace: An unusual cause of phytophotodermatitis mimicking burn injury. J Burn Care Res 28(5):767–769

Garty BZ, Mimouni M, Varsano I (1983) Penile tourniquet syndrome. Cutis 31(4):431–432

Giusti R, Tunnessen WW (1997) Picture of the month: Chilblains (pernio). Arch Pediatr Adolesc Med 151(10):1055–1056

Goette DK (1990) Chilblains (perniosis). J Am Acad Dermatol 23(2 Pt 1):257–262

Golant A, Nord RM, Paksima N et al (2008) Cold exposure injuries to the extremities. J Am Acad Orthop Surg 16(12):704–715

Golshevsky J, Chuen J, Tung PH (2005) Hair-thread tourniquet syndrome. J Paediatr Child Health 41(3): 154–155

Gordon EM, Bernat JR, Ramos-Caro FA (1998) Urticaria pigmentosa mistaken for child abuse. Pediatr Dermatol 15(6):484–485

Green S (2009) Charges: Woman caused frostbite by making boy stick hand out window. Portage Daily Register, http://portagedailyregister.com/news/local/article_38cc0956-1376-11de-a474-001cc4c002e0.html. Accessed on 2010

Greig AV, Harris DL (2003) A study of perceptions of facial hemangiomas in professionals involved in child abuse surveillance. Pediatr Dermatol 20(1):1–4

Gruson LM, Chang MW (2002) Berloque dermatitis mimicking child abuse. Arch Pediatr Adolesc Med 156(11):1091–1093

Gustavson E, Levitt C (1996) Physical abuse with severe hypothermia. Arch Pediatr Adolesc Med 150(1): 111–112

Hack M, Brish M (1972) A finger equivalent of the toe tourniquet syndrome. Pediatrics 50(2):348–349

Haene RA, Loeffler M (2007) Hair tourniquet syndrome in an infant. J Bone Joint Surg Br 89B(2):244–245

Harris CR, Evans D, Mariano C (1984) Blue jean hands syndrome. Ann Emerg Med 13(1):67

Hill PF, Pickford M, Parkhouse N (1997) Phytophotodermatitis mimicking child abuse. J R Soc Med 90(10):560–561

Hobbs CJ, Hanks HGI, Wynne JM (1993) Physical abuse. In: Hobbs CJ, Hanks HGI, Wynne JM (eds) Child abuse and neglect – a clinician's handbook. Churchill Livingstone, Edinburgh, pp 47–75

Hobbs CJ, Hanks HGI, Wynne JM (1999) Physical abuse. In: Hobbs CJ, Hanks HGI, Wynne JM (eds) Child abuse and neglect – a clinician's handbook, 2nd edn. Churchill Livingstone, London/New York, pp 63–104

Hussain HM (2008) A hair tourniquet resulting in strangulation and amputation of penis: case report and literature review. J Paediatr Child Health 44(10):606–607

Irvine A (2006) Section 19.12 ectodermal dysplasias. In: Harper J, Oranje A, Prose N (eds) Textbook of pediatric dermatology, 2nd edn. Blackwell Publishing, Oxford, pp 1412–1466

Jacobs AH, Walton RG (1976) Incidence of birthmarks in the neonate. Pediatrics 58(2):218–222

Jaddoe VC, Oranje AP (2008) [Diagnostic image (388). A boy with blue ears]. Ned Tijdschr Geneeskd 152(36):1972

Jenny C, Reece RM (2009) Cutaneous manifestations of child abuse. In: Reece RM, Christian CW (eds) Child abuse, medical diagnosis and management, 3rd edn. American Academy of Pediatrics, Elk Grove Village, pp 18–51

Johnson CF (1988) Constricting bands. Manifestations of possible child abuse Case reports and a review. Clin Pediatr (Phila) 27(9):439–444

Kirschner RH, Stein RJ (1985) The mistaken diagnosis of child abuse. A form of medical abuse? Am J Dis Child 139(9):873–875

Klusmann A, Lenard HG (2004) Tourniquet syndrome – accident or abuse? Eur J Pediatr 163(8):495–498

Kornberg AE (1992) Skin and soft tissue injuries. In: Uit Ludwig S, Kornberg AE (eds) Child abuse – a medical reference, 2nd edn. Churchill Livingstone, New York, pp 91–104

Kos L, Shwayder T (2006) Cutaneous manifestations of child abuse. Pediatr Dermatol 23(4):311–320

Krishna S, Paul RI (2003) Hair tourniquet of the uvula. J Emerg Med 24(3):325–326

Kumaravel S (2008) Chronic nonhealing ulcer in a finger of a toddler–a rare presentation of the hair thread tourniquet syndrome. Int J Dermatol 47(11):1174–1176

Kung AC, Stephens MB, Darling T (2009) Phytophotodermatitis: bulla formation and hyperpigmentation during spring break. Mil Med 174(6):657–661

Kuo JH, Smith LM, Berkowitz CD (2002) A hair tourniquet resulting in strangulation and amputation of the clitoris. Obstet Gynecol 99(5 Pt 2):939–941
Labbe L, Perel Y, Maleville J et al (1996) Erythema nodosum in children: a study in 27 patients. Pediatr Dermatol 13(6):447–450
Lacour M, Le Coultre C (1991) Spray-induced frostbite in a child: a new hazard with novel aerosol propellants. Pediatr Dermatol 8(3):207–209
Lagey K, Duinslaeger L, Vanderkelen A (1995) Burns induced by plants. Burns 21(7):542–543
Laming H (2003) The Victoria Climbié inquiry. Report of an inquiry. Presented to Parliament by the Secretary of State for Health and the Secretary of State for the Home Department by Command of Her Majesty, January 2003 http://www.victoria-climbie-inquiry.org.uk/
Lantner RR, Ros SP (1991) Blue jeans thighs. Pediatrics 88(2):417
Lawrence EJ (2005) The clinical presentation of Ehlers-Danlos syndrome. Adv Neonatal Care 5(6):301–314
Leaute-Labreze C, Mortureux P, Taieb A (2006) Section 9.1 urticaria. In: Harper J, Oranje A, Prose N (eds) Textbook of pediatric dermatology, 2nd edn. Blackwell Publishing, Oxford, pp 689–702
Lee ACW (2008) Bruises, blood coagulation tests and the battered child syndrome. Singapore Med J 49(6):445–450
Legrain V, Taieb A (2006) Section 26.4 acute hemorrhagic oedema of the skin in infancy. In: Harper J, Oranje A, Prose N (eds) Textbook of pediatric dermatology, 2nd edn. Blackwell Publishing, Oxford, pp 1897–1901
Leiferman KM, Gleich GJ (1991) The case of the blue boy. Pediatr Dermatol 8(4):354
Leung AK, Kao CP (1999) Extensive Mongolian spots with involvement of the scalp. Pediatr Dermatol 16(5):371–372
Leung AK, Robson WL (2008) Superimposed Mongolian spots. Pediatr Dermatol 25(2):233–235
Levin AV, Selbst SM (1988) Vulvar hemangioma simulating child abuse. Clin Pediatr 27(4):213–215
Lohana P, Vashishta GN, Price N (2006) Toe-tourniquet syndrome: a diagnostic dilemma! Ann R Coll Surg Engl 88(4):W6–W8
Long WB, Edlich RF, Winters KL et al (2005) Cold injuries. J Long Term Eff Med Implants 15(1):67–78
Look KM, Look RM (1997) Skin scraping, cupping, and moxibustion that may mimic physical abuse. J Forensic Sci 42(1):103–105
Lovejoy FH, Marcuse EK, Landrigan PJ (1971) Two examples of purpura factitia. Clin Pediatr (Phila) 10(3):183–184
Mackey S, Hettiaratchy S, Dickinson J (2005) Hair-tourniquet syndrome–multiple toes and bilaterality. Eur J Emerg Med 12(4):191–192
Maroon MS, Hensley D. Pernio (2009) eMedicine http://emedicine.medscape.com/article/1087946-overview. Accessed on 2011
Mayes C, Macleod C (1999) Lesson of the week: when 'NAI' means not actually injured. BMJ 318(7191):1127–1128
Mehta MN (1982) Physical abuse of abandoned children in India. Child Abuse Negl 6(2):171–175
Menter A (1987) Symmetrical purpura doesn't mirror child abuse. JAMA 257(4):486
Mhiri MN, Midassi H, Mezghanni M et al (1987) [Strangulation of glans penis by hair or penis tourniquet syndrome] [Article in French]. Pediatrie 42(5):351–353
Miller K, Hunt R, Chu J et al (2011) Erythema ab igne. Dermatol Online J 17(10):28–29
Newcomer VD, Young EM Jr (1993) Unique wounds and wound emergencies. Dermatol Clin 11(4):715–727
Nong The Anh (1976) 'Pseudo-battered child' syndrome. JAMA 36(20):2288
Oates RK (1984) Overturning the diagnosis of child abuse. Arch Dis Child 59(7):665–666
Okeke LI (2008) Thread embedded into penile tissue over time as an unusual hair thread tourniquet injury to the penis: a case report. J Med Case Reports 2:230
Oranje AP (2010) Management of urticaria and angioedema in children: new trends. G Ital Dermatol Venereol 145(6):771–774
Oranje A, Bilo RAC (2011) Skin signs in child abuse and differential diagnosis. Minerva Pediatr 63(4):319–325
Osburn K, Schosser RH, Everett MA (1987) Congenital pigmented and vascular lesions in newborn infants. J Am Acad Dermatol 16(4):788–792
Pantuck AJ, Fleisher MH, Barone JG (1997) Genital hair strangulation in an uncircumcised boy. Can J Urol 4(4):455
Pomeranz M, Schachter B, Capua T et al (2009) Hair-thread tourniquet syndrome of labia minor. J Pediatr Adolesc Gynecol 22(5):e111–e113
Predescu O (2004) Blue limbs (the importance of history and examination). BMJ 329:349
Primosch RE, Young SK (1980) Pseudobattering of Vietnamese children (cao gio). J Am Dent Assoc 101(1):47–48
Ragosta K (1989) Pediculosis masquerades as child abuse. Pediatr Emerg Care 5(4):253–254
Ravanfar P, Dinulos JG (2010) Cultural practices affecting the skin of children. Curr Opin Pediatr 22(4):423–431
Reed MH (1988) Growth disturbances in the hands following thermal injuries in children. 2. Frostbite. Can Assoc Radiol J 39(2):95–99
Ribeiro CS, Rodrigues F, Ribeiro C, Magalhães T (2010) A case report for differential diagnosis: integrative medicine vs child abuse. Leg Med (Tokyo) 12(6):316–319
Rich M, Keating M (1999) Hair tourniquet syndrome of the clitoris. J Urol 162(1):190–191
Rose SJ (1985) Recognition of child abuse and neglect. Gower Medical Publishing, London
Rosenblat J, Hong P (1989) Coin rolling diagnosed as child abuse. Can Med Assoc J 140(4):417
Sandler AP, Haynes V (1978) Nonaccidental trauma and medical folk belief: a case of cupping. Pediatrics 61(6):921–922
Scaramuzza A, Pezzarossa E, Zambelloni C et al (1997) Case of the month: a girl with edema and purpuric eruption. Diagnosis: acute haemorrhagic oedema of infancy. Eur J Pediatr 156(10):813–815

Schmitt BD (1987) The child with non accidental trauma. In: Uit Helfer RE, Kempe RS (eds) The battered child, 4th edn. The University of Chicago Press, Chicago, pp 178–196

Sekula SA, Tschen JA, Duffy JO (1986) Epidermal nevus misinterpreted as child abuse. Cutis 37(4):276–278

Serour F, Gorenstein A, Dan M (2007) Tourniquet syndrome of the clitoris in a 4-year-old girl. J Emerg Med 33(3):283–284

Sheinfeld J, Cos LR, Erturk E et al (1985) Penile tourniquet injury due to a coil of hair. J Urol 133(6):1042–1043

Simon TD, Soep JB, Hollister JR (2005) Pernio in pediatrics. Pediatrics 116(3):e472–e475

Speight N (1992) Bruises and burns: accidental or non-accidental. In: Sibert J (ed) Accidents and emergencies in childhood. RCP publications, London, pp 97–103

Stewart GM, Rosenberg NM (1996) Conditions mistaken for child abuse: part II. Pediatr Emerg Care 12(3):217–221

Strahlman RS (2003) Toe tourniquet syndrome in association with maternal hair loss. Pediatrics 111(3):685–687

Sudhan ST, Gupta S, Plutarco C (2000) Toe-tourniquet syndrome – accidental or intentional? Eur J Pediatr 159(11):866

Swerdlin A, Berkowitz C, Craft N (2007) Cutaneous signs of child abuse. J Am Acad Dermatol 57(3):371–392

Tanner JL, Dechert MP, Frieden IJ (1998) Growing up with a facial hemangioma: parent and child coping and adaptation. Pediatrics 101(3):446–452

Thakur BK, Kaplan AP (1996) Recurrent 'unexplained' scalp swelling in an eighteen-month-old child: an atypical presentation of angioedema causing confusion with child abuse. J Pediatr 129(1):163–165

Thomas AE (2004) The bleeding child: is it NAI? Arch Dis Child 89(12):1163–1167

Thomas AJ, Timmons JW, Perlmutter AD (1977) Progressive penile amputation. Tourniquet injury secondary to hair. Urology 9(1):42–44

Toguri AG, Light RA, Warren MM (1979) Penile tourniquet syndrome caused by hair. South Med J 72(5):627–628

Tournel G, Desurmont M, Bécart A et al (2006) Child barbarity and torture: a case report. Am J Forensic Med Pathol 27(3):263–265

Van Wie D (2008) Popsicle panniculitis. University of Maryland Educational Pearls http://www.umem.org/res_pearls_referenced.php?p=539. Accessed on 2010

Vázquez Rueda F, Núñez Núñez R, Gómez Meleno P et al (1996) [The hair-thread tourniquet syndrome of the toes and penis] [Article in Spanish]. An Esp Pediatr 44(1):17–20

Wang M, Schott J, Tunnessen WW (2001) Picture of the month. Hair-thread tourniquet syndrome. Arch Pediatr Adolesc Med 155(4):515–516

Waskerwitz S, Christoffel KK, Hauger S (1981) Hypersensitivity vasculitis presenting as suspected child abuse: a case report and literature review. Pediatrics 67(2):283–284

Watemberg N, Urkin Y, Witztum A (1991) Phytophotodermatitis due to figs. Cutis 48(2):151–152

Weston WL, Morelli JG (2000) Childhood pernio and cryoproteins. Pediatr Dermatol 17(2):97–99

Wheeler DM, Hobbs CJ (1988) Mistakes in diagnosing non-accidental injury, 10 years' experience. Br Med J 296:1233–1236

Wikipedia (2011) Tui na http://en.wikipedia.org/wiki/Tui_na. Accessed on 2012

Yeatman GW, Dang VV (1980) Cao gio (coin rubbing). Vietnamese attitudes toward health care. JAMA 244(24):2748–2749

Yeatman GW, Shaw C, Barlow MJ, Bartlett G (1976) Pseudobattering in Vietnamese children. Pediatrics 58(4):616–618

Zurbuchen P, LeCoultre C, Calza AM et al (1996) Cutaneous necrosis after contact with calcium chloride: a mistaken diagnosis of child abuse. Pediatrics 97(2):257–258

7 Blunt-Force Trauma: Other Cutaneous Manifestations

7.1 Introduction

The most common traumatic skin lesions in accident-related blunt-force trauma and child abuse are bruises. In child abuse, blunt-force trauma may also lead to injuries such as erythema, abrasions, and lacerations, but these are less common than bruises.

In accidents, bruises are often accompanied by other skin injuries, mainly abrasions. Bruises sustained as a result of child abuse are less frequently accompanied by other skin abnormalities such as abrasions (Reece and Grodin 1985).

7.2 Erythema

Erythema is defined as redness of the skin and/or mucous membranes caused by dilatation of the underlying capillaries (RCPCH 2008). It is a nonspecific sign, which occurs with any skin injury, infection, or inflammation (Figs. 7.1, 7.2 and 7.3). Trauma includes friction, rubbing, local pressure, response to chemical irritants, and burns and scalds from a variety of causes. Contrary to bruises, erythema does blanch under diascopy. Erythema is a vital reaction and therefore can only be found in the living. The reaction will vanish within minutes to hours.

Erythema is rarely seen in child abuse cases, unless the child is examined by a physician within hours after the incident that caused the erythema. If found in child abuse cases, erythema is most commonly seen following inflicted burns and scald injuries. It may also be encountered not uncommonly in the genital and anal area when children are interfered with sexually e.g., in dry intercourse.

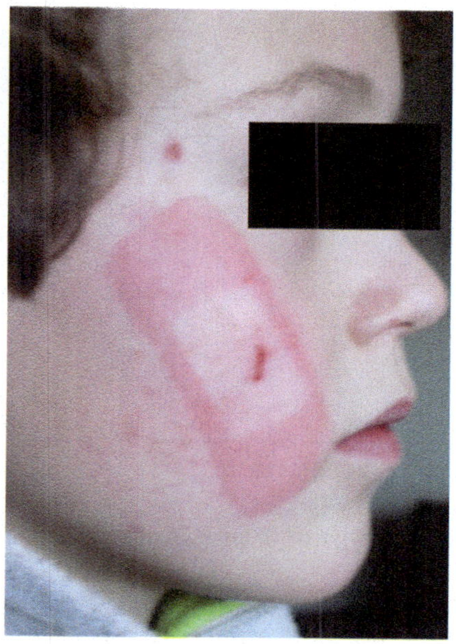

Fig. 7.1 Erythema caused by the application of a patch

R.A.C. Bilo et al., *Cutaneous Manifestations of Child Abuse and Their Differential Diagnosis*,
DOI 10.1007/978-3-642-29287-3_7, © Springer-Verlag Berlin Heidelberg 2013

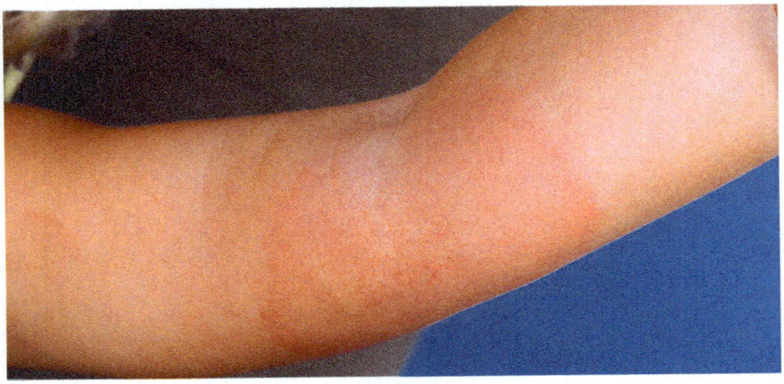

Fig. 7.2 Erythema migrans in a patient with Lyme disease

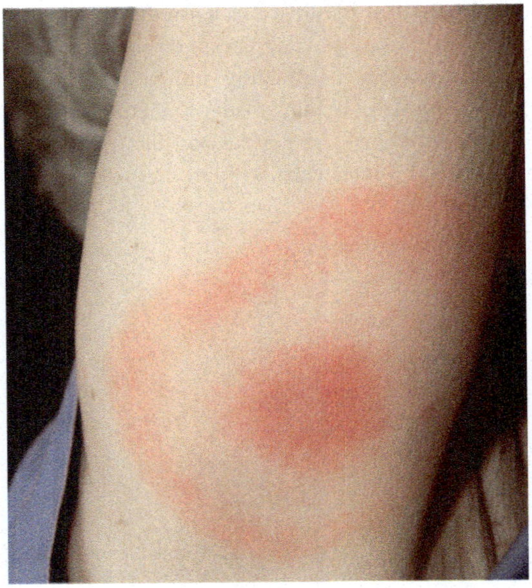

Fig. 7.3 Erythema migrans in a patient with Lyme disease (CDC, 2007)

7.3 Abrasions

7.3.1 Defining Abrasions

An abrasion is a superficial injury to the skin, which is characterized by the traumatic removal, detachment, or destruction of the epidermis (Pollak and Saukko 2000) (Fig. 7.4). Generally, abrasions are the result of friction/shearing movement (tangential or lateral force) against a rough surface (rubbing, sliding, scraping, chafing, sweeping) but may also be caused by compression/crushing (perpendicular or vertical force) or by a combination of friction and compression. Abrasions are located at the exact point of contact between the object and the body (Watson 1990).

According to their depth, abrasions can be divided into superficial abrasions or erosions (graze, scuff, or brush abrasions) and deeper abrasions or excoriations. Abrasions can be divided in three grades. Grade 1 is a focal defect limited to the epidermis of the skin; no hemorrhages are visible (sometimes referred to as erosions) (Figs. 7.5 and 7.6). Grade 2 is a somewhat deeper defect with a few pinpoint hemorrhages. The hemorrhages are caused by damage to the capillaries and venules in the dermis (Figs. 7.7 and 7.8). It is rare for the full thickness of the dermis to be abraded (grade 3) (Figs. 7.9, 7.10 and 7.11). Abrasions may be surrounded by ring-shaped erythema (especially in the acute phase) or ring-shaped inflammation. When healing is not complicated by other factors, abrasions will heal without scarring.

Abrasions may be a sign of severe internal injury. The underlying organs may sustain damage at the point of impact of the abrasion. The abrasion may even be the only indication of internal injury (Watson 1990).

Fig. 7.4 Superficial abrasion

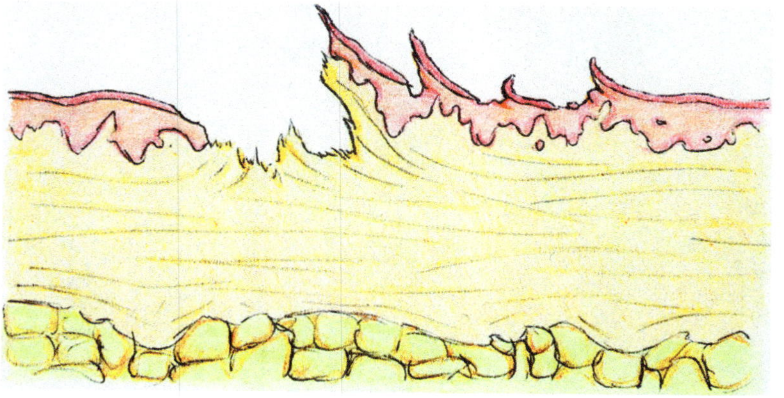

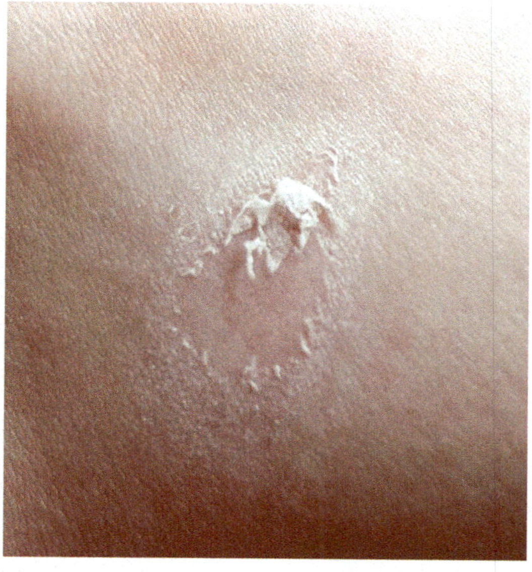

Fig. 7.5 Grade 1 abrasion: no hemorrhages visible

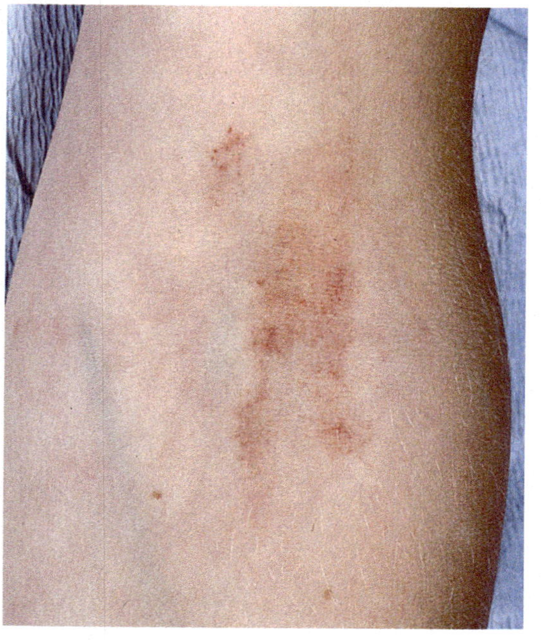

Fig. 7.6 Grade 1 abrasions: superficial scratch marks in atopic dermatitis

7.3.2 Clinical Features

Abrasions may be seen on the skin, on the mucous membranes, and at sites with non-cornified epithelium (lips and oral mucous membrane, vulva and vagina, penis). Because of the loss of waterproof epidermis, the underlying tissue will desiccate rapidly, leading to the typical shiny, semitranslucent appearance (Robinson 2000). Abrasions sustained during life are reddish brown in color and will generally heal without scarring. When they occur shortly before death, they are brown in color and will have a stiff, leathery, and parchment-like appearance (Saukko and Knight 2004). This is seen in, for example, a ligature mark caused by hanging or strangulation. If they occur postmortem, the abrasions will be yellow and translucent without any color change at the edge (Saukko and Knight 2004).

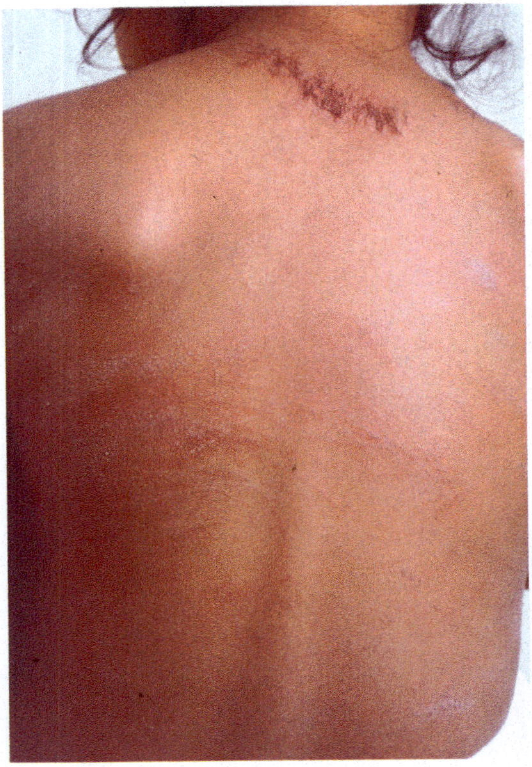

Fig. 7.7 Grade 2 abrasions: deeper scratch marks in atopic dermatitis

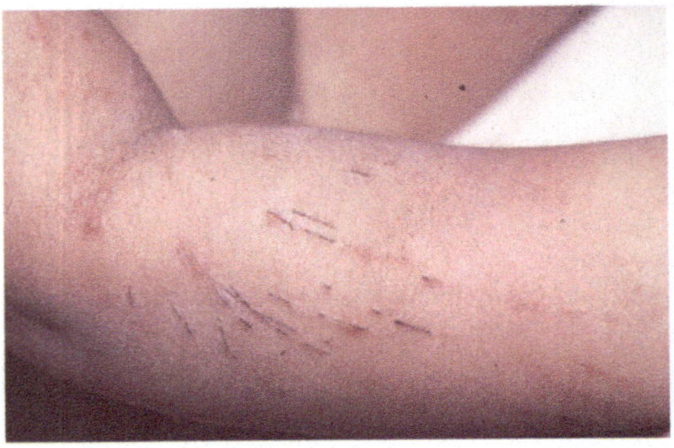

Fig. 7.8 Grade 2 abrasions: deeper scratch marks in atopic dermatitis

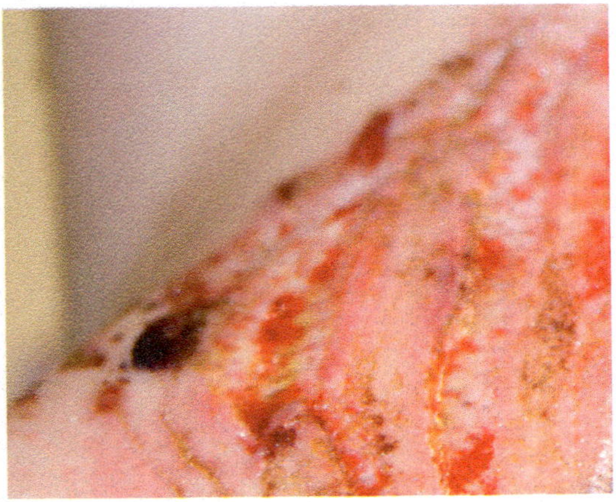

Fig. 7.9 Grade 3 abrasion: deep full-thickness abrasion

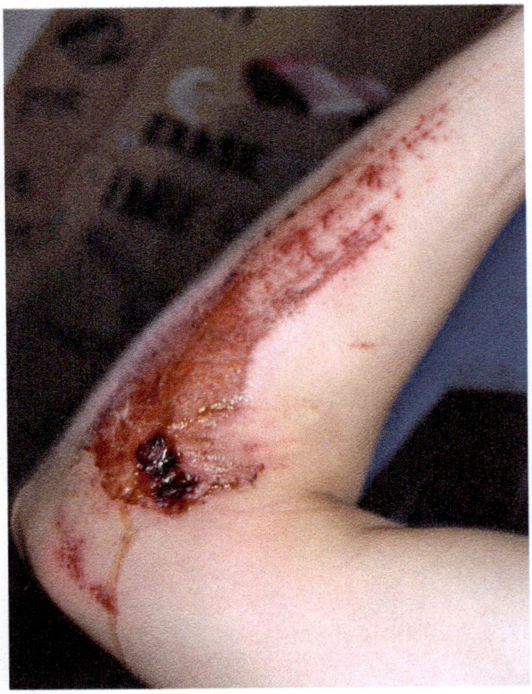

Fig. 7.10 Combined grade 2 and 3 abrasions: untreated 7-day-old healing road abrasion (Fallerd, 2007 from Wikimedia Commons, 2011: Scar.jpg)

7.3.3 Types of Abrasions

According to their origin, two types of abrasions can be distinguished: abrasions caused by a tangential force or by a compressive/crushing force (Pollak and Saukko 2000; DiMaio and DiMaio 2001).

In tangential abrasions, the superficial layers of the skin are scraped off by a blunt object (Figs. 7.12 and 7.13). Tangential abrasions are also known as graze, scuff, or brush abrasions. This type of abrasions also includes sharp abrasions.

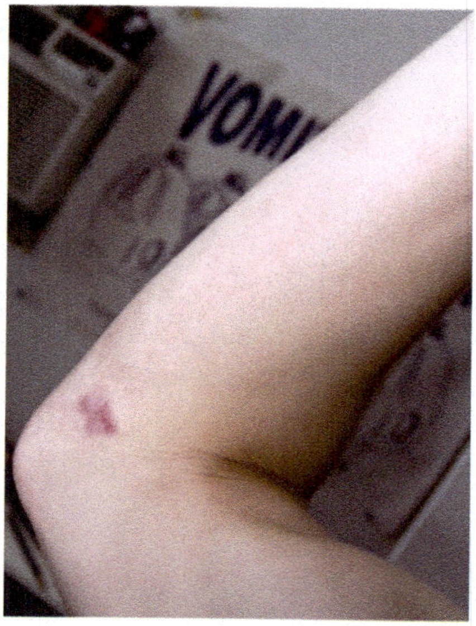

Fig. 7.11 Scar of the abrasion in Fig. 7.10: 1 year later (Fallerd 2007 from Wikimedia Commons 2011: Scar.jpg)

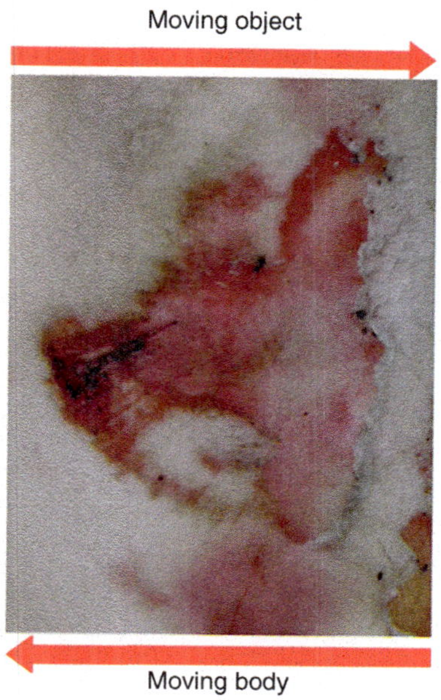

Fig. 7.13 Tangential abrasion – mechanism

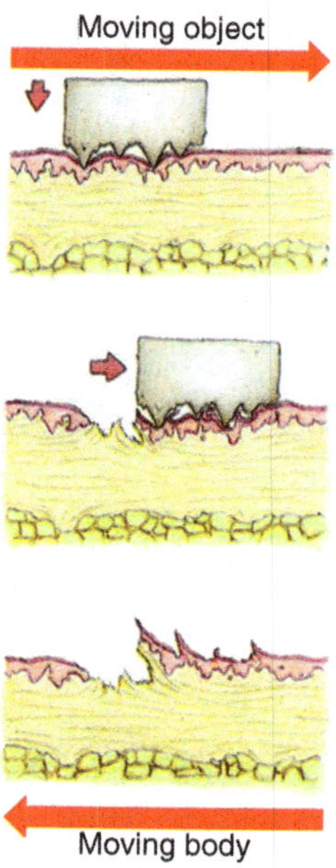

Fig. 7.12 Tangential abrasion – mechanism

Tangential abrasions may be sustained in three manners:

- An object moving along the body surface (e.g., a rough object that is pulled over the skin or in pedestrian versus motor vehicle accidents – sometimes with a pattern) (Fig. 7.14).
- The body surface moving along the object (e.g., accidental; in childhood falls or inflicted when a child is dragged over a rough surface by another person) (Figs. 7.15, and 7.16).
- A simultaneous movement of object and body surface which may occur in an accident (in the same or opposite direction).

When the abraded surface is examined within a few hours after the abrasion was sustained, it may provide an indication of the direction of the applied force, in other words, the direction of the friction between the skin and the abrading object. If one end of a fresh graze has margins with raised skin tags, the tangential force originated from the opposite side (Figs. 7.12 and 7.13) (Watson 1990; Dix 2000). However, only rarely, the direction can be established. Most tags are very small and will be lost easily, for example, by contact with clothing (Fig. 7.5). Furthermore, within a couple of hours, the abrasion will be covered with serosanguineous fluid, which dries quickly forming a brownish scab (Sect. 7.3.4).

A specific type of tangential abrasions is the sharp abrasion or scratch in which a rough, sharp object is pushed against and pulled along the surface of the skin. The shape is usually linear or

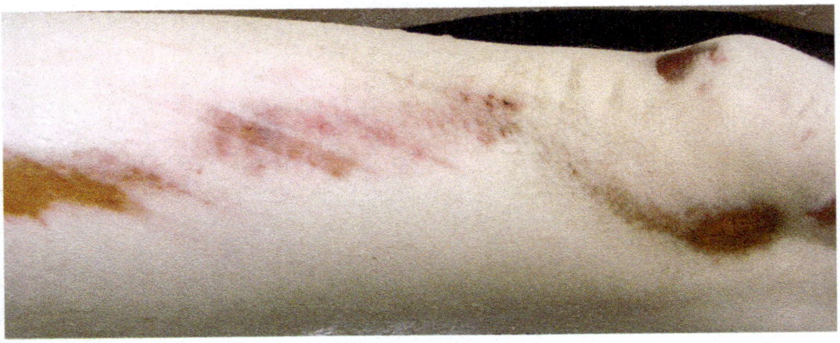

Fig. 7.14 Accidental abrasion with pattern caused by an object dragged along the body surface plus dirt marks caused by the object

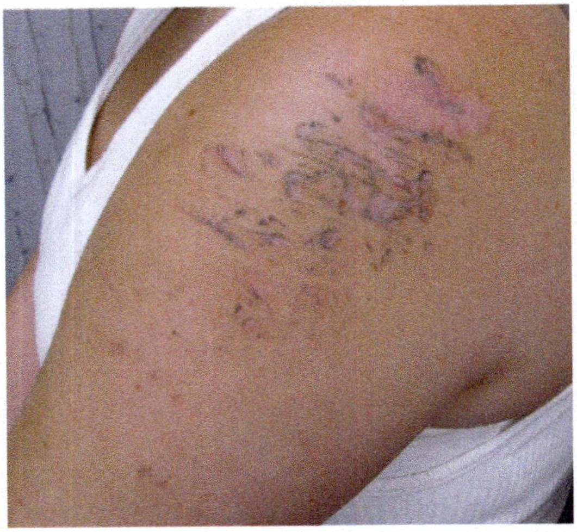

Fig. 7.15 Almost healed abrasion with "tattooing" caused by sliding on asphalt during an accident

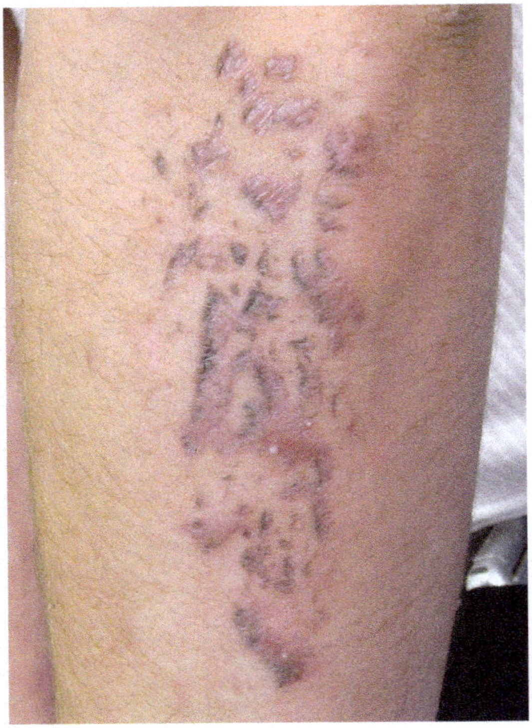

Fig. 7.16 Same person as in Fig. 7.15

curved and the lesions may be isolated or multiple (Fig. 7.17). Generally, they will show a regular and converging pattern and the scratches will have similar depth. A linear abrasion may be continuous or interrupted. Sharp abrasions may be caused by fingernails, barbed wire, the point of a weapon (e.g., a knife), the point of a nail, a piece of broken glass, or the claws of a pet, particularly cats.

When caused by fingernails, the width and depth of the abrasion will depend on the width and sharpness of the fingernail and the degree of pressure the fingernail exerted on the skin during the movement, which may lead to broader and usually somewhat deeper scratches (Figs. 7.18 and 7.19) or to more linear and usually more superficial "point" scratches (Fig. 7.20).

If only pressure is applied and there is no pulling movement, the skin will only be injured superficially, leading to a superficial linear or curved (crescentic) removal of the epidermis, with a length of 1.5 cm, without incising or lacerating the skin. This will result in a typical fingernail imprint (Figs. 7.21 and 7.22), also

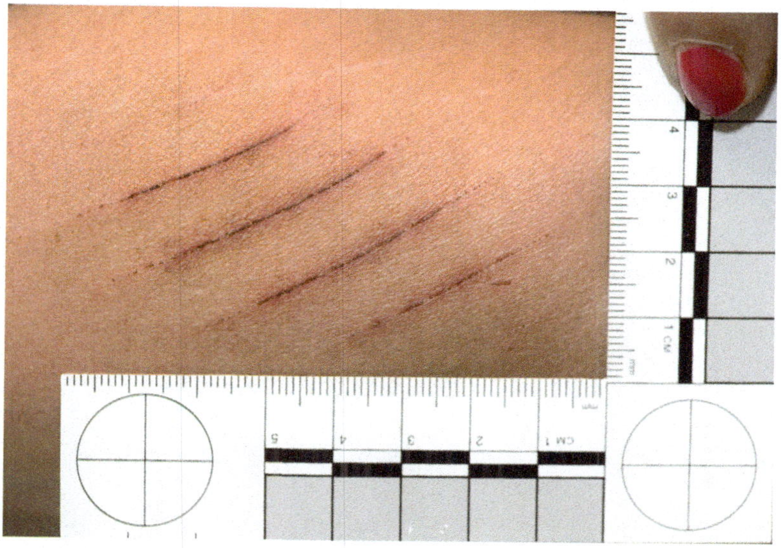

Fig. 7.17 Accidental sharp abrasions (scratches due to chicken wire)

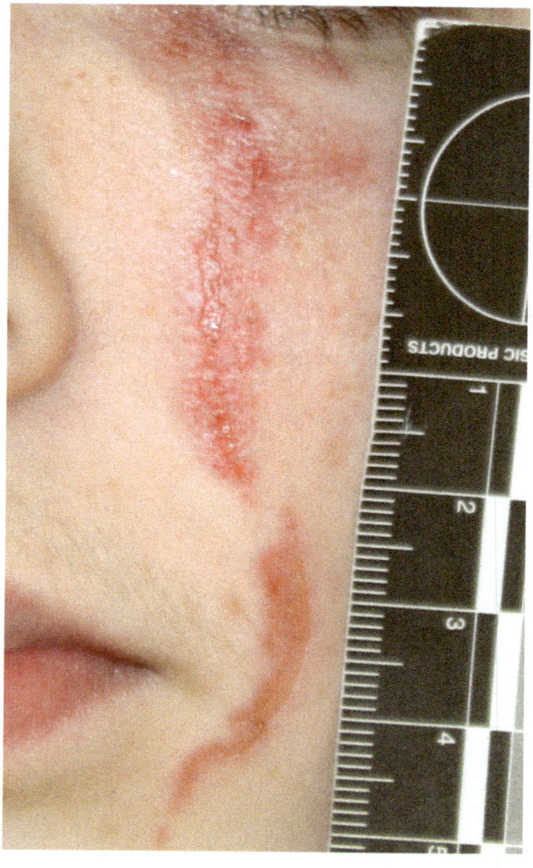

Fig. 7.18 Broad and somewhat deeper scratch marks in the face, due to fighting between two adolescent girls

known as a "static fingernail abrasion or imprint" (Saukko and Knight 2004).

Shapiro et al. (1962) showed that the orientation of the curvature in an imprint does not necessarily proof the orientation of the imprinting fingertip/fingernail (Fig. 7.22). The orientation is mainly determined by the degree of tension on and distortion of the skin during the imprint:

- Absent or minimal tension and distortion: the curvature of the imprint will correlate to the curvature of the imprinting fingernail;
- Increasing tension and distortion: the curvature of the imprint will be predominantly linear or even be reversed to the curvature of the imprinting fingernail.

If possible, sharp linear abrasions should be differentiated from superficial incisions. Superficial incisions may be caused by the point of a knife, for example, in self-mutilation. However, differentiation is difficult and sometimes even impossible.

A compression/crushing abrasion is caused by a more or less perpendicular impact to the skin (Pollak and Saukko 2000). It is generally seen at sites where bone is covered by only a thin layer of skin (forehead, elbows, wrists, knees). Compression abrasions are also known

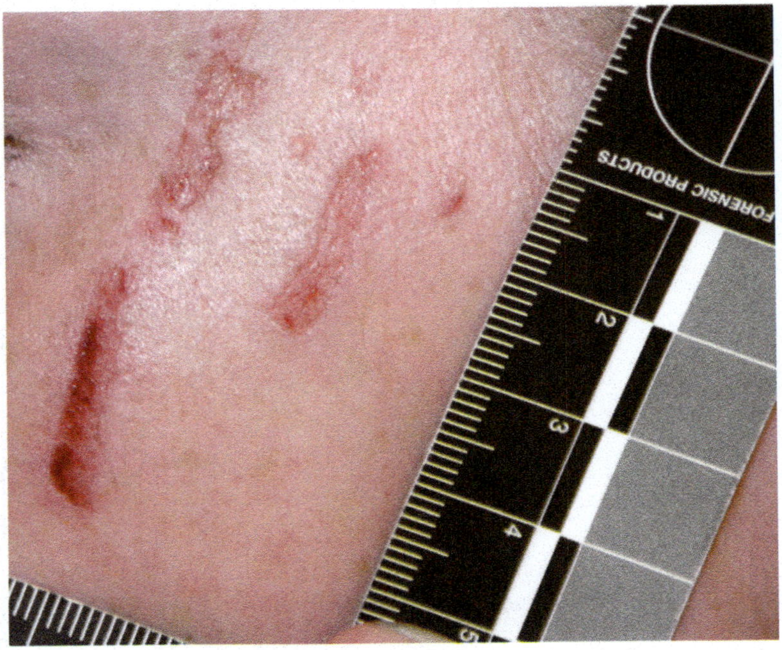

Fig. 7.19 Broad and somewhat deeper scratch marks in the face, due to fighting between two adolescent girls

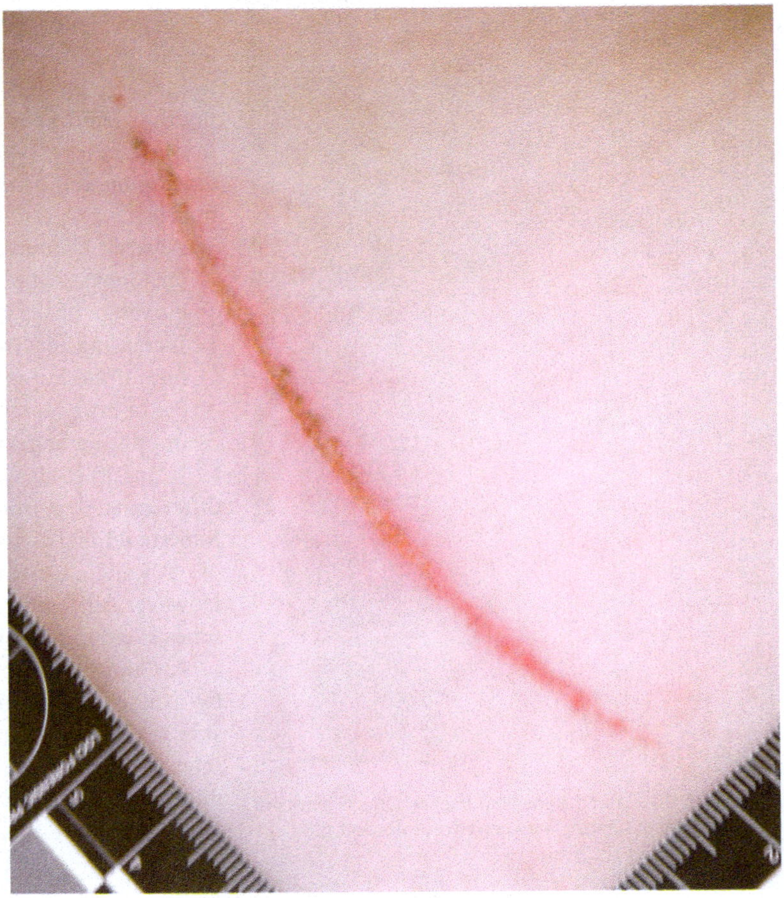

Fig. 7.20 Superficial, linear scratch

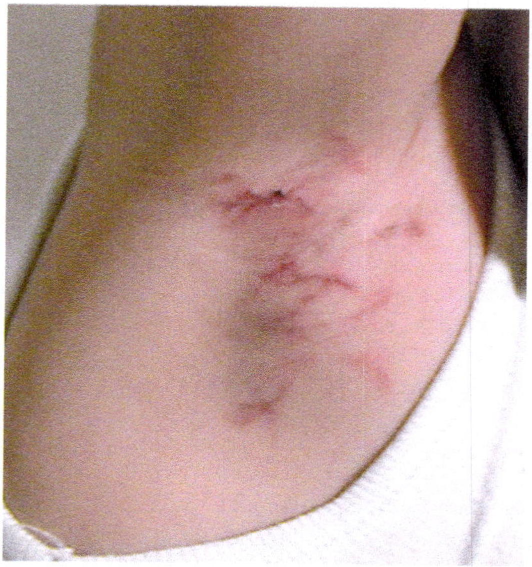

Fig. 7.21 Static fingernail imprint (multiple imprints in the right armpit, one imprint plus several superficial abrasions in the left armpit of an abused young child)

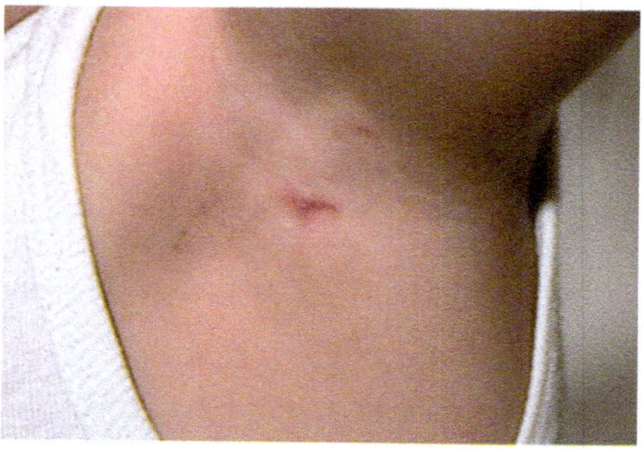

Fig. 7.22 Same child as in Fig. 7.21

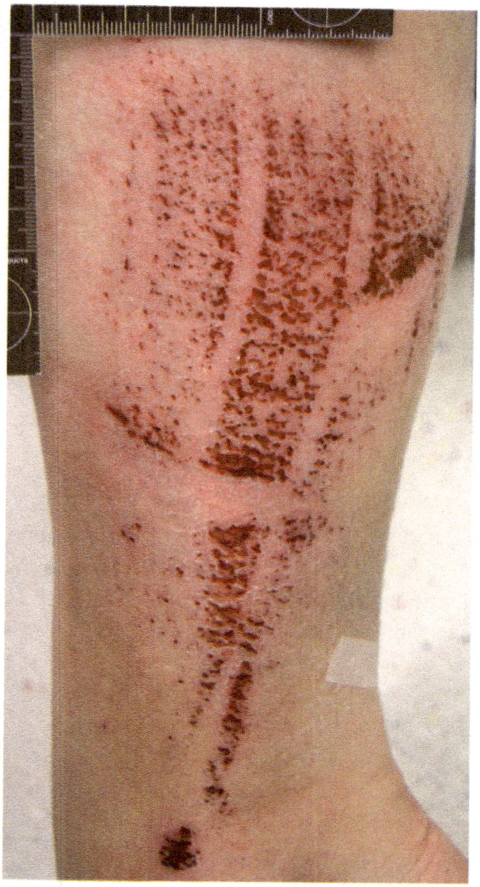

Fig. 7.23 Pattern abrasion

as contact abrasions, pressure, or crushing abrasions. The blunt force impacts the skin almost perpendicularly, which leads to "crushing" of the skin with a limited tangential movement. The injuring object may be reflected by the shape of the skin injury (Pollak and Saukko 2000; Saukko and Knight 2004), which results in a so-called patterned or imprint abrasion: a pattern or an imprint of the object, or of the clothing present between the object and the skin, arises through the "crushing" effect after a blow with a blunt object. An erythematous or inflamed zone may surround the imprint, and an area of bruising may underlie the imprint. Recognizable patterns may fade quickly (Watson 1990) (Fig. 7.23).

7.3.4 Dating of Abrasions

In case of a superficial abrasion, healing without scarring will take place in a couple of days. (Deeper) abrasions can be dated by interpreting their externally visible characteristics or by histopathological characteristics (Table 7.1 and

Table 7.1 Dating of abrasions based on clinical and histopathological findings (Robertson and Hodge 1972)

Timing	Clinical and histopathological findings
Initial hours	Clearly visible graze covered with serosanguineous fluid
Initial hours to days	Crust forming
From 30 h after the development of superficial grazes, clearly visible in most excoriations from 72 h onward	Regeneration of the epithelium
From day 5–8, most conspicuous from day 9–12 after the injury was sustained	Sub-epithelial granulation and hyperplasia of the epithelium
From day 12 onward	Regression of the epithelium and the granular tissue
30 min	16 h and 45 min
Almost 2 days	Almost 3 days
13 days	13.5 days
Almost 17.5 days	18.5 days
Almost 22 days	Ca 30 days

Figs. 7.24, 7.25, 7.26, 7.27, 7.28, 7.29, 7.30, 7.31, 7.32 and 7.33). However, as in the dating of bruising, it can be concluded that at present there is no scientific basis for an accurate dating of abrasions. This type of dating is only indicative.

7.3.5 Abrasions and Child Abuse

Generally, abrasions are caused by accidents and are rarely seen in physical abuse. Babies may scratch themselves on the cheeks, the ears, the nose, and sometimes the conjunctivae during the first months. This is caused by long fingernails, and the scratching will disappear if the parents keep the nails short. In fact, this is probably the only injury that an immobile child can inflict on itself.

Abrasions caused by abuse are often found in the orofacial area (head, face, mouth, and neck) (Cairns et al. 2005) and on the upper arms and forearms (Saukko and Knight 2004). Sharp linear or imprint abrasions caused by fingernails are probably the most prevalent abrasions in child abuse (Figs. 7.20, 7.21, 7.34 and 7.35). According to Saukko (2004), predominantly women are associated with causing fingernail imprints or abrasions since they tend to have longer and sharper fingernails (Figs. 7.17 and 7.18).

If fingernail imprints and/or scratches or broader more or less linear abrasions are found in or the neck, this could be suspicious of (attempted) strangulation. The fingernail abrasions may be caused by the perpetrator but may also be made by the victim in an attempt to protect him/herself by tearing away the ligature or the hands of the perpetrator (Saukko and Knight 2004).

If this type of abrasion is found predominantly on the upper arms, one should consider child sexual abuse, in which the child is held in a fixed position by the perpetrator. In such cases, they can be accompanied by grip marks ("fingerprint" bruises).

Imprint abrasions, often combined with linear bruises, can be found in children who have been whipped with a rope, an electrical cord, or a belt (Nathanson 2000). If instead of the "soft" part of the belt the buckle is used for whipping, one may find a typical imprint abrasion, but also a laceration caused by tearing of the skin (Figs. 7.36 and 7.37).

Abrasions caused by tangential friction can be found in children who have been tied with a rope around the ankles and/or wrists (Fig. 7.38) or have been strangulated with a rope (Figs. 7.39 and 7.40). In rare occasions, lesions occurring on the wrist can lead to confusion, for example, in children with a contact dermatitis resulting from a hospital identification band (Figs. 7.41 and 7.42).

Sometimes abrasions are seen that are the result of biting and present as a hematoma with an elliptical or circular shape in which individual teeth marks can be recognized as separate imprint bruises and/or abrasions (Chap. 8).

Self-induced abrasions in false (rape) allegations, habit disorders, and self-mutilation

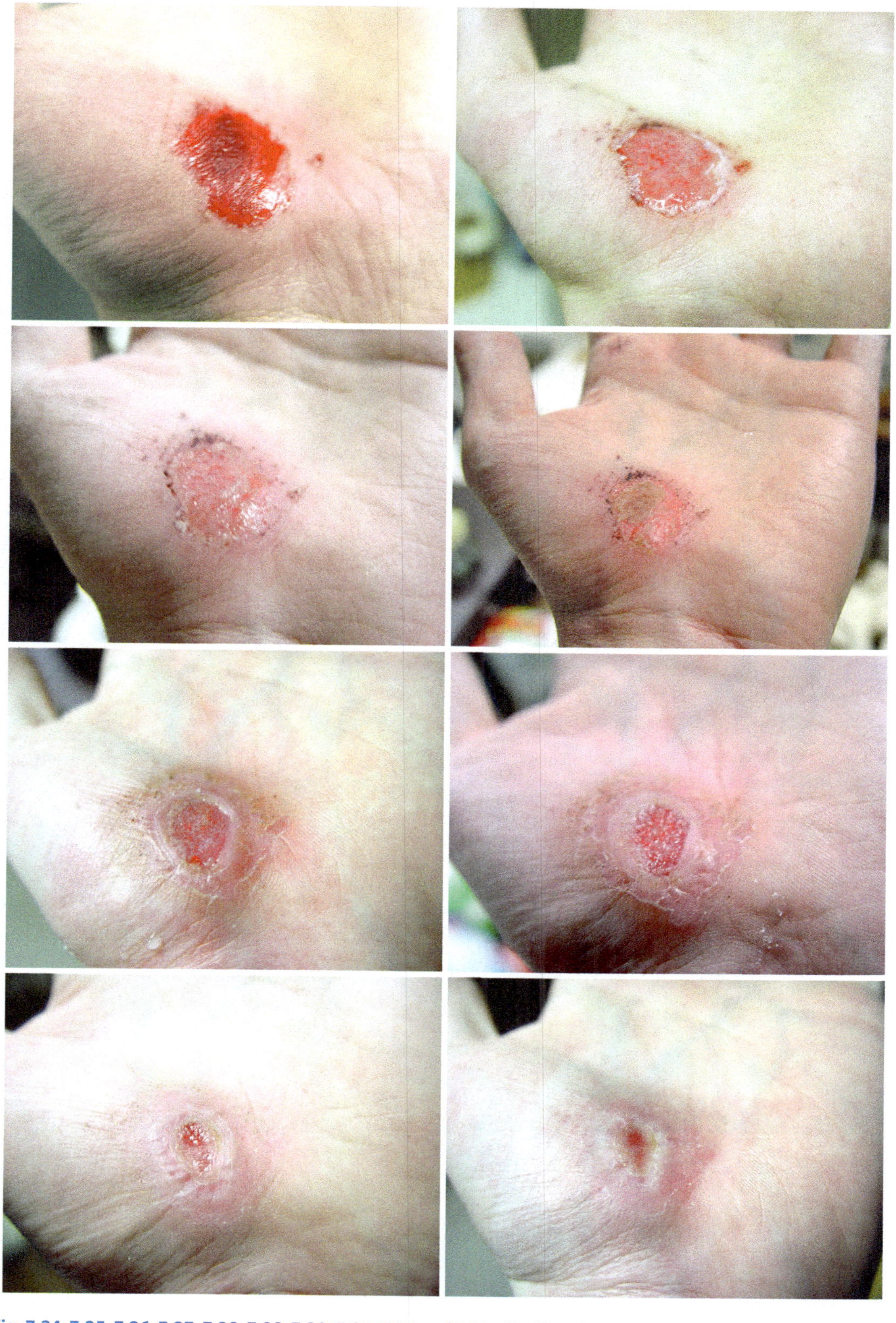

Fig. 7.24, 7.25, 7.26, 7.27, 7.28, 7.29, 7.30, 7.31, 7.32 and 7.33 Healing of an abrasion (Jpbarrass 2008 – Wikipedia http://en.wikipedia.org/wiki/Abrasion_(medical))

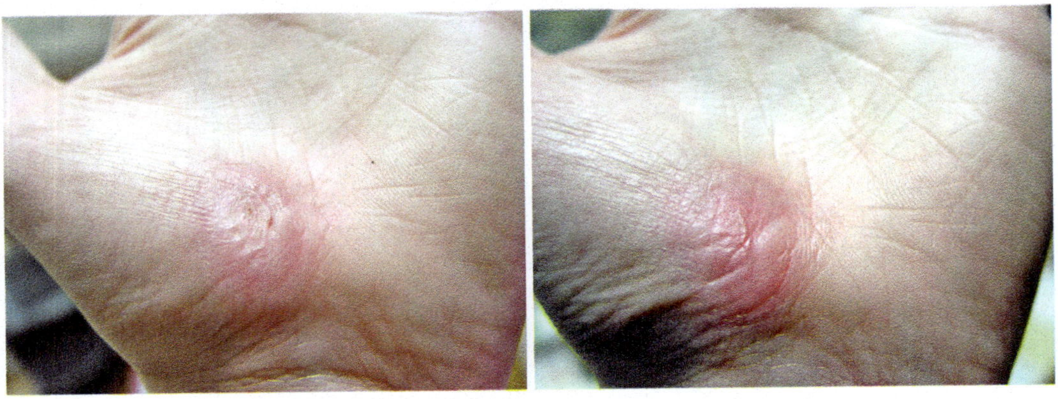

Fig. 7.24, 7.25, 7.26, 7.27, 7.28, 7.29, 7.30, 7.31, 7.32 and 7.33 (continued)

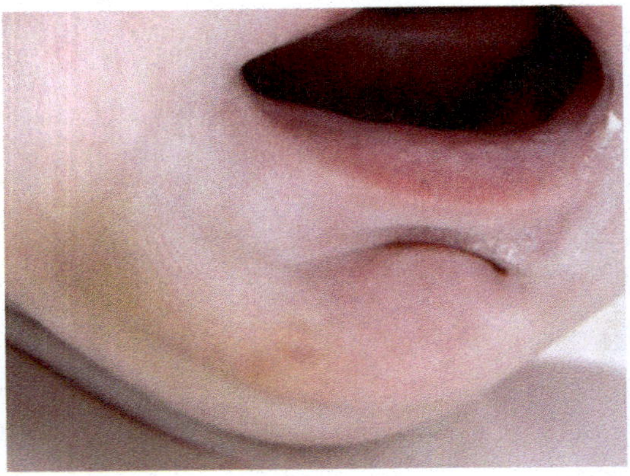

Fig. 7.34 Single “static” fingernail imprint plus bruising

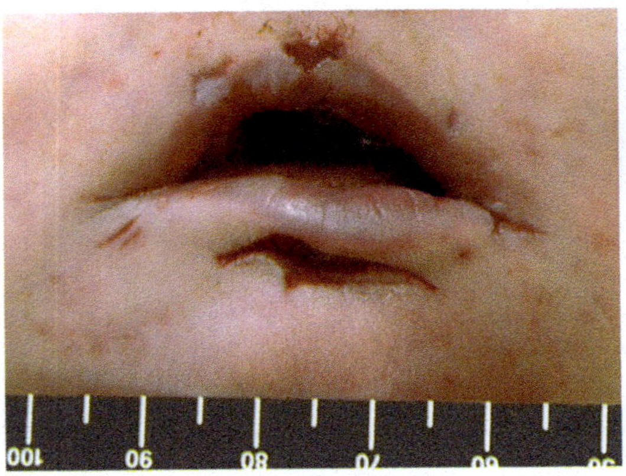

Fig. 7.35 Double “static” fingernail imprint

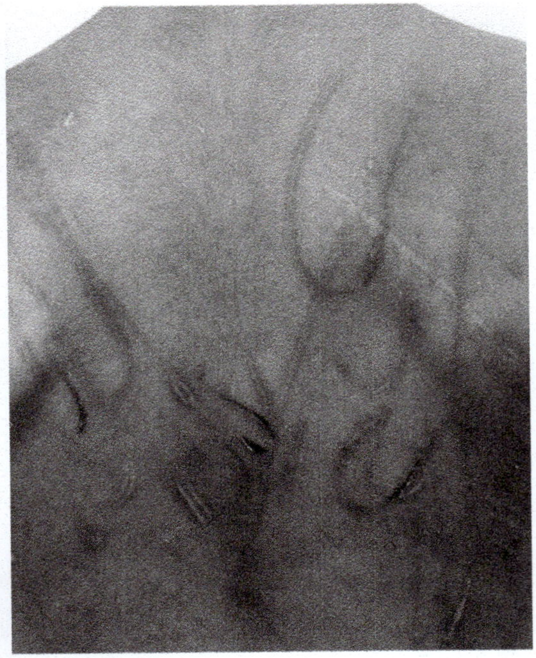

Fig. 7.36 Multiple imprint abrasions and loop marks

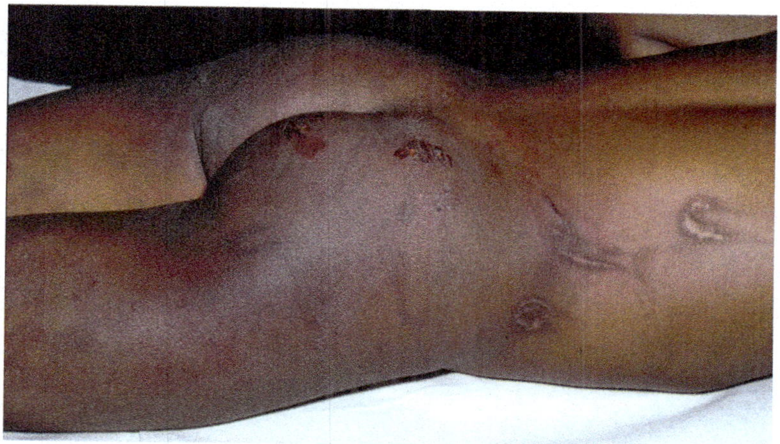

Fig. 7.37 Multiple abrasions and loop marks with scarring due to laceration of the skin (= Fig. 3.46)

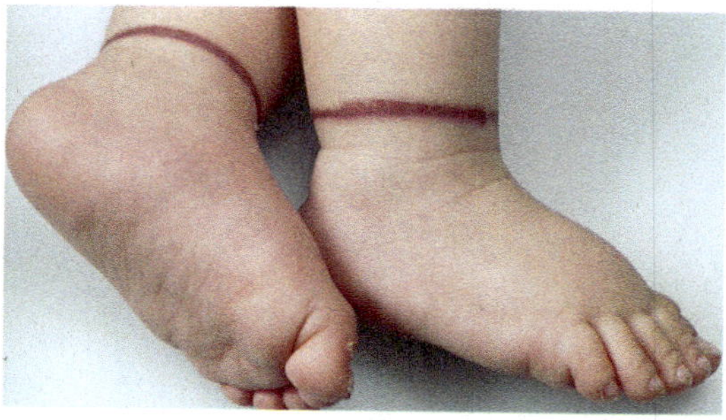

Fig. 7.38 Marks due to being tied with a rope to the bed

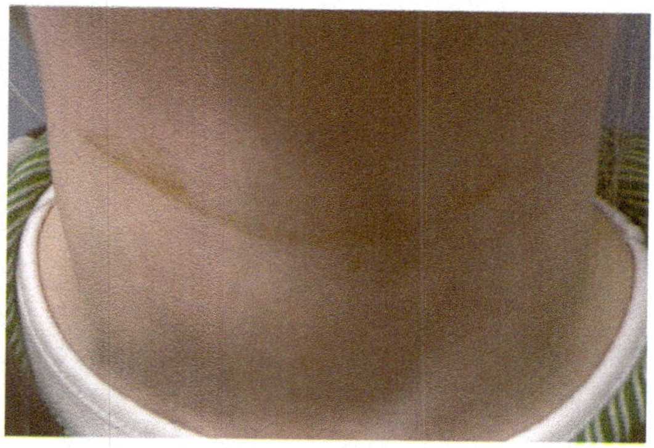

Fig. 7.40 Juvenile linear xanthogranuloma as differential diagnosis of a healing strangulation mark

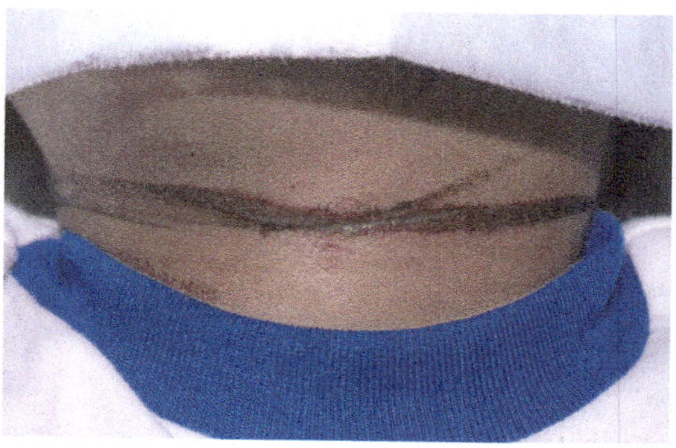

Fig. 7.39 Mark in the neck of a child who survived a strangulation attempt with a rope

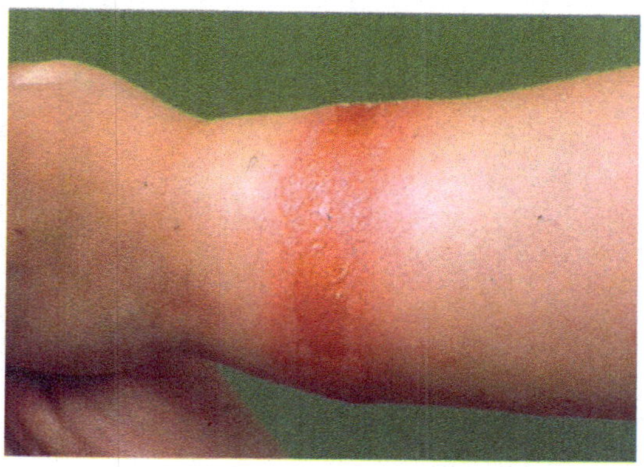

Fig. 7.41 Toxic contact dermatitis resulting from a hospital identification bracelet

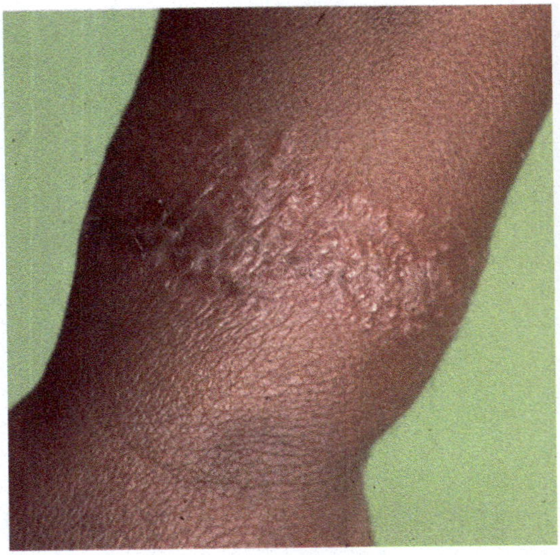

Fig. 7.42 Toxic contact dermatitis resulting from a hospital identification bracelet

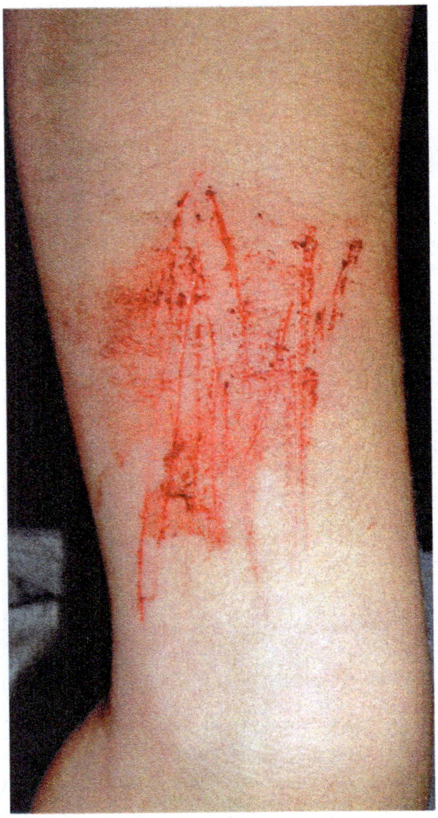

Fig. 7.43 Self-induced abrasions in a false allegation of a physical assault

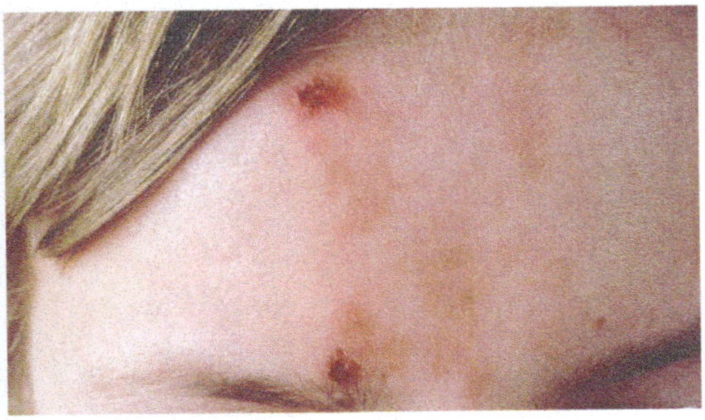

Fig. 7.44 Abrasions on the forehead due to self-mutilation

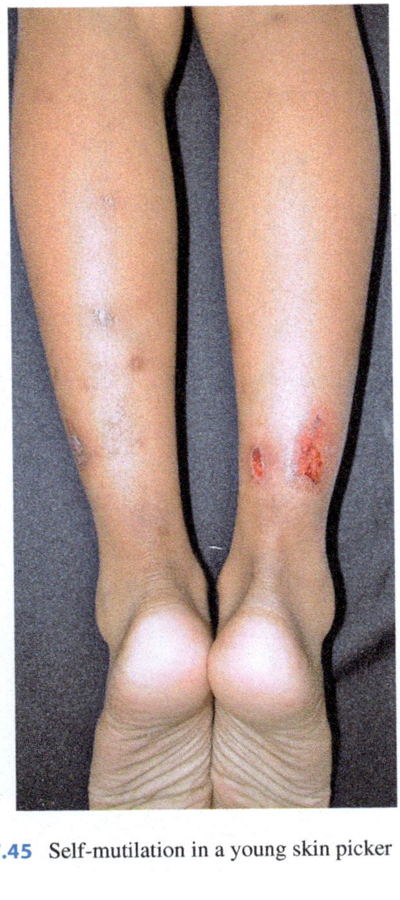

Fig. 7.45 Self-mutilation in a young skin picker

(Figs. 7.43, 7.44 and 7.45) can be found in abused children (and adults who were abused in their youth) or in children with psychological or psychiatric problems; these abrasions will have to be carefully differentiated from abrasions caused by the abuse itself. These abra-

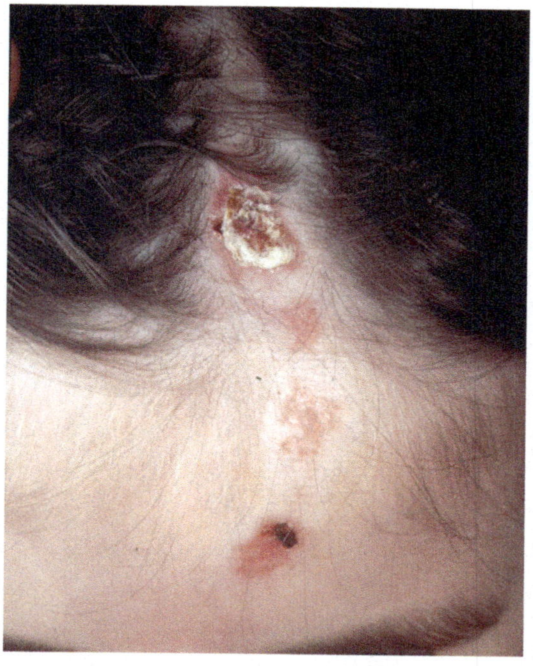

Fig. 7.46 Abrasion-like findings on the forehead: morphea

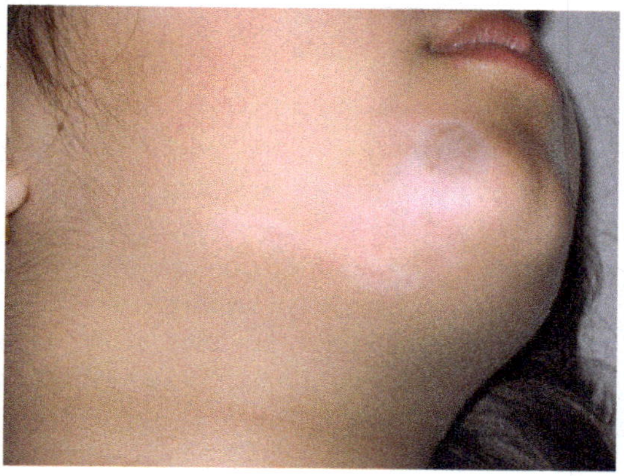

Fig. 7.47 Scarring in morphea

sions should also be differentiated from diseases with abrasion-like findings, like morphea (also known as localized scleroderma, characterized by excessive collagen deposition leading to thickening of the dermis, subcutaneous tissues, or both) (Nguyen 2010) (Figs. 7.46, 7.47 and 7.48), inflammatory linear verrucous epidermal nevus (ilven) (Fig. 7.49), nevus verrucosus (Fig. 7.50), or necrobiosis lipoidica diabeticorum (Fig. 7.51).

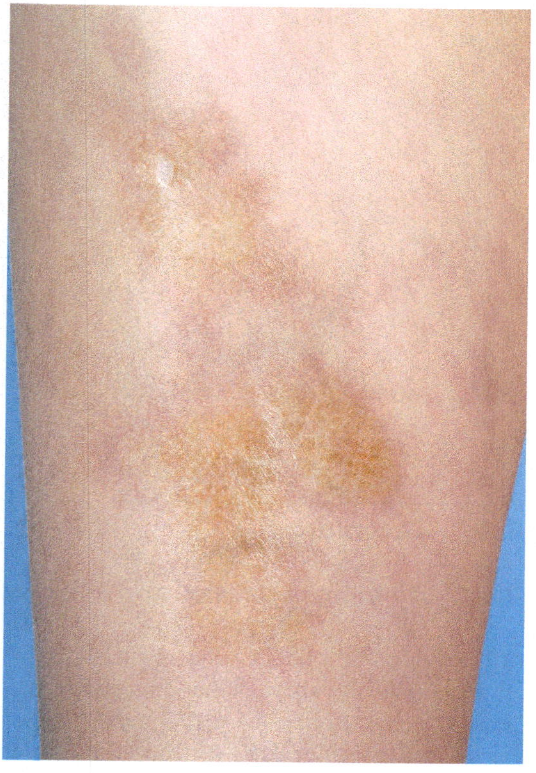

Fig. 7.48 Scarring in morphea

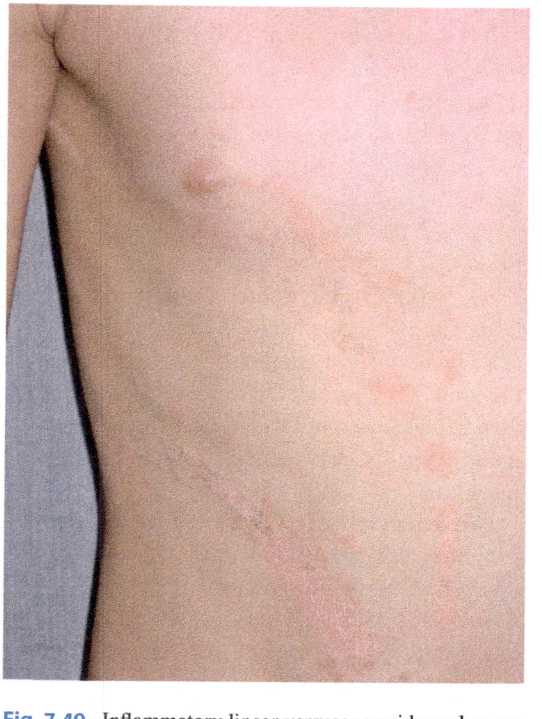

Fig. 7.49 Inflammatory linear verrucous epidermal nevus

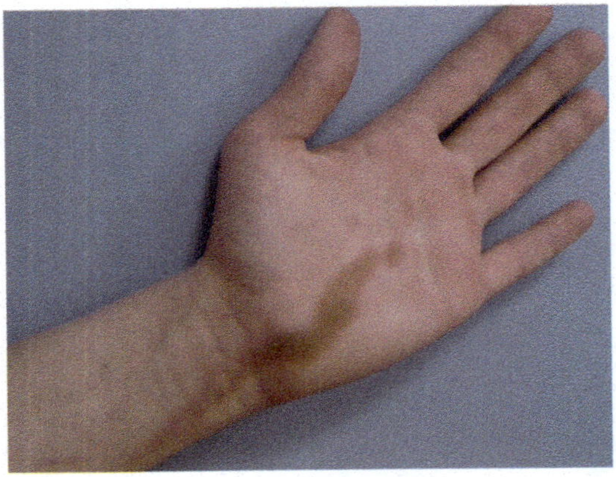

Fig. 7.50 Verrucous nevus

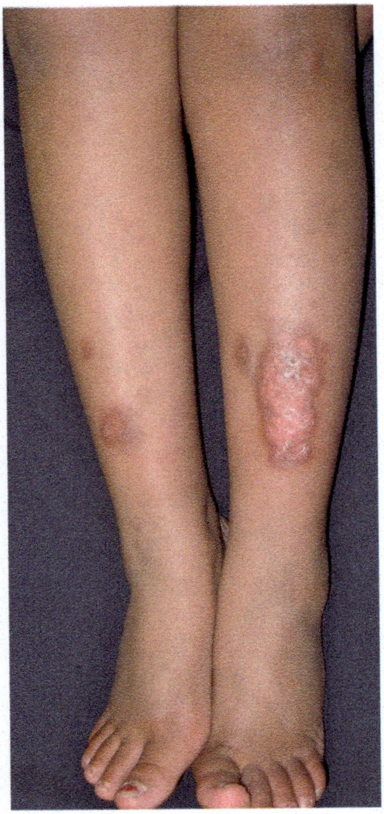

Fig. 7.51 Necrobiosis lipoidica diabeticorum

7.4 Laceration

7.4.1 Defining Laceration and Avulsion

A laceration of the skin is a full-thickness injury of the skin and subcutaneous tissues which is generally characterized by tearing of tissues in a frayed and irregular pattern (tear wound) with bruised and abraded edges and crushing of the margins of the wound (Watson 1990; Pollak and Saukko 2000; DiMaio and DiMaio 2001; RCPCH 2008). A laceration may show bridges of undamaged blood vessels, tendons, and/or nerves within the tear, reaching from one side of the tear to the other side. Bridging develops because tissues consist of components with varying resistance to stretching; for example, vessels and nerves are more resistant to stretching than other parts of the skin.

According to the depth of the injury, lacerations can be divided into (1) superficial lacerations involving only the most superficial layers of the skin, (2) deep lacerations involving all skin layers, and (3) complicated lacerations involving underlying tissues such as internal organs or muscles.

An avulsion (skin flap) refers to a laceration in which skin and subcutaneous tissues are not just separated but torn away from the underlying tissues (Fig. 7.53). When the force causing the laceration did not impact the skin perpendicularly, but oblique, an avulsion can be incurred. A closed avulsion or pocket avulsion is a specific type of avulsion that is the result of shearing forces in which the skin stays intact but the subcutaneous tissues are torn from the underlying fascia or connective tissue, leading to a subcutaneous pocket that may be filled with blood (DiMaio and DiMaio 2001). Closed avulsions have been described in pedestrian versus motor vehicle accidents.

7.4.2 Clinical Features

Lacerations may occur in:

- The skin (especially over bony prominences where the distance between skin and underlying bony structures is limited or where the skin is fixed to the bony tissue and the skin does not move easily): face, skull, back of hand, and shins (Figs. 7.52 and 7.53)
- Mucous membranes (mouth, anus, vulva, and vagina) (Figs. 7.54, 7.55, 7.56 and 7.57)

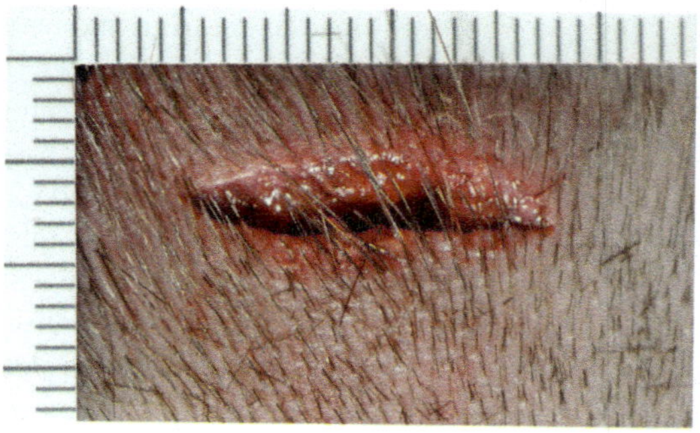

Fig. 7.52 Laceration of the scalp

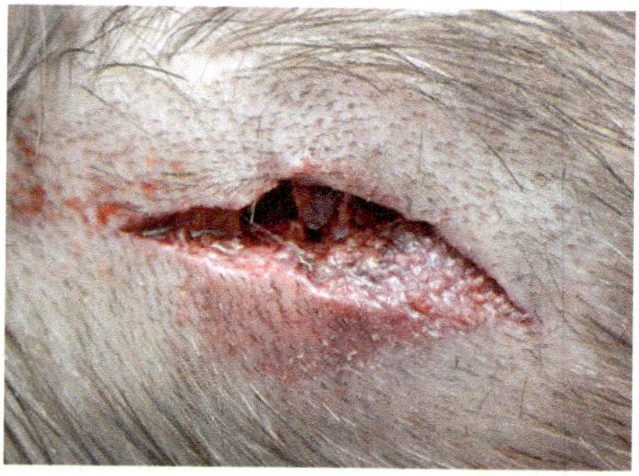

Fig. 7.53 Laceration of the scalp with tissue bridges of vessels and/or nerves within the tear

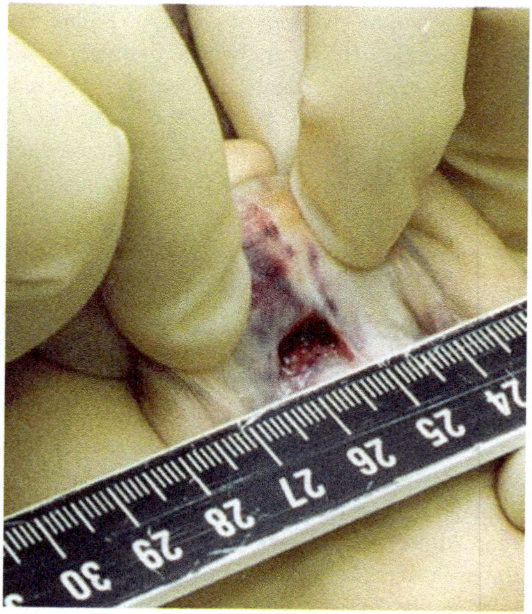

Fig. 7.54 Laceration of the inside of the upper lip next to the frenum

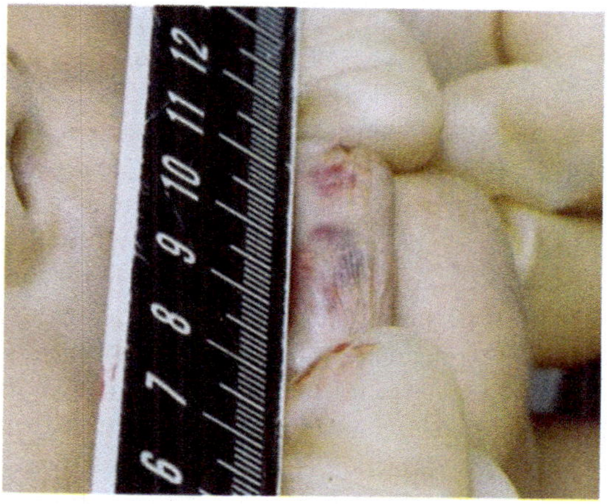

Fig. 7.55 Same child as in Fig. 7.54: simultaneously inflicted bruising of the lower lip visible as an imprint of the maxillary teeth (blunt-force trauma)

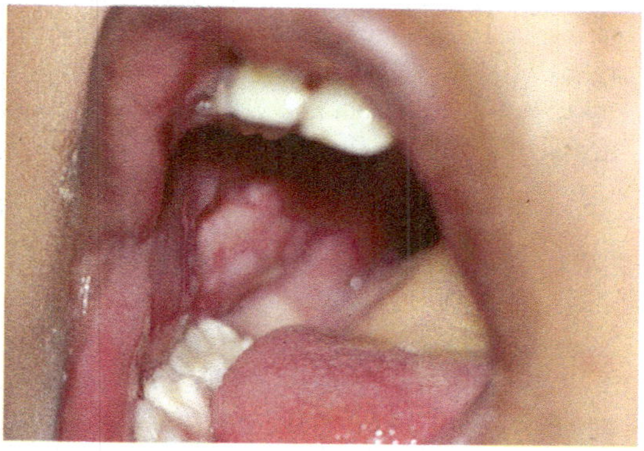

Fig. 7.56 Laceration of the inside of the cheek

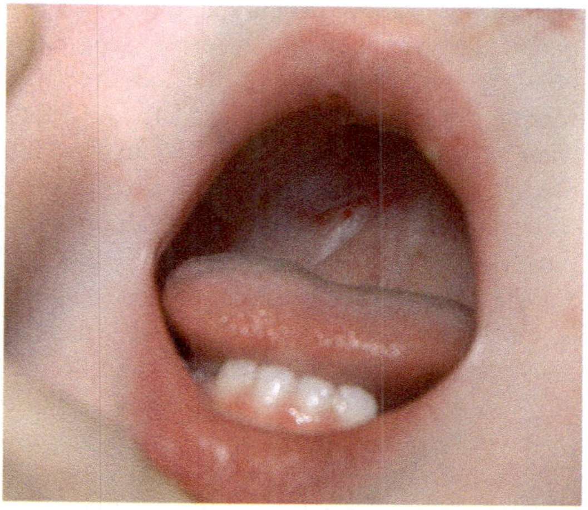

Fig. 7.57 Incision-like laceration of the palatal mucosa

- Internal organs (liver, spleen, lungs, heart, brains, and intestines), blood vessels, nerves, ligaments, tendons, and muscles

Lacerations may bleed profusely, especially when tissues with a rich vascular supply are involved such as scalp or frenum (Purdue 2000). However, the blood loss caused by the laceration is not necessarily substantial, which is probably due to two reasons: hemostasis is supported by two typical characteristics of a laceration, namely, the irregularity of the torn vessels and an almost immediate vascular spasm. Hereby, the chance of a secondary infection is higher than in a wound with more blood loss, for example, in incised wounds. Often the laceration is larger than the surface of the inflicting object. In a laceration of the skin, damage to the underlying structures, such as a skull fracture, a transverse fracture of one of the long bones, or damage to the internal organs, should always be considered (Watson 1990; Pollak and Saukko 2000; DiMaio and DiMaio 2001).

7.4.3 Types of Lacerations

Lacerations are sustained when the applied force exceeds the maximum stress-absorbing capacity of the skin. Generally, lacerations of the skin are the result of the same mechanisms that cause abrasions, namely, tangentially applied blunt forces, leading to either shearing and tearing of the skin (oblique forces), or perpendicularly applied blunt forces, leading to compression (crushing) of the skin (vertical forces), for example, in blows, falls, or pedestrian versus motor vehicle collisions. In children, tangentially and perpendicularly applied forces can be incurred in three different ways, namely:

- When the child is stationary and hit with/by a moving blunt object, for example, when the child is beaten with a stick, a bottle, or a hammer
- When the object is stationary and the child is moving, for example, when the child falls or is thrown from the stairs or against furniture
- When the child and the object are both moving, for example, in a traffic accident

Oblique forces will lead to shearing and tearing of the skin and the subcutaneous tissues (a tear or a tear wound), especially when the skin is fixed to the underlying bone structures, such as skull and shinbones. Depending on the angle at which the skin is impacted, an avulsion may occur (Figs. 7.58 and 7.59). In case of a tangential/oblique impact and depending on the impact angle, unilateral avulsive undermining of the skin will be found, which indicates the direction of the impact. According to DiMaio and DiMaio (2001), the impact side of the blunt force will be beveled, bruised, and/or abraded. A specific type of shearing and tearing is found in animal bites, for example, in children who are bitten by dogs. Generally, these lacerations are deep and/or contaminated and/or complicated (Chap. 8).

More or less perpendicular (or vertical) forces will lead to compression, crushing, and splitting/bursting of the skin (in German, a "Platzwund"). In crushing, the skin and subcutaneous tissues are compressed/crushed between the compressing object and the underlying bony structures until the skin tears/bursts and splits sideways (until the skin lacerates). In crushing lacerations (and sometimes in shearing), the abrasion surrounding the wound may mirror the shape and dimensions of the object used (or in case of a fall to the ground – the area of contact) (Pollak and Saukko 2000). However, the type of object or the mechanism causing the injury can rarely be recognized or deduced from the shape of the laceration. Generally, long, thin, often narrow-edged objects/instruments (such as pipes and cues) will cause linear lacerations, whereas objects with a flat surface will cause irregular lacerations with frayed edges or Y-shaped or star-shaped lacerations (Pollak and Saukko 2000; DiMaio and DiMaio 2001).

A third mechanism which, besides oblique and vertical forces, causes laceration can be seen in overstretching of the skin, for example, in accidents in which a person is overrun by a motor vehicle. Overstretching is also seen in children (and adults) who are sexually assaulted, namely, the overstretching of tissues surrounding orifices, such as the hymen or the perianal skin, during penetration (see 7.4.7).

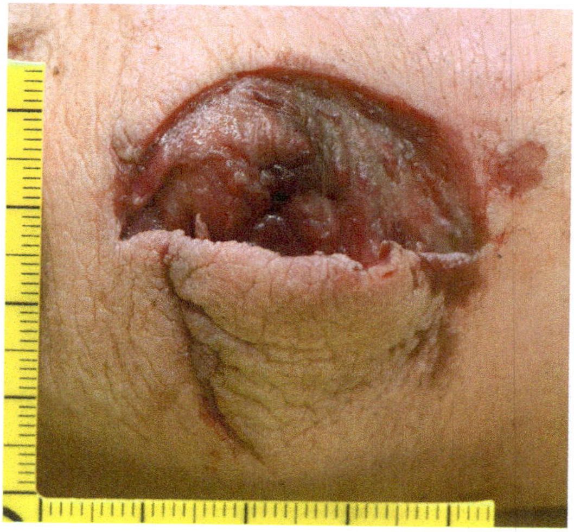

Fig. 7.58 Avulsion with sharp wound margins

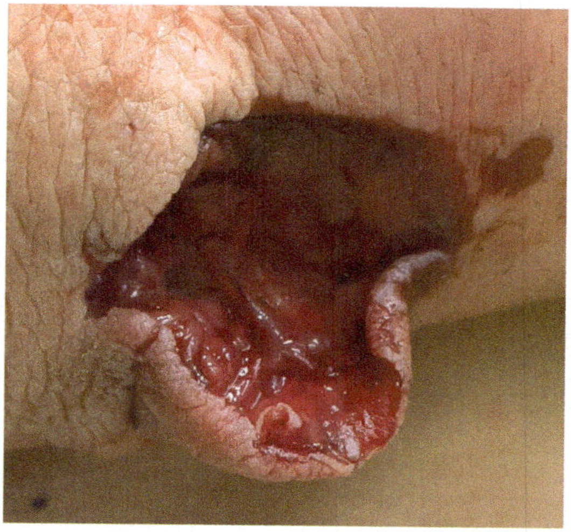

Fig. 7.59 Avulsion

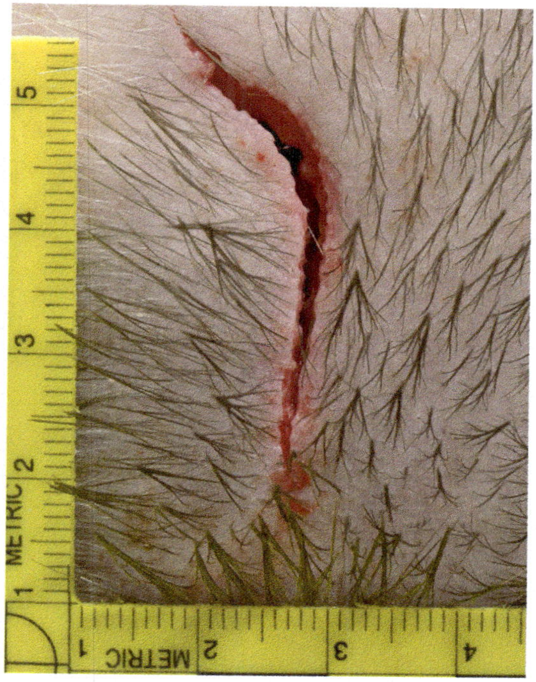

Fig. 7.60 Irregular wound edges: laceration or incised wound with, e.g., a bread knife or saw?

7.4.4 Incision-Like Lacerations

Sometimes lacerations can resemble an incised wound, especially when they are caused by an impact with a heavy object that has a relatively sharp edge, such as an axe, machete, sword, or a meat cleaver, so-called incision-like lacerations or chop(per) wounds. Using this type of instrument will normally lead to severe injuries with extensive damage to the underlying tissues, for example, bony structures or the brain. Depending on how sharp the chopping implement is, the appearance of the resulting injury will vary from a typical laceration with irregular bruised and abraded edges (e.g., a blunt axe) to a typical incision with regular edges (a sharpened machete). However, most of these injuries will show the characteristics of both a laceration and an incision. Incisions made with a bread knife, a saw, or an unsharp knife may show the characteristics of lacerations, for example, irregular abraded wound edges (Fig. 7.60).

From a clinical point of view, differentiating between lacerations, incisions, and incision-like lacerations may not always be relevant, but it is very important from a forensic point of view because it will provide an indication of the instrument used; however, sometimes differentiation will not be possible (Table 7.2).

Incision-like lacerations are also known as "cut-like" lacerations (DiMaio and DiMaio 2001) (Figs. 7.61 and 7.62). Using the term "cut-like" is

Table 7.2 Differentiating lacerations, incision-like lacerations, and incisions (Purdue 2000; DiMaio and DiMaio 2001; Forensic Medicine Resources 2007)

	Laceration	Incision-like laceration	Incision
Cause	Blunt-force trauma	Combination of blunt-force and sharp penetrating trauma	Sharp-force trauma
Wound edges	Irregular with signs of compression or crushing	Incision-like: little damage (some abrasion or bruising) to the surrounding tissue	Sharply demarcated and regular (from the top to the bottom of the incision)
Bruises and/or abrasions	Yes	Some abrasion at the wound edge	Possibly
Tissue bridging	Yes	Yes	No
Depth	Irregular	Irregular	Often uniform
Overlaying hair	Mostly intact		Cleanly divided
Location	Often underlying bony structures	Any location, often skull	Any location
Bony injuries	Possibly associated fractures	Associated fractures (skull) (axe) or linear transection of bony structures (ribs) (machete)	Possibly linear defect in or chipping of underlying bone
Foreign bodies inside the wound	Often (carefully inspect bottom of injury)	Variable	Usually clean (unless caused by breaking glass)
Healing	Generally irregular and extensive scarring	Variable	Generally fine scarring

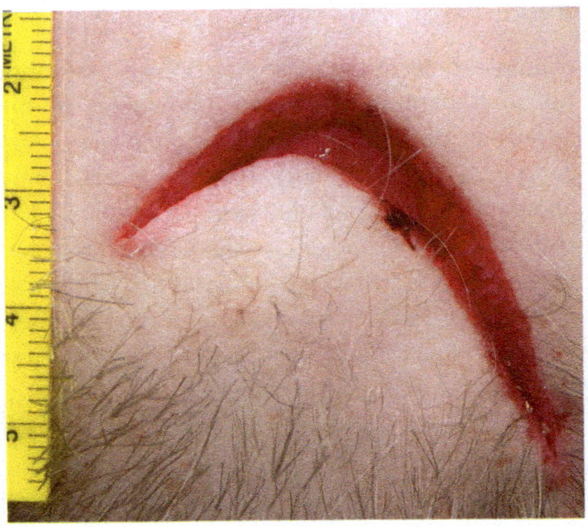

Fig. 7.61 Incision-like laceration on the scalp

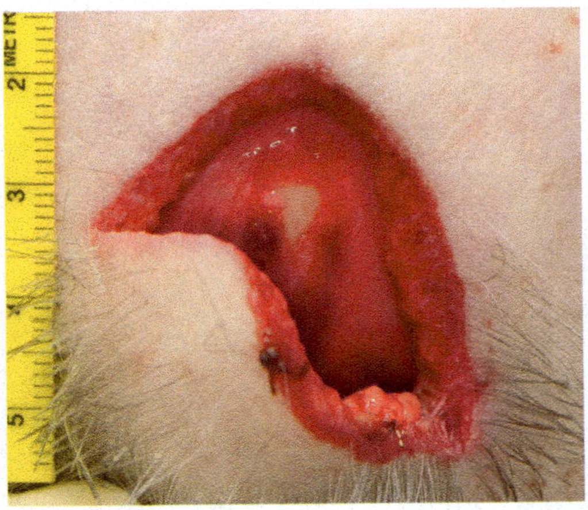

Fig. 7.62 Incision-like laceration on the scalp: no tissue bridges visible

confusing since it suggests that these lacerations have the appearance of cuts, although the definition of a cut varies from author to author. Sometimes the term is used as a synonym for incision/incised wound (DiMaio and DiMaio 2001; Purdue 2000). Saukko w uses the term "cut" as a synonym for a laceration as well as for an incised wound. Payne-James (2003) uses the term as a collective name for wounds in which the integrity of the skin is compromised. He states that cuts can be divided in cuts caused by blunt-impact force (laceration) or by sharp penetrating trauma (incision).

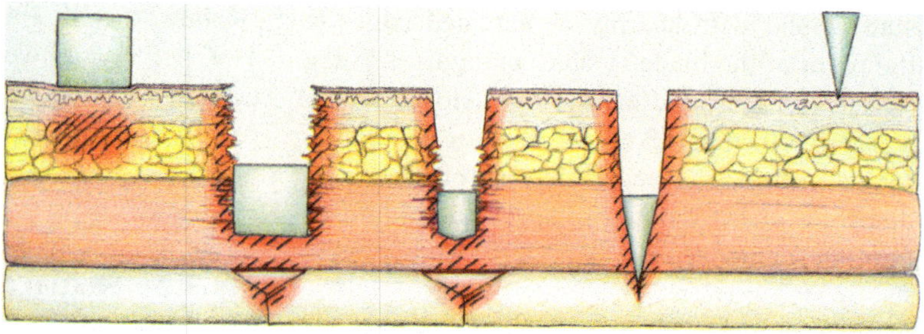

Fig. 7.63 From left to right: blunt-force trauma without penetrating, blunt penetrating trauma (2×), sharp penetrating trauma, superficial sharp trauma, e.g., scratch

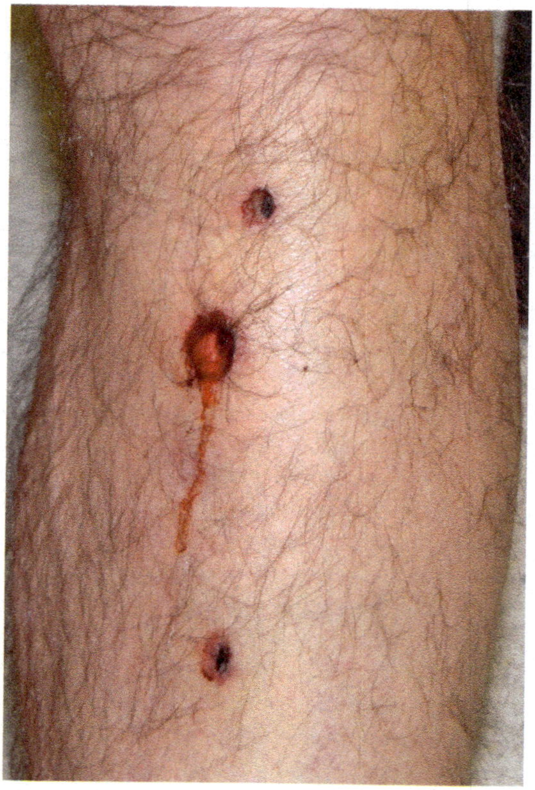

Fig. 7.64 Blunt penetrating trauma due to stamping with stiletto heels

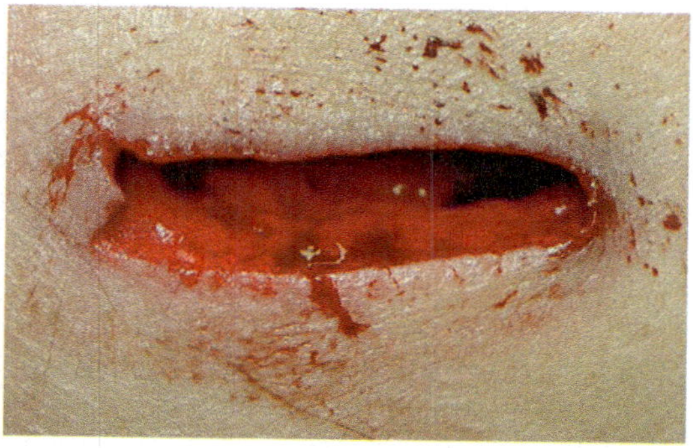

Fig. 7.65 Sharp penetrating trauma: stab wound with a sharp object, probably a single-edged knife because of the fishtailing on one side of the wound and the sharp angle on the other side of the wound (= Fig. 2.15)

7.4.5 Blunt Penetrating Injuries

A blunt penetrating injury or blunt puncture wound is caused by a more or less pointed object which pierces the skin (Fig. 7.63). The diameter of the penetrating object varies from a few millimeters (e.g., a wooden splinter, pin, nail, fork, screw driver, stiletto heel) up to more than 10 cm (e.g., a wooden stake). The result of the piercing varies from deep narrow wounds that are sometimes hard to identify due to the small entry hole without clinical consequences via the same narrow wounds with penetrating and life-threatening injuries to underlying tissues to large injuries with extensive damage to underlying organs (e.g., in a blunt penetrating trauma of the abdomen). A small puncture wound does not necessarily lead to excessive bleeding. It will close quickly, even without medical treatment.

According to Saukko and Knight (2004), this type of laceration is characterized by inversion and abrasion of the wound edges. Inversion of the edges results from the inward overstretching and tearing of the skin caused by the pressure of the object. The inversion may disappear after the piercing object has been withdrawn. Inversion of the edges will also disappear when the inflicting object is completely submerged in the subcutaneous tissue and is covered by the skin as the entry hole closes, like in wooden splinters.

Puncture wounds caused by blunt penetration (Fig. 7.64) should be differentiated from injuries caused by a sharp penetrating trauma (stab wound) (Fig. 7.65). A wound inflicted by one of the blades of a pair of scissors will result in a stab wound with sharply demarcated edges (if the point of the blade is sharp enough) (see also Sect. 2.3). A wound caused by a closed pair of scissors will most likely result in a penetrating injury with abraded and sometimes bruised edges and show characteristics of sharp and blunt penetrating trauma.

7.4.6 Dating of Lacerations

There are no reliable data available to date lacerations. If based on external characteristics, it is difficult and based mainly on the experience of the observer, as is dating of bruises and abrasion.

7.4.7 Lacerations and Child Abuse

7.4.7.1 Physical Abuse

According to Glasgow and Graham (1997), lacerations are extremely common in childhood. Most of these lacerations are relatively minor and will heal with little disability or scarring if properly treated. In physically abused children, cutaneous lacerations are seen significantly less frequently than in children who visit the emergency room for non-inflicted trauma (Pascoe et al. 1979).

In child abuse, the most common lacerations seen are probably lacerations of the frenula of the lip and tongue (Fig. 7.54) and also lacerations in the genital and anal areas of both boys and girls. Also, lacerations of the palate can be found as a result of child abuse (Naidoo 2000). Showers and Bandman (1986) describes the presence of scars and lacerations in 95% of the children ($n=78$) who had been beaten with an electric cord. The injuries and scars were found predominantly on the arm, thighs, and back (Figs. 7.36 and 7.37). Lacerations of the eyelid and periorbital area, conjunctiva, and cornea due to child abuse have been described by Giangiacomo and Frasier (2005).

Sometimes physiological striae (stretch marks) are mistaken for healing scars resulting from lacerations, especially trauma from child abuse (Robinson et al. 1994; Heller 1995; Cohen et al. 1997). Striae however are common in adolescence. They occur in the lumbar and gluteal regions, the upper thighs, breast, lower abdomen, and back (Cohen et al. 1997) (Figs. 7.66, 7.67, 7.68, and 7.69).

7.4.7.2 Sexual Abuse

The most common physical finding in child sexual abuse is a laceration of the posterior fourchette and fossa navicularis (overstretching of the fourchette probably caused by forceful spreading of the labia). However, minor lacerations of the posterior fourchette can also be found as a result of forceful separation of the labia during physical examination. Furthermore, lacerations of the hymen and anal ring may occur as a result of penetration in sexually abused children (overstretching over the hymenal and perihymenal tissues) (Hobbs et al. 1999).

Lacerations in the anogenital region can also be due to a variety of reasons, which are not related to sexual abuse. Scheidler et al. (2000) evaluated the data of 358 girls (0–16 years of age) who experienced perineal trauma. Motor vehicle crashes accounted for the majority of injuries in all age groups. Falls and bicycle-related injuries were significantly more prevalent in children under the age of 9 years. Sexual assaults were the most prevalent cause in children under the age of 4 years. Boos et al. (2003) described the occurrence of anogenital injuries in children run over by slow-motor motor vehicles (two children with perianal lacerations, two with hymenal lacerations). In each case, the wheel of the vehicle passed longitudinally over the child's torso. In cases like these, sexual abuse can only be excluded after a comprehensive investigation.

The majority of anorectal impalements in children is either caused by accidental falls during play or by abusive anal penetration (Jona 1997).

Accidental perineal impalements are rare, although before accepting the accidental circumstances one should always exclude child abuse in all cases of genital or anal trauma (Sugar and Feldman 2007). Most accidental perineal impalements occur in the home, espe-

Fig. 7.66 Striae on the back

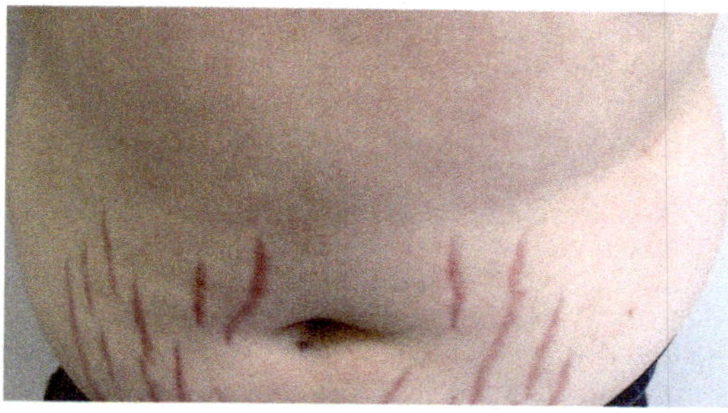

Fig. 7.67 Same person as in Fig. 7.64: striae on the lower abdomen

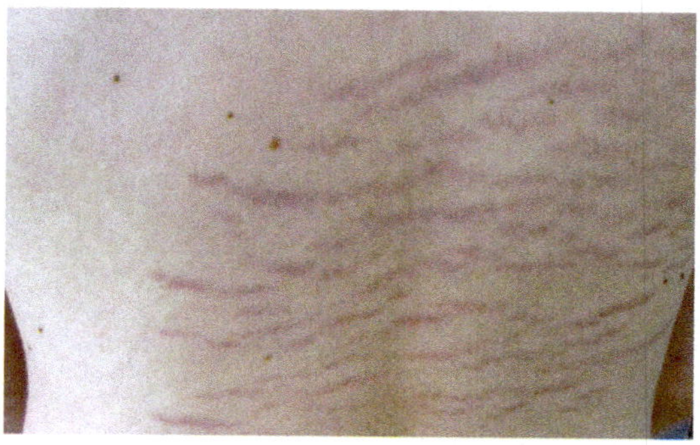

Fig. 7.68 Striae on the back

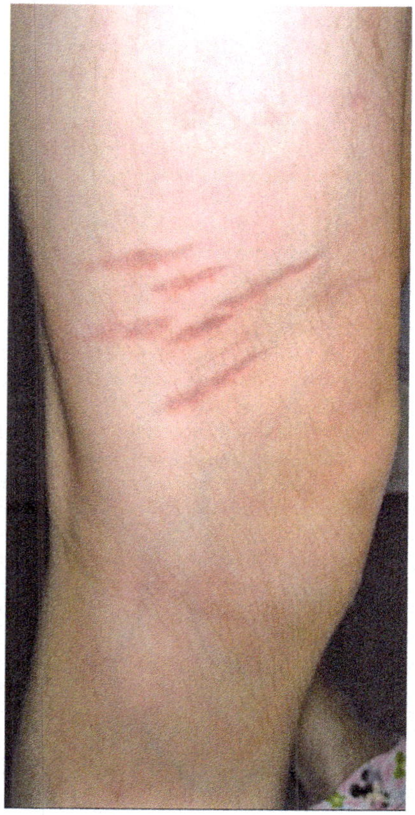

Fig. 7.69 Striae on the leg

cially in the bathroom. According to Sugar and Feldman 2007, the following items should be evaluated extensively before accepting the possibility of an accidental injury:

- History from supervising adults and from other child witnesses
- Examination of the impaling object
- Investigation of the scene

References

Boos SC, Rosas AJ, Boyle C, McCann J (2003) Anogenital injuries in child pedestrians run over by low-speed motor vehicles: four cases with findings that mimic child sexual abuse. Pediatrics 112(1Pt1):e77–e84

Cairns AM, Mok JY, Welbury RR (2005) Injuries to the head, face, mouth and neck in physically abused children in a community setting. Int J Paediatr Dent 15(5):310–318

Centers for Disease Control and Prevention 2007 Public Health Image Library 9875. http://phil.cdc.gov/phil/details.asp?pid=9875

Cohen HA, Matalon A, Mezger A et al (1997) Striae in adolescents mistaken for physical abuse. J Fam Pract 45(1):84–85

DiMaio VJ, DiMaio D (2001) Chapter 4. Blunt trauma wounds. In: DiMaio VJ, DiMaio D (eds) Forensic pathology, 2nd edn. CRC Press, Boca Raton, pp 91–116

Dix J (2000) Chapter 3. Blunt trauma. In: Dix J (ed) Color atlas of forensic pathology. CRC Press, London

Forensic Medicine Resources (2007) Sharp force trauma. http://eforensicmed.googlepages.com/sharpforcetrauma. Accessed on 2010

Giangiacomo J, Frasier LD (2005) Chapter 5. Ophthalmic manifestations. In: Giardino AP, Alexander R (eds) Child maltreatment, a clinical guide and reference, 3rd edn. GW Medical, St Louis, pp 83–89

Glasgow JFT, Graham HK (1997) Chapter 6. Lacerations. In: Glasgow JFT, Graham HK (eds) Management of injuries in children. BMJ Publishing Group, Plymouth, pp 138–175

Heller D (1995) Lumbar physiological striae in adolescence suspected to be non-accidental injury. Br Med J 311(7007):738

Hobbs CJ, Hanks HGI, Wynne JM (1999) Chapter 9. Clinical aspects of sexual abuse. In: Hobbs CJ, Hanks HGI, Wynne JM (eds) Child abuse and neglect, a clinician's handbook, 2nd edn. Churchill Livingstone, New York, pp 191–272

Jona JZ (1997) Accidental anorectal impalement in children. Pediatr Emerg Care 13(1):40–43

Naidoo S (2000). A profile of the oro-facial injuries in child physical abuse at a children's hospital. Child Abuse Negl 24(4):521–34.

Nathanson M (2000) Chapter 11. The physically and emotionally abused child. In: Mason JK, Purdue BN (eds) The pathology of trauma, 3rd edn. Arnold, London, pp 155–175

Nguyen JV (2010) Morphea. eMedicine Medscape, http://emedicine.medscape.com/article/1065782-overview#a0101. Accessed on 2011

Pascoe JM, Hildebrandy HM, Tarrier A et al (1979) Patterns of skin injury in nonaccidental and accidental injury. Pediatrics 64:245–247

Payne-James J (2003) Chapter 36. Assault and injury in the living. In: Payne-James J, Busuttil A, Smock W (eds) Forensic medicine, clinical and pathological aspects. Greenwich Medical Media, London, pp 543–563

Pollak S, Saukko PJ (2000) Causes of death: blunt injury. In: Siegel J, Knupfer G, Saukko P (eds) Encyclopedia of forensic sciences. Academic, London, pp 316–325

Purdue BN (2000) Chapter 9. Cutting and piercing wounds. In: Mason JK, Purdue BN (eds) The pathology of trauma, 3rd edn. Arnold, London, pp 123–140

Reece RM, Grodin MA (1985) Recognition of nonaccidental injury. Pediatr Clin North Am 32(1):41–60

Robertson I, Hodge PR (1972) Histopathology of healing abrasions. Forensic Sci 1(1):17–25

Robinson S (2000) Chapter 10. The examination of the adult victim of assault. In: Mason JK, Purdue BN (eds) The pathology of trauma, 3rd edn. Arnold, London, pp 140–154

Robinson AL, Koester GA, Kaufman A (1994) Striae vs scars of ritual abuse in a male adolescent. Arch Fam Med 3(5):398–399

RCPCH (Royal College of Paediatrics and Child Health) (2008) The physical signs of child sexual abuse – an evidence-based review and guidance for best practice. RCPCH, London, pp 153–157

Saukko P, Knight B (2004) Chapter 4. The pathology of wounds. In: Saukko P, Knight B (eds) Knight's forensic pathology, 3rd edn. Arnold, London, pp 136–173

Scheidler MG, Schultz BL, Schall L, Ford HR (2000) Mechanisms of blunt perineal injury in female pediatric patients. J Pediatr Surg 35(9):1317–1319

Shapiro Ha, Gluckman J, Gordon I (1962) The significance of finger nail abrasions of the skin. J Forensic Med 9:17–19

Showers J, Bandman RL (1986) Scarring for life: abuse with electric cords. Child Abuse Negl 10(1):25–31

Sugar NF, Feldman KW (2007) Perineal impalements in children: distinguishing accident from abuse. Pediatr Emerg Care 23(9):605–616

Watson AA (1990) Injuries and wounds [In Dutch] In: Cohen BAJ, Leliefeld HJ (eds). Introduction into forensic medicine [In Dutch] Kerckebosch BV Zeist, 2e druk, 279–296

Bitemarks

8

8.1 Introduction

> Carnivorous animals, like dogs or tigers, use their teeth in two distinct ways. They kill their prey primarily using their canines and they tear and slice the flesh to produce digestible fragments. Human teeth are designed principally to cut and grind food which is usually previously prepared. Some people appear to revert to more primitive instincts and use their canines and incisors to inflict bites on unsuspecting victims. (Whittaker 2004)

A bitemark is defined as a physical alteration in a medium caused by the contact of teeth or as a representative pattern left in an object or tissue by the dental structures of an animal or human (ABFO 2011). According to (Revis et al. 2009), in humans there are two types of injuries caused by the contact of teeth: occlusive bites and clenched-fist injuries.

Occlusive bites occur when teeth bite a part of a body (Revis et al. 2009). This may lead to bitemarks, in which bruising is seen and the skin is not broken (closed injury) or to open bite injuries with visible damage to the skin (lacerations and avulsions) (Sect. 2.3.1). Occlusive bites regularly occur in children as a result of animal bites. Dogs are the most prevalent biters (Lessig et al. 2006). Children are also bitten by other animals like cats, ferrets, rodents (rats and mice), apes, reptiles, and others. Only a minority of bitemarks presented for medical evaluation and treatment in children is caused by humans (Lessig et al. 2006; MacBean et al. 2007). (Revis et al. 2009) states that occlusive bites are probably most common between toddlers placed in crowded day care centers. Most of these bites are superficial. Human bitemarks are the only injury, which may assist to identify the biter (Ligthelm and van Niekerk 1994; Kemp et al. 2006), although in suspected child abuse cases bitemarks, the clarity of the mark does not always permit the identification of the bite or the biter.

Bitemarks, whether human or animal, can be found on any part of the body (Vale and Noguchi 1983; Pretty and Sweet 2000; Freeman et al. 2005). In some cases of animal bites, the possibility of neglect needs to be considered. If a child is bitten by a human, it is always non-accidental and consciously inflicted with the intention to cause pain. Intentional biting is also seen in self-mutilation (Warnick et al. 1987).

Occlusive bitemarks can be offensive injuries, present in a victim and inflicted during the attack by the perpetrator, or defensive injuries, present in a perpetrator and inflicted during the defense by the victim (Sweet and Pretty 2001). Offensive bitemarks can be found all over the body of the victim (Sect. 8.2.2), while defensive bitemarks are often found on the hands and arms of the attacker (Sweet and Pretty 2001). When a bitemark is found in either a victim or a suspect, both should be carefully examined for the presence of other bitemarks since in 43% of cases, more than one bite wound was present (Freeman et al. 2005).

Clenched-fist injuries occur as a person's closed fist strikes the teeth of another person with enough force to create a open small injury of the skin, often at dorsal surface of the middle finger metacarpophalangeal joint of the dominant hand

R.A.C. Bilo et al., *Cutaneous Manifestations of Child Abuse and Their Differential Diagnosis*,
DOI 10.1007/978-3-642-29287-3_8, © Springer-Verlag Berlin Heidelberg 2013

(usually 3–8 mm in length) and sometimes even leading to joint penetration, metacarpal fracture, and a laceration of the underlying extensor tendon (Revis et al. 2009). This type of injury is usually the result of a fist fight. Sometimes, this type of injury is referred to as a reverse bite injury, a closed fist injury or a fight bite (Wikipedia, 2011a). Clenched-fist injuries are typical attack injuries and may indicate the perpetrator in domestic violence or child abuse. Clenched-fist injuries are mostly seen in males between adolescence and the fourth decade of life (Revis et al. 2009).

8.2 Epidemiology

8.2.1 Human and Animal Bites

8.2.1.1 Incidence

In the United States, bite injuries constitute about 1% of all visits to the emergency room. After dog and cat bites, human bites are the third category (Pretty et al. 1999). MacBean et al. (2007) investigated the occurrence of mammal (human and animal) bites in Victoria, Australia, and did find similar data. In the period 1998–2004, a total of 12,982 bite injuries were treated in living patients (0.8% of treated patients on the participating EDs). Younger patients predominated, with 1,528 (11.8%) children between 1 and 4 years. Dogs (79.6%), humans (8.7%), and cats (7.2%) were responsible for 95.6% of all bite injuries. One-third of the dog bites occurred in children <14 years old. Around 2% of children <14 years old appeared to have human bites. Schweich and Fleisher (1985) evaluated 40 children between the age of 4 months and 18 years who were examined at the emergency room for bite injuries. The incidence of human bites was 1 per 600 visits. The most prevalent site appeared to be the face (superficial abrasions inflicted by another child). Baker and Moore (1987) evaluated 322 human bites in children over a period of 6 years and found almost the same incidence as Schweich: one human bitemark per 615 emergency room visits.

Rawson et al. (1984) investigated the occurrence of bite injuries in children in residential facilities over a period of 3 months and found 1,545 bite injuries per 100,000 admitted children (approximately one bite injury per 60 admitted children). Garrard et al. (1988) evaluated the data of 224 children in a day care center over a 1-year period. Forty-six percent of the children were bitten once or more than once by other children. The incidence of human bitemarks seems to be the highest in children in residential facilities (Rawson et al. 1984), in abused children, and in children with a mental handicap (Gold et al. 1989).

The foregoing data are likely to underestimate the exact incidence of bitemarks, whether human or animal, because many bites do not require medical attention. The exact incidence of intentional human biting, resulting in bitemarks, in children is obviously not known for the same reason but also because biting parents will avoid medical care as long as the bitemark can be recognized as such and as long (Leung and Robson 1992).

8.2.1.2 Age and Sex

Bite rates vary with age. Toddlers suffer the highest rate (1.4 bites per 100 child days of enrollment in a day care center) followed by infants and preschoolers (Garrard et al. 1988). Another peak is seen in the 11–16 years age group (Baker and Moore 1987). Boys are bitten more often than girls (Marr et al. 1979; Baker and Moore 1987; Merchant et al. 2005).

8.2.1.3 Season and Time of Day

Human bites marks in children are found more often during summer months (71%), probably due to a relative lack of protective clothing during warmer summer months (May–October) (Baker and Moore 1987). A large majority (86%) of human bites seem to be inflicted between 2 p.m. and 11 p.m. with only 4% between midnight and noon (Baker and Moore 1987).

8.2.2 Anatomical Location of Bitemarks Caused by Human Biting

Freeman et al. (2005) studied the etiology, anatomical location, victim characteristics, and legal dispositions of bitemark cases. Freeman evaluated a total of 259 cases with 778 bite injuries. Of the bitemarks, 46.7% were found in victims of sexual assault, 39.4% in homicide victims, and 32.8% in victims of child abuse (Table 8.1). The sum of the percentage distribution of the individual offenses is more than 100%. The reason for this is that in some cases, more than one type of offense was involved. It appeared that women were bitten more often than men. On the average, male victims appeared to be younger than female victims. Furthermore, male victims appeared to be either very young or very old. Often, the perpetrators appeared to be males. Most bite injuries were seen on the arms, followed by the breasts. When gender was included in the analysis, it appeared that men were bitten more often on the arms, whereas women were bitten more often on the breasts. Freeman also found a relationship between, on the one hand, the anatomical location and number of bite injuries and, on the other hand, the type of offense and the age of the victim. Freeman concluded, like Sweet and Preety (2001), that bitemarks may be found anywhere on the body, may be single or multiple, and occur in both the victims and the perpetrators of violence. They further concluded that the distribution pattern varied greatly and that distribution was determined, at least partially, by:

1. The type of offense (Table 8.1)
2. The age of the victim
3. The gender of the victim
4. The occurrence of the bite wound in either the victim or the perpetrator
5. The age and the gender of the perpetrator

According to Schweich and Fleisher (1985), Baker and Moore (1987), and Merchant et al. (2005), in children, the head and neck are the most common sites in 30–45%, followed by the extremities in 30–36%.

8.3 Clinical Features of Human Bitemarks

8.3.1 Severity and Forensic Significance of Bitemarks

As stated before, bitemarks vary in severity and forensic significance from mild injuries in the form of a minimal, hardly recognizable imprint mark from teeth without bruising, which vanish quickly, and perhaps a few abrasions via a typical and easy to recognize pattern injury to severe injuries such as lacerations or avulsions of the skin, which without a clear history often cannot be recognized as bite injuries, and damage to

Table 8.1 Distribution of bite wounds according to the type of offense

Overall		Sexual assault 46.7%		Homicide 39.4%		Child abuse 32.8%	
Arms	22.4%	Breasts	18.6%	Arms	24.3%	Arms	28.6%
Legs	12.1%	Arms	15.9%	Legs	14.3%	Legs	18.9%
Breasts	11.2%	Face	13.3%	Breasts	12.7%	Back	8.5%
Face	10.7%	Legs	9%	Face	10.6%	Buttocks and face simultaneously	7.3%
Shoulders	8.2%	Shoulders	8.5%	Shoulders	9%	Shoulders	6.1%
Back	6.9%	Back	6.9%	Back	6.9%	Belly	5.3%

Freeman et al. (2005)

Table 8.2 The bitemark severity and forensic significance scale

Severity scale	Forensic significance
1. Very mild bruising, no individual tooth marks present, diffuse arches visible	Low
2. Obvious bruising with individual, discrete areas associated with teeth, skin intact	Moderate
3. Very obvious bruising with superficial abrasions associated with teeth on the most severe aspects of the injury, likely to be assessed as definite bitemark	High
4. Numerous areas of abrasion, with some bruising, some areas of the wound may be incised. Unlikely to be confused with any other injury mechanism	High
5. Partial avulsion of tissue, some lacerations present indicating teeth as the probable cause of the injury	Moderate
6. Complete avulsion of tissue, possibly some scalloping of the injury margins suggesting that teeth may have been responsible for the injury. May not be an obvious bite injury	Low

After Pretty (2008)

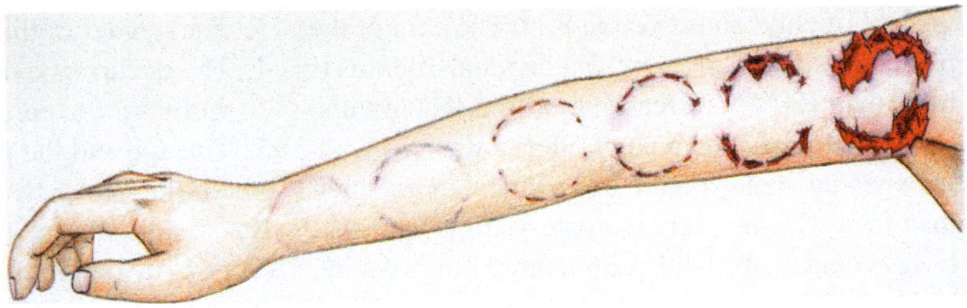

Fig. 8.1 Severity scale from 1–6 (from left to right)

Table 8.3 Possible conclusions after evaluation of a suspicious injury

Probability	Description
Excluded	The injury is not a bitemark
Possible	An injury showing a pattern that may or may not be caused by teeth, could be caused by other factors but biting cannot be ruled out
Probable	The pattern strongly suggests or supports origin from teeth but could conceivably be caused by something else
Definite	There is no reasonable doubt that teeth created the pattern

ABFO, cited from Pretty (2008)

brain, joint, and bones (Table 8.2 and Fig. 8.1). The "prototypical" human bitemark in a child, which is typically inflicted by an adult, will be a circular or oval (doughnut) (ring-shaped) patterned injury consisting of two opposing (facing) symmetrical, U-shaped arches separated at their bases by open spaces. The arches consist of a series of individual bruises, abrasions, and/or lacerations, reflecting the size, shape, arrangement, and distribution of the contacting surfaces of the human dentition (ABFO 2011). The ABFO (American Board of Forensic Odontology) also defines a range of conclusions whether or not a physical finding is a bitemark (Table 8.3, cited from Pretty 2008) (Figs. 8.2, 8.3, 8.4, 8.5, and 8.6). Variations of the prototypical human bitemark include additions, subtractions, and distortions. If the integrity of the skin is compromised, abrasions are the most prevalent injury (about 75%). Punctures are found in about 13% and lacerations in almost 12% (Baker and Moore 1987).

8.3.2 Appearance of Bitemarks in Human Biting

8.3.2.1 Physical Factors Influencing the Appearance

Human biting may lead to complex injuries (bruises, abrasions, and sometimes lacerations in various combinations, see Table 8.2). This is the result of the simultaneous action of:

- Perpendicular compressive forces on the skin by the closing and compressing of the jaws during biting
- Forces that arise through the simultaneous perpendicular and parallel cutting by the incisors and the horizontal to and fro movement by the teeth on the skin's surface and the underlying structures

The types of injury that arise by biting and the exact appearance of the corresponding bruising depend on the following factors (Sognnaes 1977; McLay 1990; Bernat 1992; Richardson 1993):

- The force of the bite and/or the applied pressure
- The duration of the occlusive pressure
- The resistance and the elasticity of the skin
- The curvature of the body surface
- The resistance by the victim
- The movement of the skin between the teeth
- The time lapse between the time of the injury and the examination

Three mechanisms play a role in the developing of bitemarks: imprint, suction, and pressure (Bernat 1992).

8.3.2.2 Imprint

Ultimately, the imprint of the dental elements (together with the shape of the jaws) on the skin will lead to bitemarks. These are generally characterized by conspicuous crescent-shaped

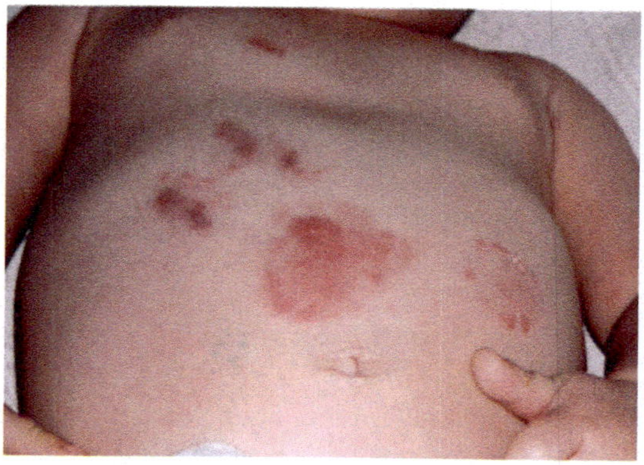

Fig. 8.2 Several injuries suggestive for bitemarks: severity scale 3 – superficial abrasions associated with teeth on the most severe aspects of the injury – definite bitemark, low to moderate forensic significance (no measuring scale, low quality of picture)

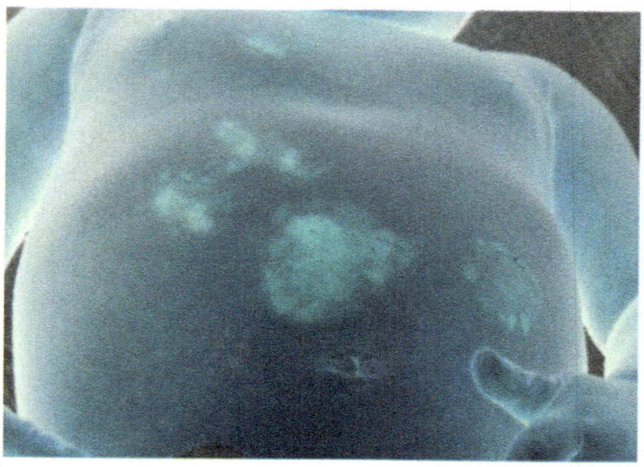

Fig. 8.3 Several injuries suggestive for bitemarks (color negative): severity scale 3

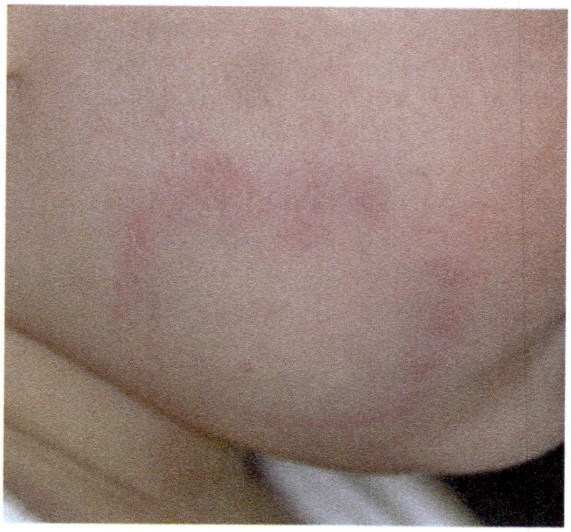

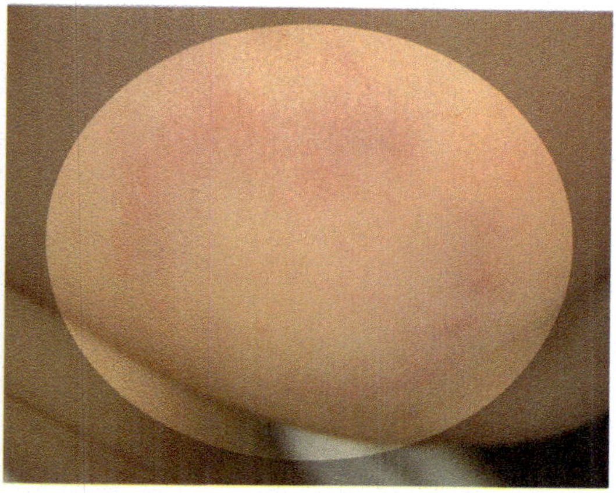

Fig. 8.5 Adapting of levels (see also Chap. 9) – possibly/probably a bitemark (= Fig. 9.16)

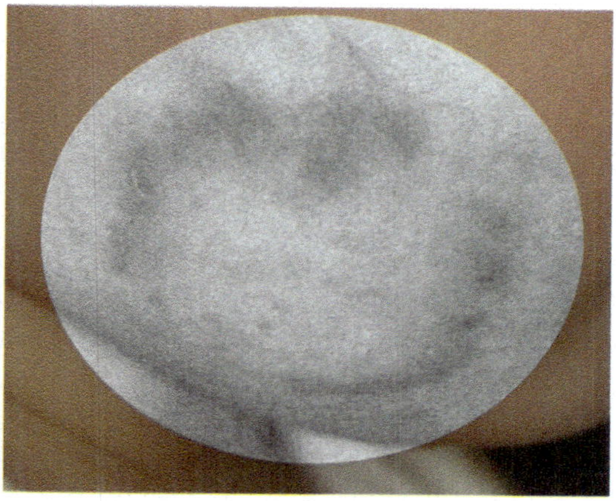

Fig. 8.6 Uncoloring: black/white conversion (see also Chap. 9) – probably a bitemark, severity scale 2, low to moderate forensic significance (no measuring scale, low quality of picture) (= Fig. 9.17)

(crescentic) or U-shaped bruising. In these bruises, individual teeth imprints can be distinguished. Sometimes, a complete ring is visible when the upper and lower arch are not separated but joined at their edges. Sometimes, only partial bitemarks can be distinguished, for example, one arch, one tooth, or a few teeth or unilateral marks. The imprint of the maxillary teeth arch generally leads to diffuse bruising, whereas the mandibular arch often displays individual

Fig. 8.4 Original picture: hardly recognizable pattern injury – severity scale 1, possibly a bitemark (= Fig. 9.15)

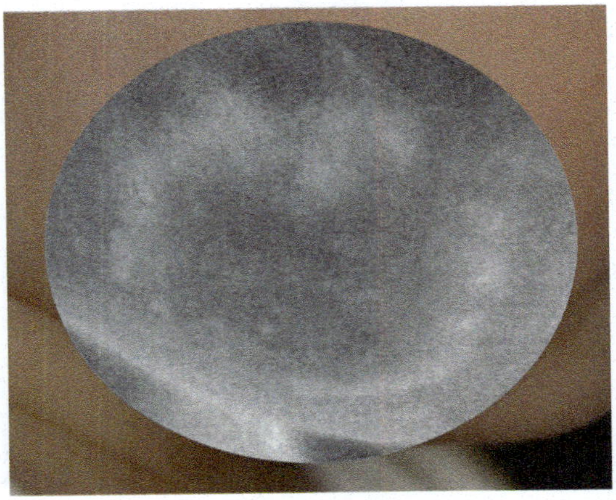

Fig. 8.7 Uncoloring: black/white negative (see also Chap. 9) – probably a bitemark, severity scale 2, low to moderate forensic significance (no measuring scale, low quality of picture) (= Fig. 9.18)

elements (Levine 1984). These bruises develop as a result of positive pressure when the teeth are closed with disruption of small vessels (Kellogg 2005).

In a human bitemark, the canines are less conspicuous than in an animal bite with well-developed canines (McLay 1990). When compared with the canines of, for example, a cat, the human canines are relatively blunt and proportionally broader so that the chance of puncture wounds (point-shaped wounds, whereby the skin is damaged) is small. Human canines leave round or ovoid marks and rarely penetrate the skin.

8.3.2.3 Suction

Biting may be used to maintain a grip on the skin during sucking. Hereby, an area of negative pressure develops in the central part of the bitemark, leading to the formation of suction petechiae (sometimes called hickey or lovebite, see Sect. 3.3.3). The effect of the sucking is enhanced by tongue thrusting. If the sucking and thrusting is severe, outlines of the palatal and lingual surfaces of the teeth may become evident within the outlines of the petechial hemorrhage.

8.3.2.4 Pressure

During biting, the part of the skin that is "imprisoned" by the bite between the lower and the upper jaw is pressed by the biter's tongue against the teeth or the palate, which may lead to bruising. According to Kellogg (2005), bruising on this site may also develop as a result of negative pressure. Sometimes, an imprint of the inner side of the teeth or the ridges on the hard palate may be seen in the bruise.

8.3.3 Dating of Bitemarks

The problems involved in dating on the basis of visible changes, reflecting healing of the injuries, are comparable with those involved in the dating of bruises in general (Sect. 3.3.3). Exact dating based on objective scientific data is not possible (Dailey and Bowers 1997). Dating of a bitemark is neither a scientific nor an accurate process (Bowers 2004).

Imprints of bites may vanish within several hours if the skin has not been damaged or may be visible for days when the skin has been damaged. This also depends on the site of the bite, the bite force, and the thickness of the tissue. In the thinner areas of the skin, bite injuries will remain visible for prolonged periods (Wagner 1986).

8.3.4 Infection Risk in Human Biting

Schweich and Fleisher (1985) evaluated 40 children aged between 4 months and 18 years who were seen at the emergency room for a bite injury. The aim of the study was to obtain insight into the spectrum of human bites and the incidence of infections in treated and non-treated injuries. Schweich concluded that the majority of the human bites will lead to superficial damage and that generally infections do not occur. Prophylactic antibiotic treatment of bites with only bruises or superficial abrasions, without any damage to the underlying tissues, is not required. Only if the skin is broken, antibiotics may be needed because severe infections may develop (Schweich and Fleisher 1985; McLeod 2008).

Baker (1987) evaluated 322 human bites in children over a period of 6 years (one bitemark per 615 emergency room visits). Most bites occurred during a fight (69%) or play (26%). Superficial abrasions were present in 75%, punctures in 13%, and lacerations in 11%. Infections occurred in 38% of the punctures and in 37% of the lacerations. No infection was seen in any of the children with only abrasions. Other factors that influenced the development of infection were a delay of more than 18 h in seeking medical care, a site on the upper extremities, and an injury sustained during sports. Baker (1987) showed that the risk of wound infection is very high in human bites with more than superficial damage to the skin.

Revis et al. (2009) states that approximately 10–15% of open human bite injuries will become infected.

8.3.4.1 Viral Infections

The risk of transmission of the pathogens of hepatitis B (Hamilton et al. 1976; Cancio-Bello et al. 1982; Stornello 1991; Carr 1995; Hui et al. 2005) and C (Dusheiko et al. 1990) and herpes simplex virus (HSV) (Revis et al. 2009) is low but present in a human bite.

Although according to some authors, HIV may be transmitted in human biting (Pretty et al. 1999; Andreo et al. 2004; Bartholomew and Jones 2006), Revis et al. (2009) states that this is biologically possible, although quite unlikely in biting. Stockheim et al. (2005) pointed out the risks of HIV transmission through biting in a juvenile population (Stockheim et al. 2005). They evaluated 734 bite- and blood-exposure incidents. Nine incidents involved children who were either HIV-positive or who were suspected of being HIV-positive. Although theoretically the risk of transmission by biting does exist as illustrated by Revis et al. (2009) and Stockheim et al. (2005), no proven case of biting related HIV transmission is found in medical literature.

8.3.4.2 Bacterial Infections

Infections with streptococcus and staphylococcus have been described (Carr 1995). This involved case reports in adults. Also, the transmission of *Mycobacterium tuberculosis* (tuberculosis), *Actinomyces israelii* (*Actinomycosis cutaneum*), *Clostridium tetani* (tetanus) (Revis et al. 2009), and *Treponema pallidum* (syphilis) (Fiumara and Exner 1981) has been reported, but the risk seems to be extremely low.

8.3.5 Fatal Human Biting Injuries

Human bites are probably very rarely if ever lethal (Pollak and Mortinger 1989; Lauridson and Myers 1993). There are no reports in the medical literature of children dying after a human bite. Nevertheless, bite injuries are regularly seen during autopsies of children who died as a result of child abuse. Trube-Becker (1977), for example, did find bitemarks in 11 of 48 cases of fatal child abuse (23%). Most bitemarks in these fatal cases were found on the extremities, abdomen, and cheeks.

8.4 Bitemarks and Bite Injuries in Children and Child Abuse

8.4.1 The Circumstances of Human Biting

Children are bitten by other children and by adults. Human biting is always non-accidental. The circumstances differ with age (Schweich and Fleisher 1985; Barsley and Landcaster 1987; Leung and Robson 1992). When a child is bitten by another child, it is either during play (no intention to cause pain), frustration (the inability of infants and toddlers to express themselves verbally), or quarreling (intention to cause pain or to end the argument, frustration, fights, or aggressive play) (Leung and Robson 1992). Frequent biting of children may reflect a lack of discipline at home. In older children and adolescents, biting can result from fighting (Baker and Moore 1987). Bitemarks in children and adolescents can also occur during sporting activities (Schweich and Fleisher 1985; Baker and Moore 1987). In adolescents, bitemarks may be the result of lovebites, inflicted during love making or sexual assault (sexual biting – Sect. 8.4.2).

Bites in children, inflicted by an adult, are always consciously inflicted with the intention to cause pain. The circumstances under which a child is bitten by an adult are:

- Inappropriate punishment by example: the child is bitten in order to teach the child not to bite others.
- Part of physical abuse: this may involve a single incident or a regularly recurring form of abuse. In physical abuse, many human bite-

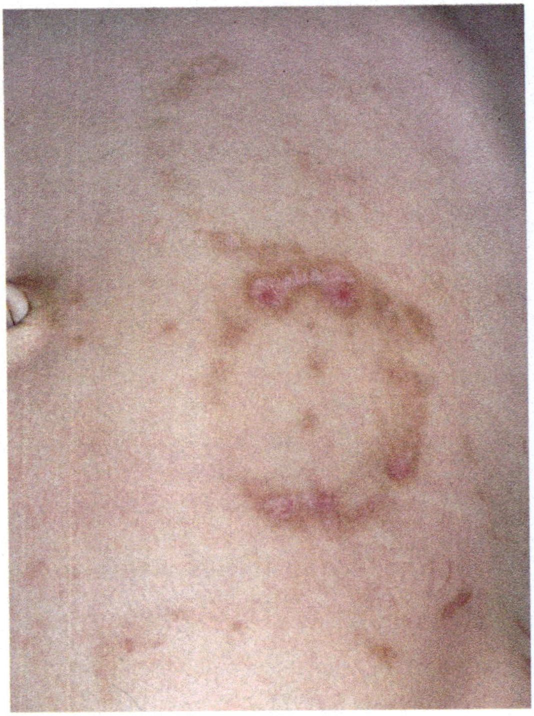

Fig. 8.8 Bitemark on the abdomen (= Fig. 3.9)

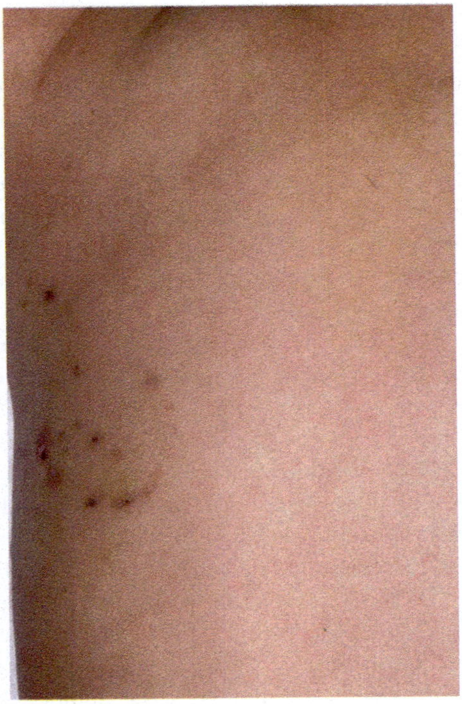

Fig. 8.9 Bitemark on the back

marks can be found on many different parts of the body. Trube-Becker (1973), for example, described a child with 17 bitemarks spread all over the body.

- Part of a sexual assault: lovebites and bitemarks are mainly found on the neck, breasts, anogenital region, and buttocks.

8.4.2 Aggressive and Sexual Biting

In child abuse cases, the motivation of biting by adults can be divided in biting with a predominantly aggressive or a predominantly sexual intention (Levine 1977; McLay 1990).

In most cases, the injuries caused by aggressive or sexual biting cannot be differentiated from each other because the resulting injury will be the same.

8.4.2.1 Aggressive Biting

In aggressive biting, teeth are used as a weapon (Figs. 8.8 and 8.9). The bite is quick and forceful.

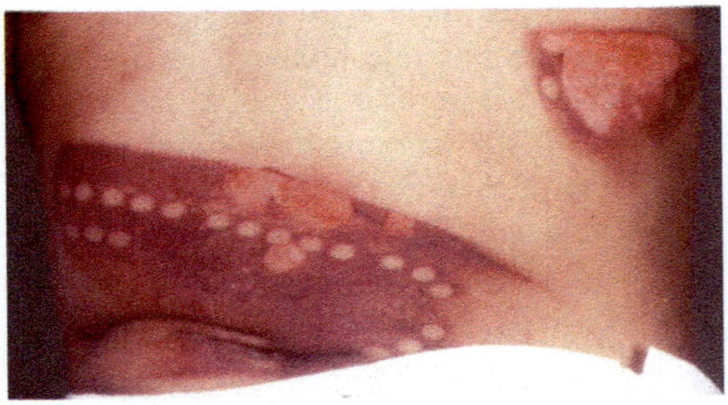

Fig. 8.10 Same child: burning with a steam iron (= Fig. 2.28)

The injuries comprise imprint injury as well as pressure injury. Generally, the site of the bite is determined by chance. Therefore, bite injuries may be found anywhere on the body. However, they are generally seen at sites such as the arms which are not (always) covered by clothing and thus easily accessible. Other sites are the legs, the hands/fingers, the chest, the cheeks, the ears, and the nose. Often, other injuries are found (Figs. 8.10, 8.11, 8.12, 8.13, 8.14, and 8.15).

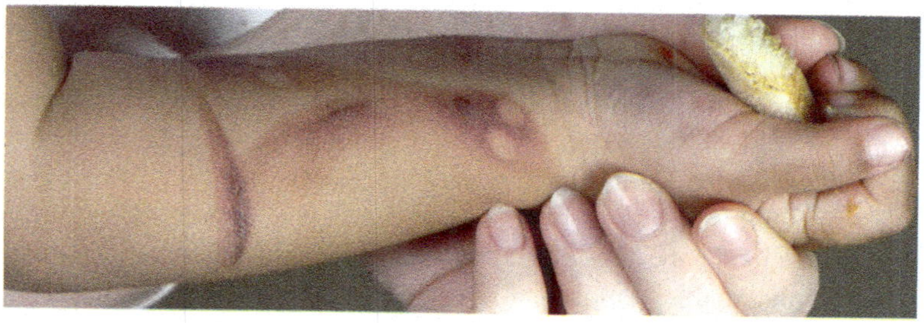

Fig. 8.11 Same child: burning with a steam iron

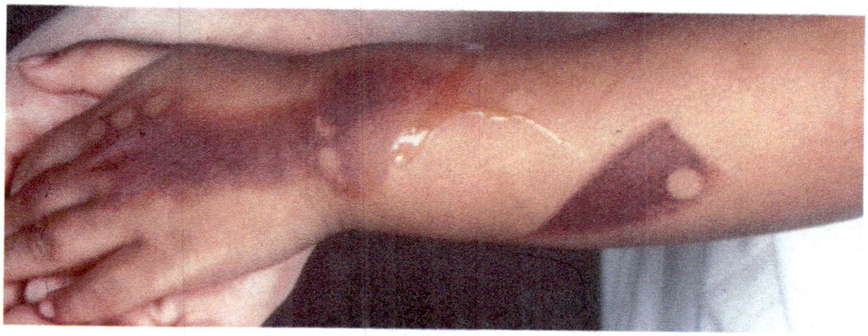

Fig. 8.12 Same child: burning with a steam iron

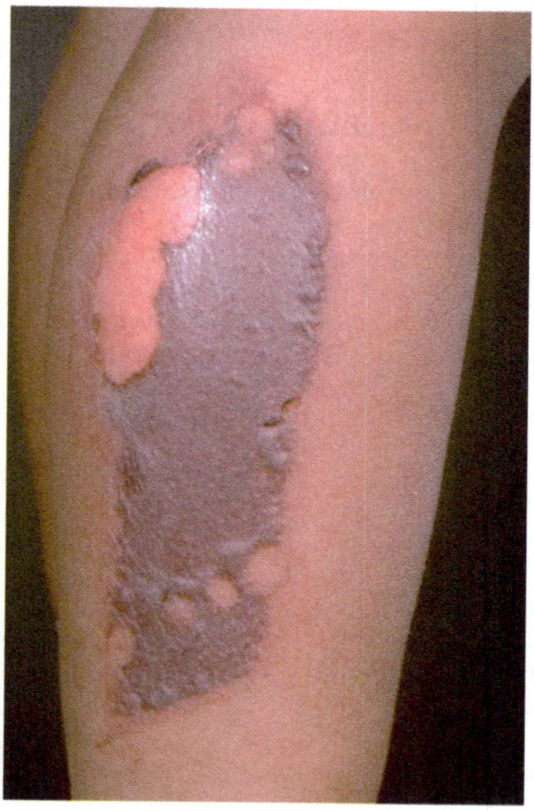

Fig. 8.13 Same child: burning with a steam iron

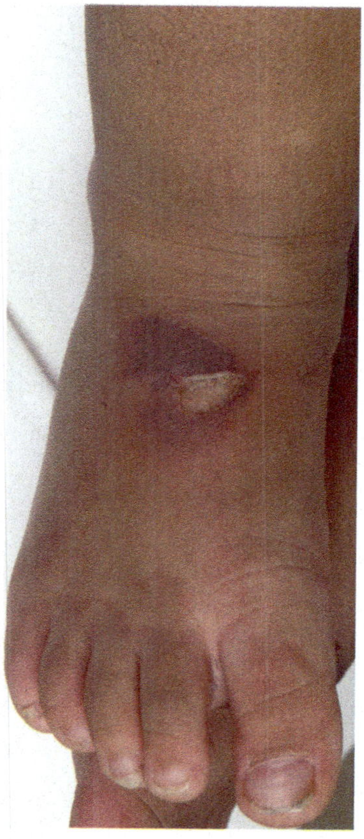

Fig. 8.14 Same child: burning with a steam iron

Sexual Biting

In sexual biting, three types of injuries are found, namely, imprint, suction, and pressure injuries. Biting with sexual intention is slow and forceful, in contrast to the bite in aggressive biting, and may not lead to a typical bitemarks. According to Levine (1977), the slow pace of the perpetrator may be regarded as almost sadistic behavior. In the absence of a (clearly) visible imprint injury, only the suction injury and the pressure injury may be visible, resembling a lovebite or hickey (Sect. 3.3.3) (Fig. 8.16). This manner of biting may involve all body sites. However, bites found in sites such as the breast(s)/nipples, the neck, the shoulders, the upper back, the thighs (Fig. 8.17), the cheeks, the belly, the anogenital region (e.g., a circular bitemark on the penis or near the penis – Fig. 8.18), and the buttocks (Figs. 8.19 and 8.20) are more suspect for this type of biting than for bites of an aggressive type. In nipple bites, there is a risk that the nipple is partially or completely bitten off.

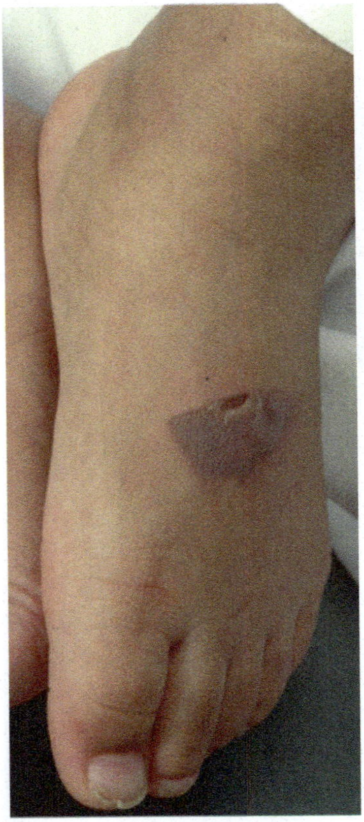

Fig. 8.15 Same child: burning with a steam iron

A perpetrator may bite the tongue of a child in a sexual as well as in an aggressive way. Differentiation with a tongue bite by the child itself is possible by looking at the curvature in the bite, if present. The tongue bite will be parallel to the own tongue arch if the child is responsible. The curve in the injury runs in the opposite direction to the tongue arch of the child when the child has been bitten (Mouden 1998; Lee et al. 2002).

8.5 Identification of the Biter

8.5.1 Imprint Characteristics and DNA

At the moment, bite injuries are the only physical injury in child abuse that may indicate or may even lead to the identification of the biter/perpetrator (Wagner 1986; Fischman 2002) because of the typical and relatively unique characteristics

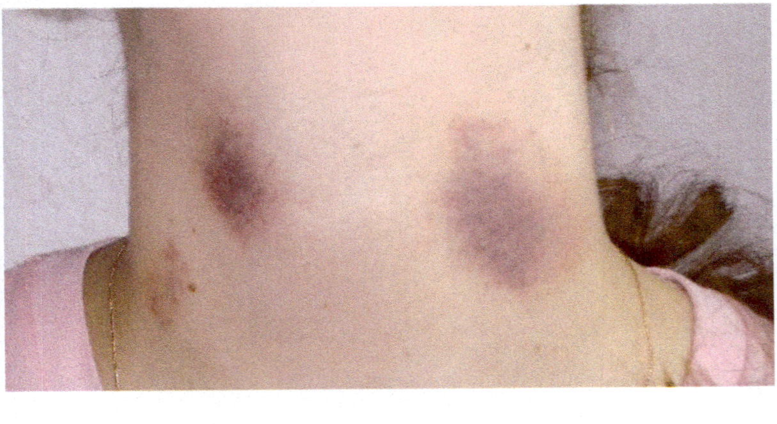

Fig. 8.16 Lovebite. (Janek B, 2008. From Wikipedia, 2011 http://en.wikipedia.org/wiki/Love-bite)(= figure 3.102)

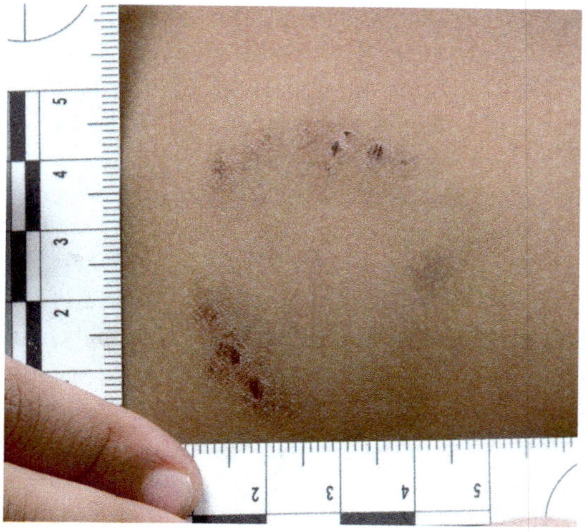

Fig. 8.17 Bitemark on the inside of the left thigh (size of the bitemark suggests biting by an adult)

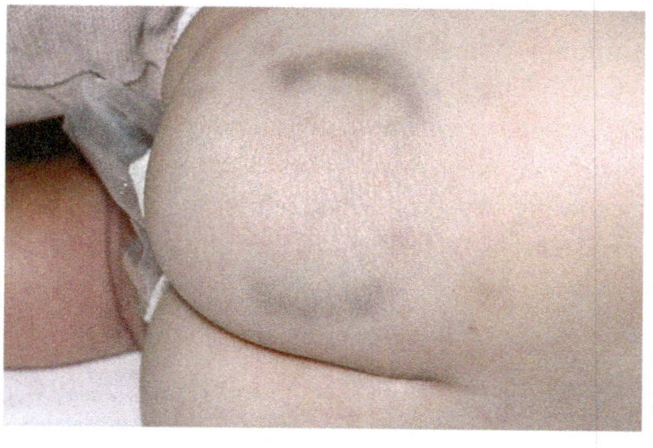

Fig. 8.18 Bitemark on the buttocks

of the dental imprints that are visible in a bitemark and/or the DNA from the saliva of the biter that was transferred onto the body of the person who was bitten.

8.5.1.1 Typical and Unique Imprint Characteristics

The unique characteristics of human bitemarks were recognized early in human history. There is a legend, which states that William the Conqueror, King of England in the eleventh century, would bite into wax used to seal official documents (Rothwell, 1995). The legend also states that his teeth were misaligned, creating a distinctive pattern which made it easy to determine the authenticity of his letters and documents (Enotes,

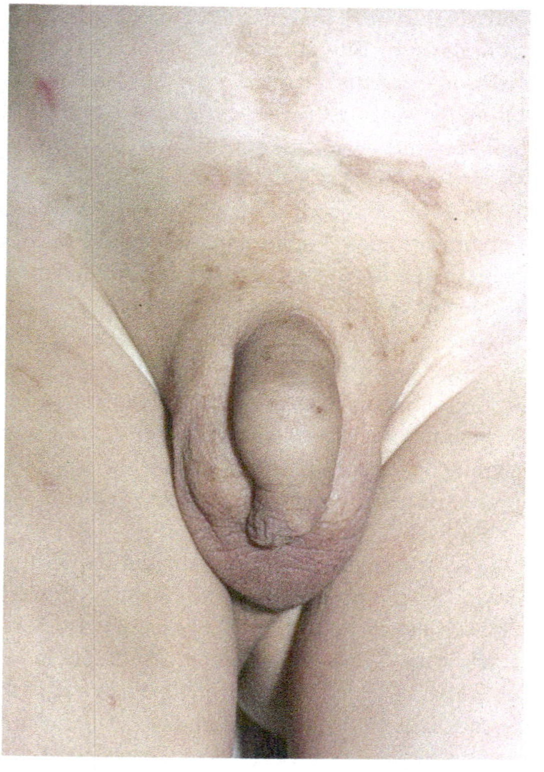

Fig. 8.19 Several injuries in the genital area, suggestive for bitemarks

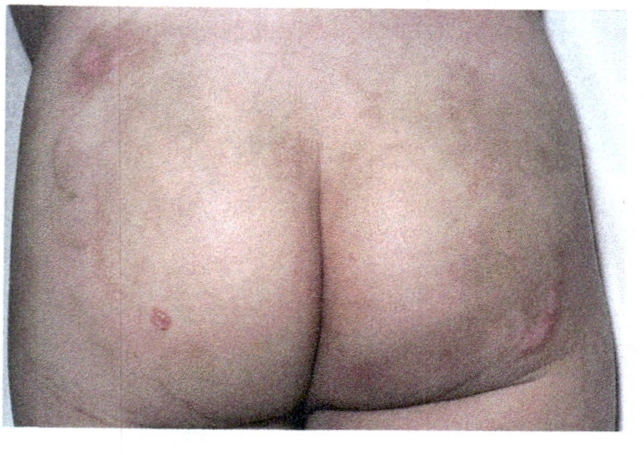

Fig. 8.20 Several injuries on the buttocks, suggestive for bitemarks

undated). Senn (2011) did not find any proof for this legend but did find other evidence that teeth were used in England in the thirteenth and fourteenth century to mark sealing wax. Another example of the use of the supposed unique characteristics of dentition is found in the seventeenth and eighteenth century (Wikipedia, 2011b). Debtors from Europe, who went to America to work as servants, verified their agreements by biting the seal on the pact instead of a signature and became known as indentured servants (Rothwell, 1995) (Figs. 8.21 and 8.22).

Probably, the earliest recorded bitemark case and first attempt to admit bitemark evidence in a court of law in the United States was Ohio versus Robinson in 1870 (Pierce et al. 1990). Ansil Robinson was charged with the murder of his mistress, Mary Lunsford. The evidence against Robinson included an attempt to match his teeth to bitemarks on the victim's arm. Robinson was acquitted after a 3-week trial despite the evidence presented in court matching his teeth to bitemarks on the victim's arm.

The analysis of bitemarks is based on the following two concepts or assumptions (Bowers 2004), namely, that the dental characteristics of anterior teeth involved in biting are unique in all individuals (the individuality of human dentition in regard to size, shape, and alignment of the teeth) and that this asserted uniqueness is transferred and recorded in the injury as a unique pattern. These typical and unique characteristics of the dental imprints may be visible in the bite injury.

In evaluating the imprint, the following characteristics should be taken into account:

- The size of the injury
- The dental class characteristics in the injury
- The presence of puncture marks
- The shape of the arch and the distance between the canines (Christian and Mouden 2001)

The fundamental step in bitemark analysis is the determination of which teeth made specific marks. This determination is based on the appearance of the tooth class and bitemark class characteristics (Bowers, 2004). The expertise of a forensic odontologist is required to identify the perpetrator by comparing these characteristic hallmarks of the bitemark with the dental imprint of the suspect (Sims et al. 1973).

In 1983, Geberth stated that a human dental imprint is probably as unique as the finger prints of an individual: "*Remember, bitemark identification represents individual characteristic evidence which can positively identify a suspect.*" However, according to Pretty and Turnbull (2001), the expectations regarding the identification based on

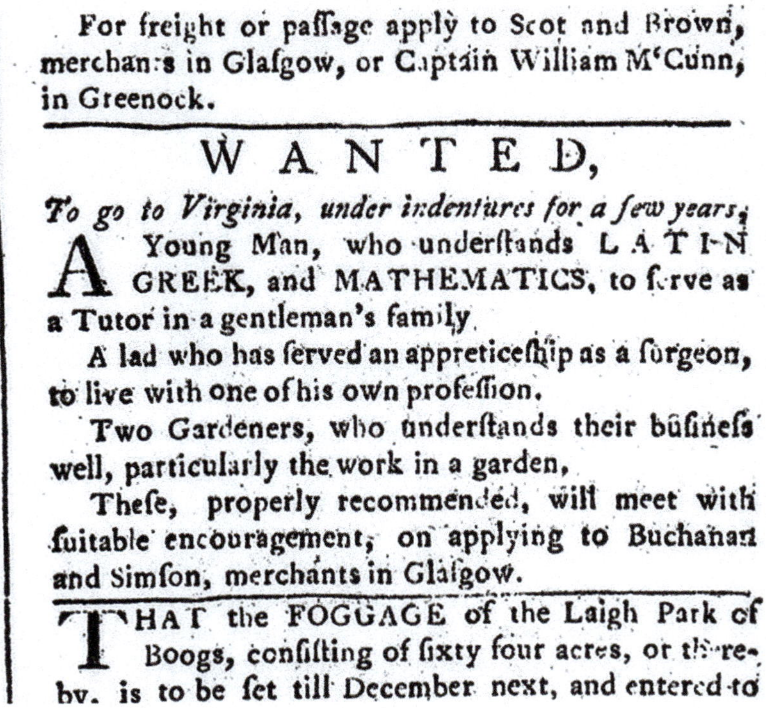

For freight or paſſage apply to Scot and Brown, merchants in Glaſgow, or Captain William M'Cunn, in Greenock.

WANTED,

To go to Virginia, under indentures for a few years,

A Young Man, who underſtands LATIN, GREEK, and MATHEMATICS, to ſerve as a Tutor in a gentleman's family.

A lad who has ſerved an appreticeſhip as a ſurgeon, to live with one of his own profeſſion.

Two Gardeners, who underſtands their buſineſs well, particularly the work in a garden,

Theſe, properly recommended, will meet with ſuitable encouragement, on applying to Buchanan and Simſon, merchants in Glaſgow.

THAT the FOGGAGE of the Laigh Park of Boogs, conſiſting of ſixty four acres, or thereby, is to be ſet till December next, and entered to

Fig. 8.21 An advertisement from the Glasgow Courant, September 4, 1760, for indentured servants to go to Virginia dental hallmarks are sometimes exaggerated. They presented a case in which there was comparable positioning of the dental elements in two suspects. Comparison of the dental hallmarks of both suspects with those of the bite injury was consistent for both the suspects.

If the transferred imprint was a perfect mirror of the configuration of dentition, combined with the shape of the arches, this would make identification of the biter indisputable. However, there are factors which make that perfect imprints are rarely found. These factors include the elasticity of human skin; the curved contours of the skin surface; the distortability of the skin, depending on underlying tissues (e.g., fat, muscle, bone); and the reactive edema immediately

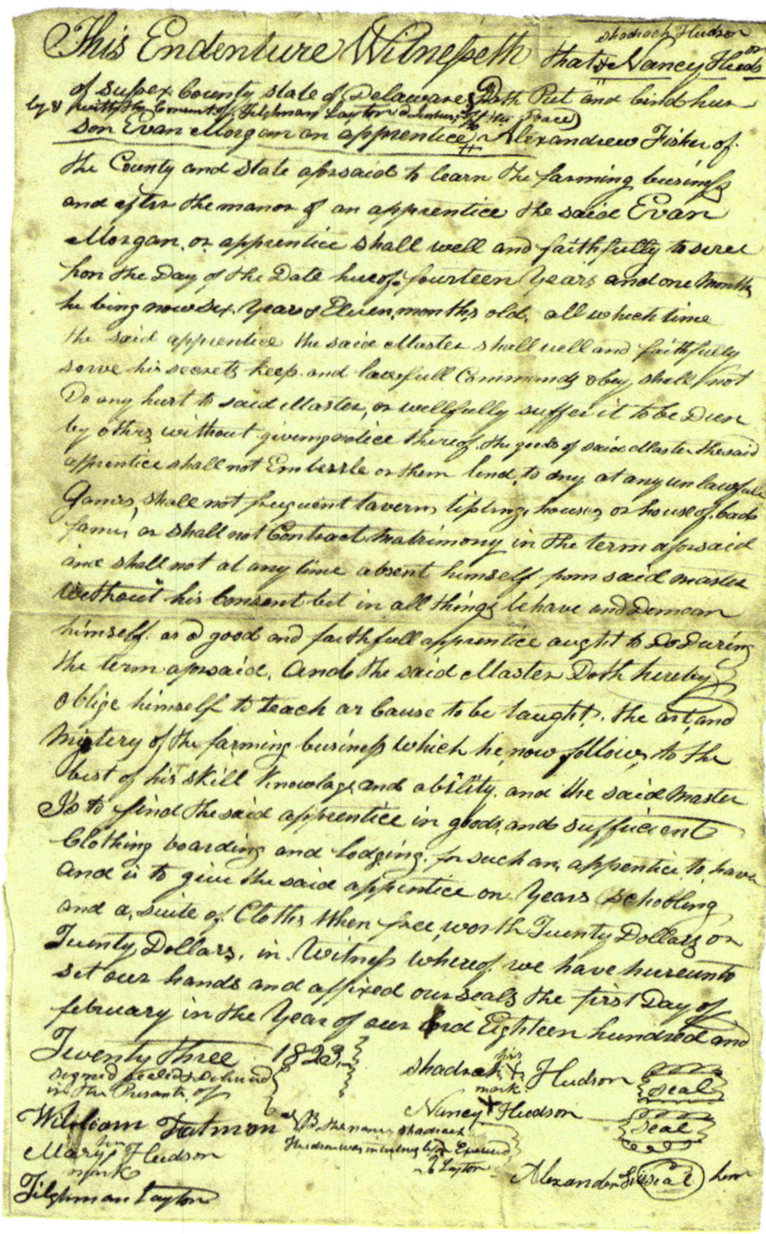

This Indenture Witnesseth that Nancy Hudson of Sussex County State of Delaware Doth Put and bind her Son Evan Morgan an apprentice to Alexander Fisher of the County and State aforesaid to learn the farming business and after the manor of an apprentice the said Evan Morgan or apprentice shall well and faithfully to serve from the Day of the Date hereof fourteen Years and one Month he being now six Years & Eleven months old, all which time the said apprentice the said Master shall well and faithfully serve his secrets keep and lawfull Commands obey, shall not Do any hurt to said Master, or wilfully suffer it to be Done by others without giving notice thereof. the goods of said Master the said apprentice shall not Embezzle or them lend to any at any unlawful Games, shall not frequent tavern, tipling houses or houses of bad fame, or shall not Contract Matrimony in the term aforesaid and shall not at any time absent himself from said Master without his consent but in all things behave and Demean himself as a good and faithfull apprentice aught to Do During the term aforesaid. And the said Master Doth hereby oblige himself to teach or cause to be taught. the art and Mistery of the farming business which he now follows to the best of his skill knowledge and ability. and the said Master Is to find the said apprentice in goods and sufficient Clothing boarding and lodging, for such an apprentice to have And is to give the said apprentice one Years Schooling and a Suite of Clothes when free, worth Twenty Dollars or Twenty Dollars, in Witness whereof we have hereunto set our hands and affixed our Seals the first Day of february in the Year of our Lord Eighteen hundred and Twenty Three 1823.

Signed Sealed & Delivered in the Presents of
William Tatman
Mary Hudson her mark
Tilghman Layton

Shadrach his mark Hudson (Seal)
Nancy her mark Hudson (Seal)
Alexander Fisher (Seal)

Fig. 8.22 Example of a indentured servitude contract of a boy of almost 7 years. *Summary*. Indenture made in Sussex County, Delaware, on February 1, 1823, for the apprenticeship and education of Evan Morgan, a child of 6 years and 11 months, to and in the service of Alex Fisher, a farmer, for a term of 14 years and one month (to age 21 years), with the endorsement of Evan Morgan, dated March 1, 1837, that the terms of the indenture had been satisfied. The Cooper Collection of U.S. Historical Documents (Wikipedia. Indentured servant. 2011 http://en.wikipedia.org/wiki/Indentured_servant)

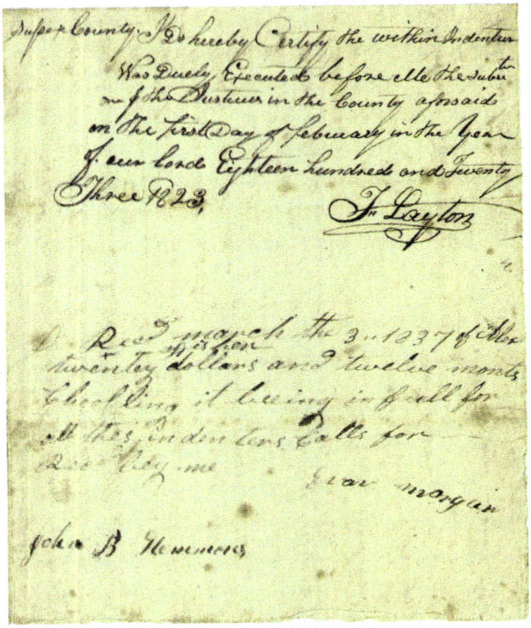
Sussex County ss I do hereby Certify the within Indenture Was Duely Executed before me the Subscriber one of the Justices in the County aforesaid on the first Day of February in the Year of our Lord Eighteen hundred and Twenty Three 1823
J. Layton

Recd March the 3.. 1837 of Alex twenty dollars and twelve months Schooling it being in full for all this indentures calls for
Recd by me
John B Hemmons

Fig. 8.22 (continued)

after biting (Sweet and Pretty 2001). Above that, the compressive force in occlusive bites and the time of exposure of the skin to the bite are important variables in determining the configuration of the bitemark. As a result, some of the unique characteristics are lost. In other words, the dentition of the biter is highly likely unique and the imprint of the dentition in human skin is less unique.

This can be summarized as the characteristics of a bitemark can no longer be regarded as undisputed evidence to identify the biter (Clement and Blackwell 2010; Pretty and Sweet 2010). Instead, if carefully evaluated, the characteristics of a bitemark can be used to exclude in some case possible suspects (Lessig et al. 2006; Bernitz et al. 2008; Pretty and Sweet 2010) or act as an indicator of the likely biter (Bernitz et al. 2008).

One scheme for the identification of a biter, based on the evaluation of a bitemark, is proposed by Pretty (2008) (see Table 8.4).

8.5.1.2 DNA Transfer During Biting

DNA is present in epithelial cells from the mouth and may be deposited along with saliva of the biter onto the body of the bitten person. Therefore, it is important to sample for the presence of saliva in and around fresh bitemarks before bathing after the incident (Sect. 8.7).

8.5.2 Age of the Biter: Milk Versus Permanent Dentition

An evaluation of the age of the biter may be obtained based on the diameter of the bitemark, the number of teeth imprints, and the tooth size, which may be optimally visible after a number of days. In milk teeth (deciduous dentition), the arch is smaller and narrower as are individual milk teeth. The distance between the canines provides an approximate indication of the age of the biter (Levine 1984; Barsley and Landcaster 1987; Bishara et al. 1997; Kemp et al. 2006):

Table 8.4 Possible conclusions after evaluation of a suspicious injury concerning the identification of the biter

Probability	Description
Excluded	There are discrepancies between the bitemark and suspect's dentition that exclude the individual from making the mark
Inconclusive	There is insufficient forensic detail or evidence to draw any conclusion on the link between the suspect's dentition and the bitemark injury
Possible	Teeth like the suspect's could be expected to create a mark like the one examined but so could other dentitions
Probable	Suspect most likely made the bite; most people in the population would not leave such a bite
Reasonable medical certainty	Suspect is identified for all practical and reasonable purposes by the bitemark – any expert with similar training and experience, evaluating the same evidence, should come to the same conclusion of certainty

Pretty (2008)

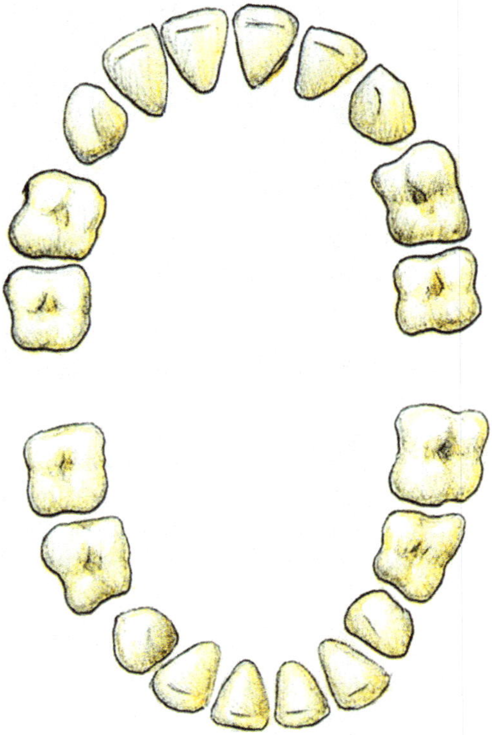

Fig. 8.23 Milk dentition

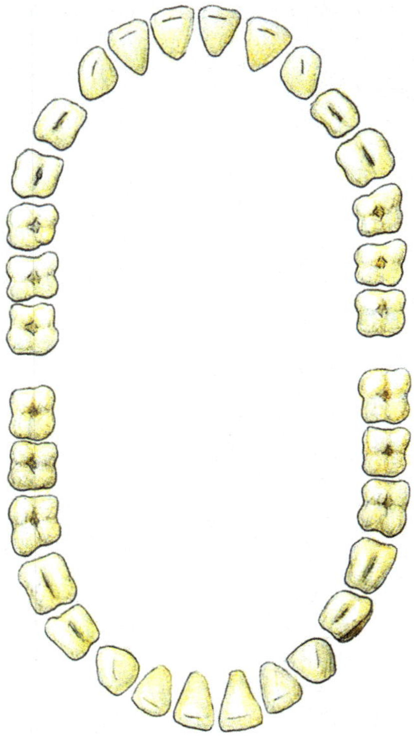

Fig 8.24 Permanent dentition

- 3–4.5 cm: it is highly likely that the bite is caused by an adult
- 2.5–3 cm: it is possible that the bite is from a child with permanent canines (most probably older than 11 years – Bishara et al. 1997) or a small adult
- Less than 2.5 cm: the bite is from a child with milk teeth (most probably younger than 8 years)

The above measurements have not been validated by clinical investigations but are based on odontological data. Although these data are useful, interindividual, interracial, and gender differences must be taken into account (Bishara et al. 1997; Bishara et al. 1998).

In an adult bite, part of the bitemark may be caused by the molars. This is less likely in a bite caused by a young child with milk teeth (Figs. 8.23 and 8.24). Sometimes, however, it will not be possible to distinguish between a bitemark made by a child and one made by an adult (Rothwell, 1995). Overviews of the time of appearance of the elements of the milk teeth and permanent teeth are shown in Tables 8.5 and 8.6.

Table 8.5 Time of appearance of milk dentition

Lower central incisors	6 months
Upper central incisors	7–8 months
Lower lateral incisors	7–12 months
Upper lateral incisors	8–10 months
1st molars	12–15 months
Canines	15–20 months
2nd molars	20–30 months

8.6 Differential Diagnosis

8.6.1 Human Bites and Self-Inflicted Injuries

Anderson and Hudson (1976) described a victim of child abuse in whom bitemarks were found on

Table 8.6 Time of appearance of permanent teeth

1st molar	6 years
Central incisors	7 years
Lateral incisors	8 years
1st premolar	9 years
2nd premolar	10 years
Canine	11 years
2nd molar	12–13 years
3 rd molar (wisdom tooth)	17 years and older

both arms at physical examination. They established that the child had bitten itself. Other authors including Hobbs and Wynne (2001) also pointed out this possibility. Self-biting usually is usually an emotional response to pain (Leung and Robson 1992) and may indicate a lot of stress in the child. Self-biting should lead to further investigation because often the child is the victim of some form of child abuse.

The relation between congenital disorders and self-injurious behavior is complex. Self-injurious behavior may be a disorder-related symptom, but in some cases, it is difficult to differentiate between disorder-specific behavior and stress-related behavior, in which the child responds to his or her social and environmental circumstances. Severe lip biting and knuckle gnawing, gouging of the eyes, scratching the face, and headbanging are specifically associated with the Lesch-Nyhan syndrome (Leung and Robson 1992). Sometimes, the biting is so severe that extraction of the teeth at a young age has to be considered (Cauwels and Martens 2005). Self-biting is also seen, for example, in children with Cornelia de Lange syndrome (especially lip biting), fragile X syndrome (often hand biting, usually at the base of the thumb in response to anxiety or excitement), and hypomelanosis of Ito (wrist and knuckle biting) (Turk 2010). Lip biting and hand biting have also been described in children with Prader-Willi syndrome (Ainsworth and Baker 2004; Butler et al. 2010).

James and Cirillo (2004) reported a situation in which a 42-year-old woman made a false allegation of sexual assault. An abnormality, initially considered to be a bitemark on the right buttock, was found at physical examination. Forensic odontological examination showed that the abnormality did not meet the criteria of a bite injury. The abnormality seemed to have been self-inflicted by the application of a corrugated bottle top.

8.6.2 Human Bites in Traditional Medicine

Bitemarks can be related to traditional folklore medicine. For example, in some Chinese populations, biting is used to stimulate respiration (Leung and Robson 1992). Leung (1985) reported a case of a 4-month-old Chinese infant who sustained multiple bitemarks on the legs, thighs, and buttocks as a resuscitation attempt by the mother to stimulate the infant to breathe has been described.

8.6.3 Animal Bites

8.6.3.1 Human Versus Animal Bites

Animals may bite in self-defense, in an attempt to predate food, or as part of normal interactions with other animals, including humans. Animal bitemarks are only rarely the subject of bitemark analysis (Lessig et al. 2006).

Whittaker (2004) states that carnivorous animals, such as dogs or tigers, use their teeth in two distinct ways in predating. Firstly, they kill their prey primarily using their canines, and secondly, they tear and slice the flesh to produce digestible fragments. According to Whittaker, human teeth are designed principally to cut and grind food which is usually previously prepared. In the biting of a child by an adult, the act is meant to cause pain, which can be reached by mere forceful compression of the skin, sometimes leading to crushing of the skin. Tearing of the skin is not necessary to inflict pain, although in very rare cases in human bites, tearing of the skin can be seen. Most of the time, the skin will remain intact. Abrasions, bruises, and sometimes lacerations may develop. The chances of the occurrence of a laceration and sometimes even an avulsion of the skin are more common in an animal bites than in human bites.

8.6.3.2 Dogs

Dog bites are the most prevalent type of bites in humans. According to the CDC (2009), 4.5 million Americans are bitten by dogs each year. Most of these bites are not serious, but one in five dog bites results in injuries that require medical attention (CDC 2009). In 2006, more than 31,000 people underwent reconstructive surgery as a result of being bitten by dogs (CDC 2009). Approximately in the USA, 10–20 dog bites each year are fatal (Brogan et al. 1995). In the USA, the rate of dog bite-related injuries is highest for children between the ages 5 and 9 years. Having a dog in the household is associated with a higher incidence of dog bites (CDC 2009). Sixty to 70% of dog bites are to children (Mathews and Lattal 1994).

About 250,000 people attend trauma units in the United Kingdom because of dog bites (Morgan and Palmer 2007). Many of them are attacks on children under the age of 5 years often in their home by the family pet or a dog known to them (Brogan et al. 1995; Besser 2007).

Dogs bite humans at a rate eight to ten times more frequently than humans bite each other, at least in bites that are brought for medical treatment (Lessig et al. 2006; MacBean et al. 2007). In dog biting, one may find many bites spread all over the entire body (Ligthelm and van Niekerk 1994). Fischer (2003) pointed at a significant difference between human and dog teeth. Humans have four incisors in each dental arch and relatively short canines. The incisors lead to rectangular injuries and the canines to round, ovoid, or triangular injuries (Sweet and Pretty 2001; Fischer and Hammel 2003). The human dental arch is elliptical or oval, in contrast to dogs that have six incisors and two long curved canines per arch. The dog's arch is elongated with a short front segment. In a dog bite, deep punctures with tearing of the skin may be seen.

The shape of the bitemark caused by a dog bite is a narrow, almost rectangular arch at the front with conspicuous pointed markings from the canines on the corners of the rectangle (McLay 1990) (Fig. 8.25). The bite of a dog is strong, the teeth are not very sharp, resulting in a crush-type injury and rarely to very severe injury of the underlying structures such as the bones, joints, tendons, brain, and nerves. A penetrating injury of the skin and sometimes also the underlying muscles may occur, leading to a laceration or avulsion. The force an adult dog can exert with its jaws corresponds to 7.5–10 kg/cm², sometimes leading to extensive bruising around the bitemark (Fig. 8.26). This may increase to 20 kg/cm² in some breeds of dog (Stump 2001). Dog bites are generally large and multiple. A differentiation between the bitemarks of different breeds normally is not possible (Lessig et al. 2006).

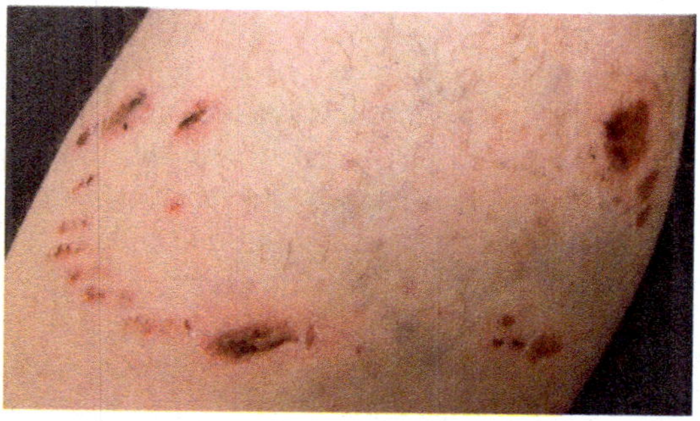

Fig. 8.25 Almost rectangular dog bite in an adult – 3 days old (Nicor – Wikipedia. Bite. 2011 http://en.wikipedia.org/wiki/Bite)

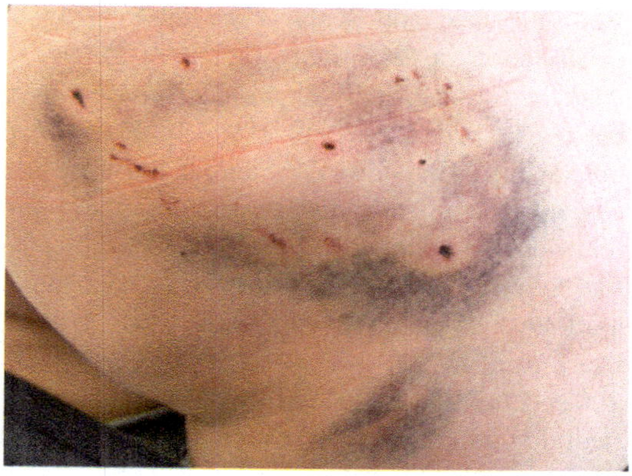

Fig. 8.26 Almost rectangular dog bite in an adolescent girl with extensive bruising around the bite

Dog bites on the face, hairy scalp, and neck are more frequently seen in children than in adults. Dog bites are particularly dangerous in children <2 years old. A bite may lead to a skull fracture, fractures of the facial bones, neck injuries, brain-tissue damage (cuts, lacerations), and infections of the central nervous system.

Therefore, it is important in every severe dog bite to evaluate whether there are any other injuries before the bite wounds are treated. Duteille et al. (2002) describes the amputation of the forearm and substantial damage to the back, shoulder, thorax, and neck in an 18-month-old child.

The risk of death from dog bites in children <12 years old is about 2.5 times higher than in adults. Most victims of fatal dog attack are under the age of 1 year (Bux and McDowell 1992). Death mostly results from bleeding and shock due to damage to major vessels (Bux and McDowell 1992). Sometimes, there may also be extensive and mutilative stripping of soft tissues from the face and scalp, even progressing to decapitation in the infant (Tsokos et al. 2007). Also, extensive fatal abdominal injuries have been described (Clark et al. 1991). In this respect, breeds like pitbull terrier, American Staffordshire terrier, Rottweiler, and German shepherd are notorious, although also more "friendly" breeds, like Siberian Husky, Chow Chow, or dachshund are known to have killed children (Wright 1985; Clark et al. 1991; Chu et al. 2006; Tsuji et al. 2008). Chu et al. (2006) describes three cases of fatal dog attacks in two 18-day-old children and one 3-month-old and raises the possibility that the use of mobile swings in very young children may trigger a predatory response in dogs, including traditionally less aggressive breeds.

Sometimes, dogs are falsely accused of attacking or biting children. Boglioli et al. (2000) reported the supposedly fatal attack by a German shepherd on a 6-day-old baby. The child was not killed by the dog, but by the father. The child urinated on the father during a diaper change. The father killed the infant, dismembered him, and fed his remains to the family's dog.

8.6.3.3 Cats

Cats have long, thin, and sharp canines. The jaw can only move vertically. This is essential for holding prey. The prey is as it were "impaled" on the canines. When a child has been bitten by a cat, a small arch with puncture injuries caused by the sharp canines is seen. Such a bite often causes penetrating injuries in which bones and joints may be damaged and deep cuts may develop. At physical examination, scratches caused by the claws are a frequently seen accompanying injury (McLay 1990). Cat bites are generally found on the hands of children.

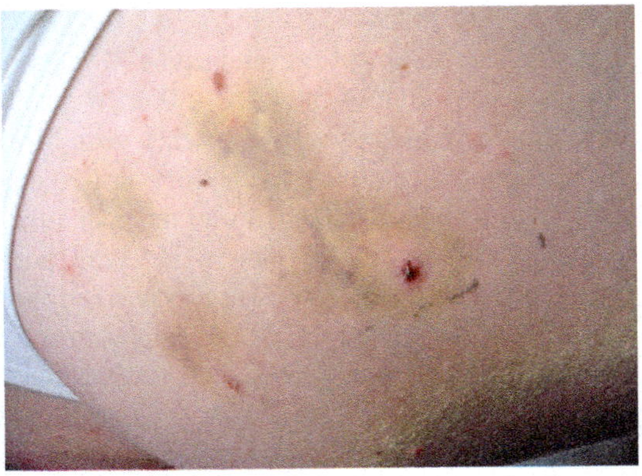

Fig. 8.27 Bitemarks caused by a playful young tiger

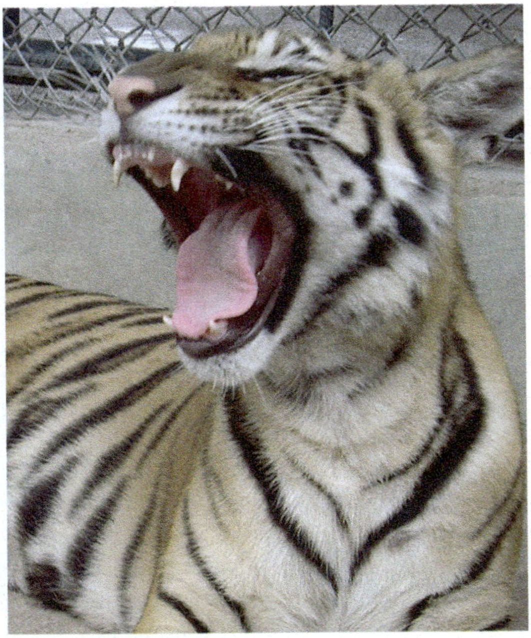

Fig. 8.28 The playful young tiger

Injuries caused by attacks by larger cat species, such as tigers and lions, are rare (Figs. 8.27 and 8.28). Clark et al. (1991) reported a boy of 12 years old, who tried to pet a circus tiger. The tiger bit off the arm of the boy at the shoulder. The child survived the attack.

Risk of Infection in Dog and Cat Bites

A bite (or scratch) from a dog or cat that breaks the skin poses the danger of infection. A cat bite is almost always infected. In dog bites, the risk of infection is relatively small. Only 15–20% of dog bite wounds are infected (Presutti, 2001). The infection rate also depends on the site and depth of the bite. Crush injuries, puncture wounds, and hand wounds are more likely to become infected than scratches or tears (Presutti, 2001). Most infections caused by mammalian bites are polymicrobial, with mixed aerobic and anaerobic species. Griego et al. (1995) isolated 28 species of aerobic organisms and 12 species of anaerobic organisms from dog bite wounds.

The child's risk of rabies and the tetanus status must always be identified in dog and cat bites, and, if necessary, immunoprophylaxis should be administered (Presutti 2001). Although most household pets are immunized against rabies, the possibility of infection still exists. It is also possible to contract an infection with *Clostridium tetani* from an animal bite. *Clostridium tetani*, the microbe that causes tetanus, lives in the top layers of soil and in the intestinal tracts of cows and horses. It easily infects wounds (particularly crushing and puncture wounds) which results in reduced oxygen flow in the tissue.

In dog bites, some strains of streptococci (*Streptococcus pyogenes*) and several other kinds of bacteria may lead to a rare but fulminant infection called necrotizing fasciitis (also known as flesh-eating bacterial infection) (Arima et al. 2005; Lee et al. 2008). For that reason, dog bite wounds should be treated prophylactically, although usually the infections caused by these bacteria are mild and include, for example, streptococcal pharyngitis or impetigo. Direct oral antibiotic administration with drugs such as amoxicillin/clavulanic acid or co-amoxyclav as combination antibiotic (amoxicillin trihydrate) is always indicated whenever the "eating bacteria" is involved.

The symptoms of necrotizing fasciitis often start suddenly with muscular pain in arms or legs after an injury. Medical care is indicated right away if pain initially improves over the first 24–36 h and then suddenly gets worse. The pain may be much worse than expected from the size of the wound or injury.

Other risk factors than dog bites for developing necrotizing fasciitis include:

- Insect and spider bites
- Traumatic injuries, for example, scratches, abrasions, burns, or cuts
- Chicken pox
- Contact with ocean water, raw saltwater fish, or raw oysters
- Handling sea animals such as crabs
- Intestinal surgery site or in tumors

Bacteria that cause necrotizing fasciitis can be passed from person to person through close contact, such as kissing, or by touching the wound of the infected person. However, a person who gets infected by the bacteria in this way is unlikely to get necrotizing fasciitis unless he or she has an open wound, chickenpox, or an impaired immune system.

8.6.3.4 Ferrets

Ferrets are carnivores, predators related to the polecat. Ferrets are popular, but risky pets. Ferrets may cause numerous and severe injuries in young children (Paisley and Lauer 1988; Applegate and Walhout 1998). A ferret uses its teeth, particularly the canines, to bite into the prey, to tear the skin, and to tear off parts of the prey (Ferret Central 1998). This leads to puncture wounds and lacerations. It is difficult to force the ferret to let go once it has bitten.

8.6.3.5 Rodents

In rodents, the central incisors are the most strongly developed teeth. These leave a relatively minor injury which may resemble a cut or puncture wounds.

There is generally little risk of infection. There are a number of case reports in which the potentially life-threatening character of rat bites in children was described. Donoso et al. (2004) reported an 8-month-old girl with rat bites on her head and hands (*Rattus norvegicus*) after she had fallen from her parents' bed while asleep. She developed hypovolemic shock that was almost fatal. For 5 days, she was in need of intensive treatment but recovered completely. Both her parents had an alcohol

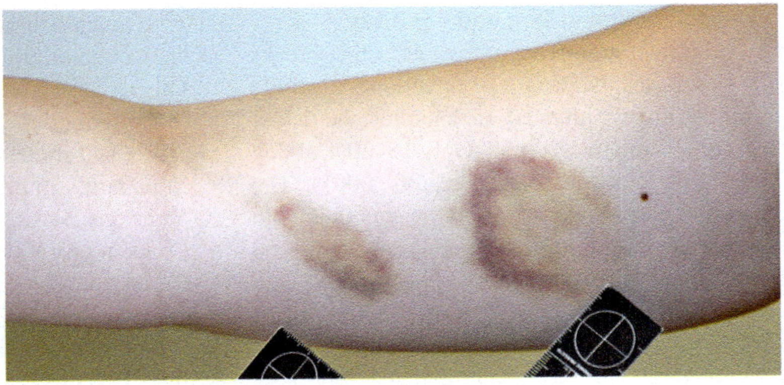

Fig. 8.29 Grip and pinch marks on the right upper arm of an adolescent

problem. Donoso drew attention to the relationship between the occurrence of rat bites in children and poor social circumstances. Yanai et al. (1999) described an 11-week-old, malnourished girl in whom rat bites were fatal. The girl slept in her mother's bed. According to Yanai, rat bites usually occur postmortem; however, postmortem rat bites are characterized by "clean" bite injuries with sharp edges and without subcutaneous blood loss. In this girl, there were clear indications that the injuries had been sustained while she was alive: her clothes were drenched in blood, and around the bites, subcutaneous hemorrhages were seen. Yanai and Donoso stress the relationship between the occurrence of rat bites in young children and severe social deprivation.

8.6.3.6 Apes

When a child has been bitten by an ape, there is a high risk of wound infection. Bitemarks by apes are similar to those by humans. Where the species have more developed canines than humans, such as the orangutan, the chance of puncture injuries and lacerations is higher.

8.6.4 Other Differential Diagnostic Considerations

In case there is doubt whether the injury is a bitemark, the following possibilities must be considered in the differential diagnosis (Gold et al. 1989; Grey 1989; Sweet and Pretty 2001; Clement 2003; James and Cirillo 2004; Brown and Kreshak 2010; Payne-James and Hinchliffe 2011):

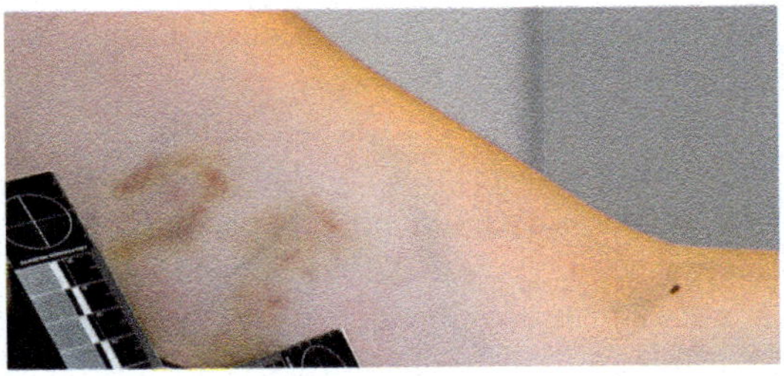

Fig. 8.30 Same adolescent: grip and pinch marks on the left upper arm

- Grip- and pinch marks (Figs. 8.29 and 8.30).
- Imprints of implements, for example, buckle, shoe (especially heel marks), patterned door knobs, bottom of a glass bottle, corrugated bottle top (described in a 42-year-old female), jewelry, children's toys, and ECG electrode applied by emergency medical personnel/defibrillator injury (described in an deceased adult patient)
- Dermatological disorders, especially annular or arciform dermatoses, like:
  - Ringworm. Gold et al. (1989) described a 2-year-old girl in whom various annular abnormalities were found. It was incorrectly assumed to be ringworm; antifungal treatment was not effective. A dermatologist finally established it to be a human bite injury.
  - Scars of linear IgA disease.
  - Subacute cutaneous lupus erythematosus (extremely rare in children): especially if the erythematosus scaly papules enlarge and become confluent to form larger annular lesions (Figs. 8.31 and 8.32).

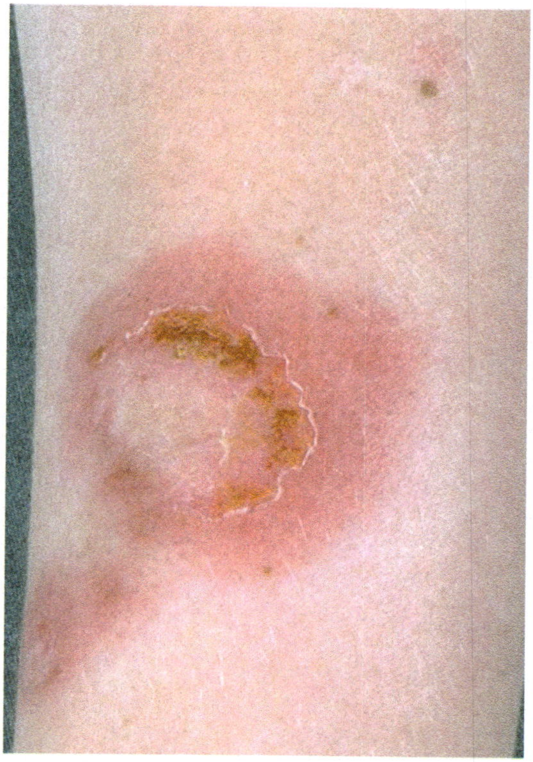

Fig. 8.31 Subacute cutaneous lupus erythematosus

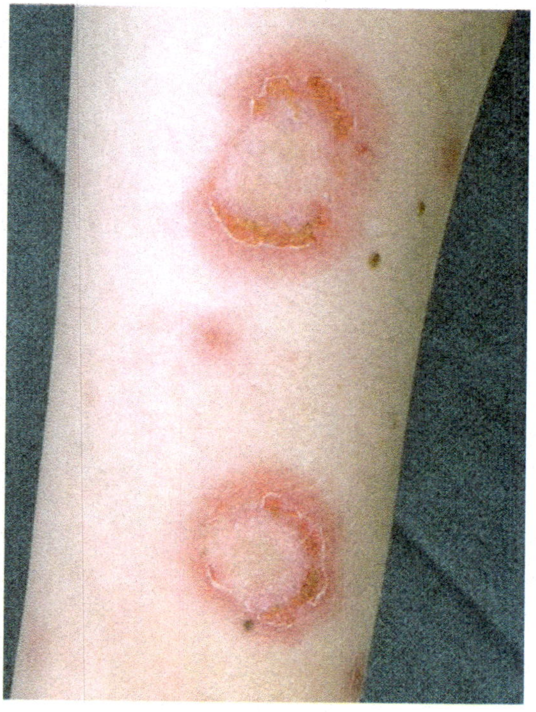

Fig. 8.32 Subacute cutaneous lupus erythematosus

- Pityriasis rosea initially: may present as an oval herald patch.
- Tinea corporis: typical annular lesion with an active erythematous border and central clearing (Figs. 8.33 and 8.34).
- Granuloma annulare: skin colored erythematous or violaceous papules that form annular configuration (Figs. 8.35, 8.36, and 8.37).
- Fixed drug eruptions: especially when a single, erythematous, well-demarcated lesion is present.
- Psoriasis (Fig. 8.38).

- Burns due to circular or semicircular heated objects, for example, in wet and dry cupping (traditional medicine) or with the end of a curling iron
- Patterned injuries with a circular or elliptical shape, for example, the end of a lead pipe

Differentiation should be possible because of the absence of the typical aspects of a bitemark. In a bite, there is no scaling, as there will be in some dermatological disorders. Most disorders will affect wider areas of the body or have other symptoms associated with the disorders.

8.7 The Examination of Bitemarks

The finding of a human bitemark in a child may have serious consequences, concerning the safety of the child. It may prove that the child has been abused. It may indicate who has bitten the child (or who did not bite the child) and why the child was bitten. Bernstein (1985) pointed out the importance of an adequate and structured examination when a patient presents with a suspected bitemark. The presence of a scale marker and color card on all photographs of suspected bitemarks is mandatory (Chap. 9). The following elements must be considered during the examination of a suspected bite wound:

1. Patient history.
2. Examination of the bite injury: pattern, size, contour, and color.

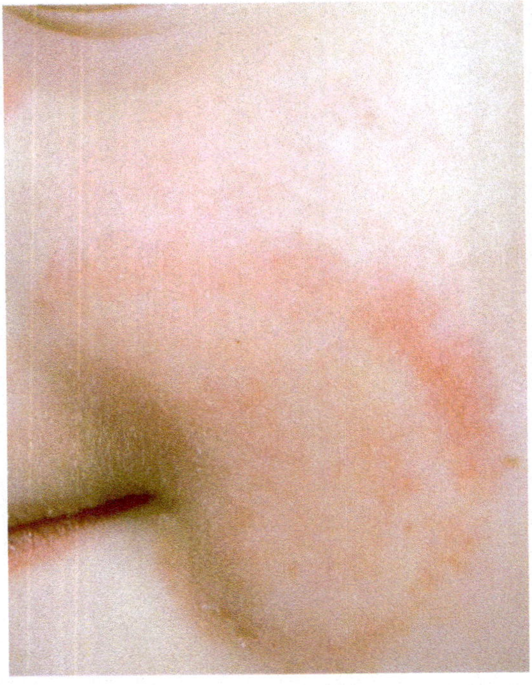

Fig. 8.33 Fungal infection: tinea faciei

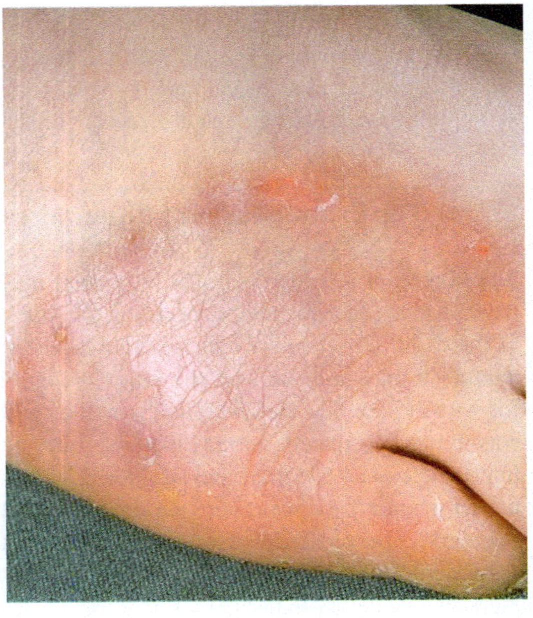

Fig. 8.34 Fungal infection: tinea pedis

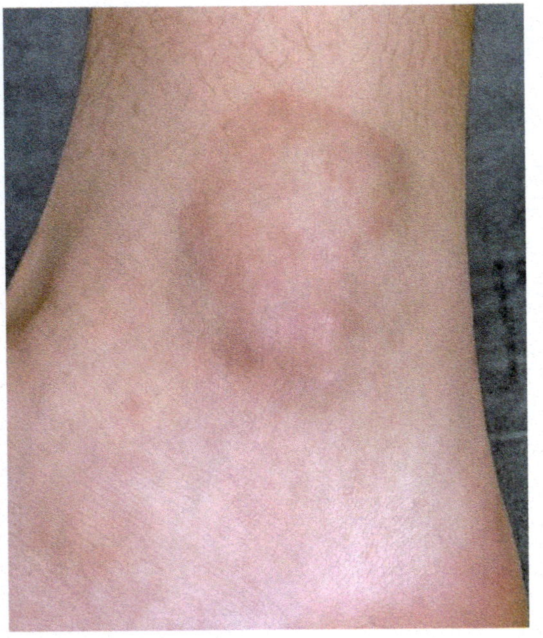

Fig. 8.35 Granuloma annulare

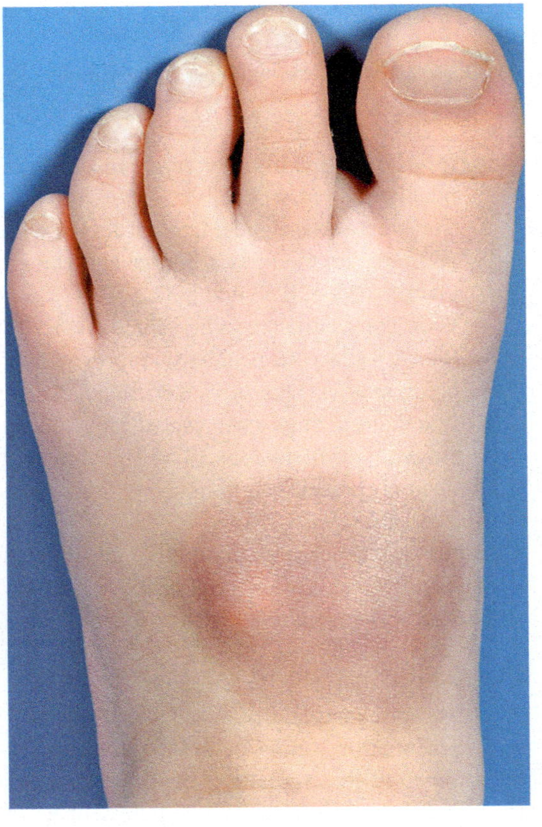

Fig. 8.36 Granuloma annulare

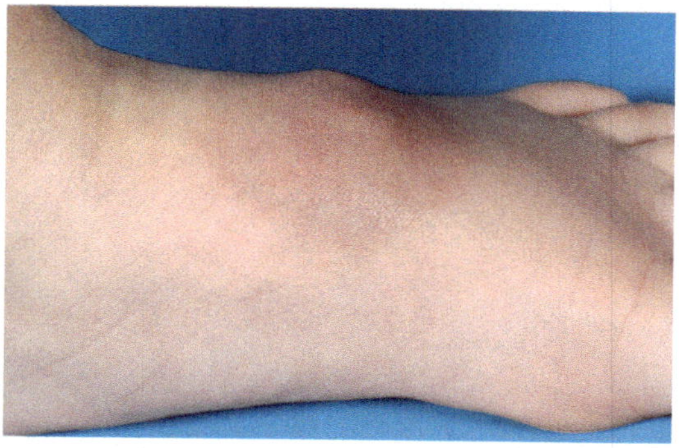

Fig. 8.37 Granuloma annulare

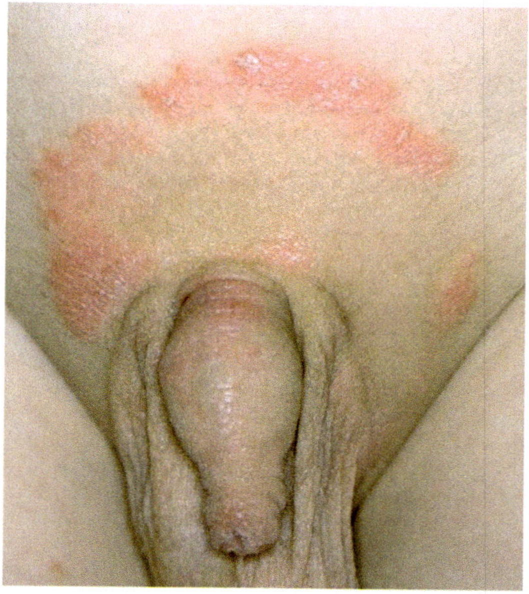

Fig. 8.38 Psoriasis

3. Documenting the bite injury.
4. Complete physical examination: during physical examination, one must look for additional injuries such as other bitemarks, considering that often there is more than one bitemark (Freeman et al. 2005).
5. Additional investigation:
   (a) Blood group typing and DNA: ABO blood group typing can be performed on the "saliva washing" from the skin around the bite. Approximately 0.3 ml of saliva is transferred during the bite (Hobbs and Wynne 2001). The disadvantage of exclusive ABO typing is that only 80% of the people with blood group A or B blood group antigens, which correspond with their blood group, secrete these antigens in their saliva (Mollison 1993). DNA is present in epithelial cells in the mouth and may be similarly transferred during the bite. Even when the saliva and the cells have dried, they may be harvested by using the double-swab technique. A sterile cotton swab is first moistened with distilled water. The site of the bite is sampled. The swab is dried and placed in a specimen tube. The same site is subsequently sampled with a dry cotton swab. This cotton swab is also placed in a specimen tube. A third swab is used as a control by harvesting material from a noninvolved site. All swabs must be sent immediately to a certified forensic laboratory for analysis (Kellogg 2005). The swabs must dry in cool air for 1 h. Vigorous swabbing may contaminate the DNA of the biter with that of the bitten person.
   (b) Dental imprint: if there are indentations, then a polyvinyl siloxane impression must be made immediately after photographing the bitemark and obtaining the DNA samples. This makes it possible to construct a three-dimensional model of the bite injury (Kellogg 2005). By using this model, it is possible to compare the teeth of the suspected biter with the bite injury.
6. Registration of the abnormality:
   (a) Body diagrams with registration of sizes: the abnormality must be always measured in 2 directions.
   (b) Photographic documentation of the injuries: Photographs should be taken at all times and before any other handling that could disturb the bitemark pattern. The ABFO no. 2 scale must be used and placed in the plane of the injury while the camera must be held directly over the abnormality, perpendicular to the plane of the injury, in order to avoid any distortions. Both black and white and color photographs must be taken from two additional directions (American Board of Forensic Odontology, not dated) for curved body surfaces and be repeated with 12–24 h

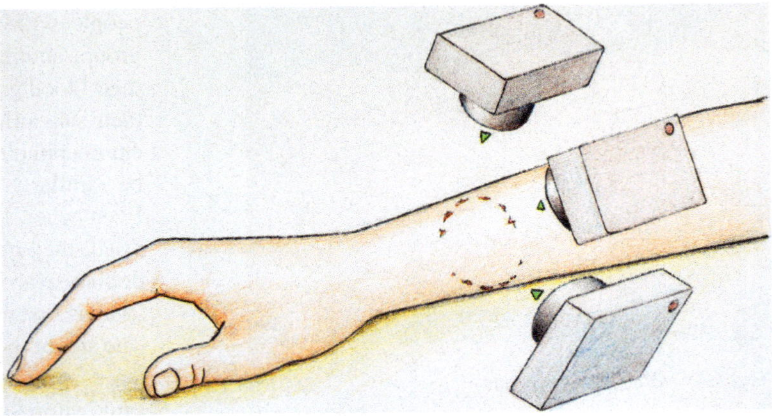

Fig. 8.39 Photography of bitemarks: perpendicular and two additional directions

intervals to register the changes in the appearance of the bitemark (Fig. 8.39).

7. Repeating (parts of) the examination: It is important to follow a child with bite injuries for a consecutive number of days. Firstly, this may clear up any doubt concerning the nature of the injury and assist in establishing it clearly as a bitemark. Secondly, through the "ripening" of the bruise, further clarification can be obtained on the shape of the teeth of the biter. Dental elements may be better identified after a certain period of time has passed than immediately after the injury was sustained.

Finally, both the British Association of Forensic Odontology (BAFO) and the American Board of Forensic Odontology (ABFO 2011) have compiled guidelines on a structured examination of bite injuries.

References

ABFO (American Board of Forensic Odontology) (2011) Diplomates reference manual http://www.abfo.org/pdfs/ABFO_Diplomate_Reference_Manual3-2011_3-18-2011revision.pdf. Accessed on 2011

Ainsworth P, Baker PC (2004) Understanding mental retardation. University Press of Mississippi, Jackson, pp 26–28

Anderson WR, Hudson RP (1976) Self-inflicted bite marks in battered child syndrome. Forensic Sci 7(1):71–74

Andreo SM, Barra LA, Costa LJ et al (2004) HIV type 1 transmission by human bite. AIDS Res Hum Retroviruses 20(4):349–350

Applegate J, Walhout M (1998) Childhood risks from the ferret. J Emerg Med 16(3):425–427

Arima H, Nagata M, Fujisaki K et al (2005) GRAFT infection of thoracic aorta due to group C beta-hemolytic streptococcus – a case report. Angiology 56(2):237–241

BAFO (British Association of Forensic Odontology) (2002) Forensic Odontology http://www.bafo.org.uk/guide.php. Accessed on 2010

Baker MD, Moore SE (1987) Human bites in children. A six-year experience. Am J Dis Child 141(12):1285–1290

Barsley RE, Landcaster DM (1987) Measurement of arch widths in a human population – relation of anticipated bite marks. J Forensic Sci 32(4):975–982

Bartholomew CF, Jones AM (2006) Human bites: a rare risk factor for HIV transmission. AIDS 20(4):631–632

Bernat JE (1992) Dental trauma and bite mark evaluation. In: Ludwig S, Kornberg AE (eds) Child abuse – a medical reference, 2nd edn. Churchill Livingstone, New York, pp 175–190

Bernitz H, Owen JH, van Heerden WF, Solheim T (2008) An integrated technique for the analysis of skin bite marks. J Forensic Sci 53(1):194–198

Bernstein ML (1985) Two bite mark cases with inadequate scale references. J Forensic Sci 30(3):958–964

Besser R (2007) Dog attacks: it's time for doctors to bite back. BMJ 334(7590):425

Bishara SE, Jakobsen JR, Treder J et al (1997) Arch width changes from 6 weeks to 45 years of age. Am J Orthod Dentofacial Orthop 111(4):401–409

Bishara SE, Jakobsen JR, Treder J et al (1998) Arch length changes from 6 weeks to 45 years. Angle Orthod 68(1):69–74

Boglioli LR, Taff ML, Turkel SJ et al (2000) Unusual infant death: dog attack or postmortem mutilation after child abuse? Am J Forensic Med Pathol 21(4):389–394

Bowers CM (2004) Recognition, recovery and analysis of bite mark evidence. In: Bowers CM (ed) Forensic dental evidence, an investigator's handbook. Elsevier Academic Press, San Diego, pp 67–105

Brogan TV, Bratton SL, Dowd MD, Hegenbarth MA (1995) Severe dog bites in children. Pediatrics 96(5pt1):947–950

Brown SW, Kreshak AA (2010) Chapter 8 Forensic bite mark evidence. In: Riviello RJ (ed) Manual of forensic emergency medicine, a guide for clinicians, 1st edn. Jones and Bartlett Publishers, Sudbury, pp 65–76

Butler M, Hanchett DM, Thompson T (2010) Chapter 1 Clinical findings and natural history in Prader-Willi syndrome. In: Butler M, Lee PDK, Whitman BY (eds) Management of Prader-Willi Syndrome. Springer, New York, pp 32–33

Bux RC, McDowell JD (1992) Death due to attack from chow dog. Am J Forensic Med Pathol 13(4): 305–308

Cancio-Bello TP, de Medina M, Shorey J et al (1982) An institutional outbreak of hepatitis B related to a human biting carrier. J Infect Dis 146(5):652–656

Carr MM (1995) Human bites to the hand. J Can Dent Assoc 61(9):782–784

Cauwels RG, Martens LC (2005) Self-mutilation behaviour in Lesch-Nyhan syndrome. J Oral Pathol Med 34(9):573–575

CDC (Centers for Disease Control and Prevention) (2009) Dog bite prevention http://www.cdc.gov/HomeandRecreationalSafety/Dog-Bites/biteprevention.html. Accessed on 2011

Christian CW, Mouden LD (2001) Maxillofacial, neck, and dental manifestations of child abuse. In: Reece RM, Ludwig S (eds) Child abuse, medical diagnosis and management, 2nd edn. Lippincott Williams & Wilkins, Philadelphia, pp 117–118

Chu AY, Ripple MG, Allan CH, Thogmartin JR, Fowler DR (2006) Fatal dog maulings associated with infant swings. J Forensic Sci 51(2):403–406

Clark MA, Sandusky GE, Hawley DA et al (1991) Fatal and near-fatal animal bite injuries. J Forensic Sci 36(4):1256–1261

Clement JG (2003) Chapter 45 Role of and techniques in forensic odontology. In: Payne-James J, Busuttil A, Smock W (eds) Forensic medicine, clinical and pathological aspects, 1st edn. Greenwich Medical Media Ltd, London, pp 689–703

Clement JG, Blackwell SA (2010) Is current bite mark analysis a misnomer? Forensic Sci Int 201(1–3):33–37

Dailey JC, Bowers CM (1997) Aging of bitemarks: a literature review. J Forensic Sci 42(5):792–795

Donoso A, Leon J, Rojas G et al (2004) Hypovolaemic shock by rat bites. A paradigmatic case of social deprivation. Emerg Med J 21(5):640–641

Dusheiko GM, Smith M, Scheuer PJ (1990) Hepatitis C virus transmitted by human bite. Lancet 336(8713):503–504

Duteille F, Hadjukowicz J, Pasquier P, Dautel G (2002) Tragic case of a dog bite in a young child: the dog stands trial. Ann Plast Surg 48(2):184–187; discussion 187–8

Enotes on forensic odontology, not dated. http://www.enotes.com/forensic-science/odontology-historical-cases

Ferret Central (1998) Ferret Natural History FAQ http://www.ferretcentral.org/faq/history.html. Accessed on 2010

Fischer H, Hammel PW (2003) Human bites versus dog bites. N Engl J Med 349:e11

Fischman SL (2002) Bite marks. Alpha Omegan 95(4):42–46

Fiumara NJ, Exner JH (1981) Primary syphilis following a human bite. Sex Transm Dis 8(1):21–22

Freeman AJ, Senn DR, Arendt DM (2005) Seven hundred seventy eight bite marks: analysis by anatomic location, victim and biter demographics, type of crime, and legal disposition. J Forensic Sci 50(6):1436–1443

Garrard J, Leland N, Smith DK (1988) Epidemiology of human bites to children in a day-care center. Am J Dis Child 142(6):643–650

Geberth VJ (1983) Identification of suspects – bite mark identification. In: Geberth VJ (ed) Practical homicide investigation – tactics, procedures, and forensic techniques. Elsevier, New York, pp 381–389

Gold MH, Roenigk HH, Smith ES, Pierce LJ (1989) Human bite marks. Differential diagnosis. Clin Pediatr (Phila) 28(7):329–331

Grey TC (1989) Defibrillator injury suggesting bite mark. Am J Forensic Med Pathol 10(2):144–145

Griego RD, Rosen T, Orengo IF, Wolf JE (1995) Dog, cat, and human bites: a review. J Am Acad Dermatol 33(6):1019–1029

Hamilton JD, Larke B, Qizilbash A (1976) Transmission of hepatitis B by a human bite: an occupational hazard. Can Med Assoc J 115(5):439–440

Hobbs CJ, Wynne JM (2001) Bites. In: Hobbs CJ, Wynne JM (eds) Physical signs of child abuse, a colour atlas, 2nd edn. WB Saunders, London, pp 47–54

Hui AY, Hung LC, Tse PC et al (2005) Transmission of hepatitis B by human bite – confirmation by detection of virus in saliva and full genome sequencing. J Clin Virol 33(3):254–256

James H, Cirillo GN (2004) Bite mark or bottle top? J Forensic Sci 49(1):119–121

Kellogg N (2005) American Academy of Pediatrics/American Academy of Pediatric Dentistry – clinical report: oral and dental aspects of child abuse and neglect. Pediatrics 116(6):1565–1568

Kemp A, Maguire SA, Sibert J et al (2006) Can we identify abusive bites on children? Arch Dis Child 91(11):951

Lauridson JR, Myers L (1993) Evaluation of fatal dog bites: the view of the medical examiner and animal behaviorist. J Forensic Sci 38(3):726–731

Lee LY, Ilan J, Mulvey T (2002) Human biting of children and oral manifestations of abuse: a case report and literature review. ASDC J Dent Child 69(1):92–95

Lee S, Roh KH, Kim CK et al (2008) A case of necrotizing fasciitis due to *Streptococcus agalactiae*, *Arcanobacterium haemolyticum*, and *Finegoldia magna* in a dog-bitten patient with diabetes. Korean J Lab Med 28(3):191–195

Lessig R, Wenzel V, Weber M (2006) Bite mark analysis in forensic routine case work. EXCLI Journal 5:93–102

Leung AK (1985) Pseudo-abusive human bite marks in a Chinese infant. Injury 16(7):503–504

Leung AK, Robson WL (1992) Human bites in children. Pediatr Emerg Care 8(5):255–257

Levine LJ (1977) Bite mark evidence. Dent Clin North Am 21(1):145–158

Levine LJ (1984) Bite marks in child abuse. In: Sanger RG, Bross DC (eds) Clinical management of child abuse and neglect: a guide for the dental professional. Quintessence books, Chicago, pp 53–59

Ligthelm AJ, van Niekerk PJ (1994) A comparative review of bitemark cases from Pretoria, South Africa. J Forensic Odontostomatol 12(2):23–29

MacBean CE, Taylor DM, Ashby K (2007) Animal and human bite injuries in Victoria, 1998–2004. Med J Aust 186(1):38–40
Marr JS, Beck AM, Lugo JA (1979) An epidemiologic study of the human bite. Public Health Rep 94(6):514–521
Mathews JR, Lattal KA (1994) A behavioral analysis of dog bites to children. J Dev Behav Pediatr 15(1): 44–52
McLay WDS (1990) Odontology and identification – the relevance of bite marks. In: McLay WDS (ed) Clinical forensic medicine. Pinter Publisher, London, pp 310–320
McLeod IK (2008) Human bites clinical presentation. eMedicine http://emedicine.medscape.com/article/881270-overview. Accessed on 2011
Merchant RC, Fuerch J, Becker BM, Mayer KH (2005) Comparison of the epidemiology of human bites evaluated at three US pediatric emergency departments. Pediatr Emerg Care 21(12):833–838
Mollison PL (1993) Blood transfusions in clinical medicine, 9th edn. Blackwell Scientific, Oxford/Boston, pp 157–158
Morgan M, Palmer J (2007) Dog bites. BMJ 334(7590):413–417
Mouden LD (1998) Oral injuries of child abuse. In: Monteleone JA, Brodeur AE (eds) Child maltreatment – a clinical guide and reference, 2nd edn. GW Medical, St. Louis, pp 59–66
Paisley J, Lauer B (1988) Severe facial injuries to infants due to unprovoked attacks by pet ferrets. JAMA 259(13):2005–2006
Payne-James JJ, Hinchliffe J (2011) Chapter 4 Injury assessment, documentation, and interpretation. In: Stark MM (ed) Clinical forensic medicine, a physician's guide, 3rd edn. Humana Press, New York, pp 133–168
Pierce LJ, Strickland DJ, Smith ES (1990) The case of Ohio vs. Robinson: an 1870 bite mark case. Am J Forensic Med Pathol 11(2):171–177
Pollak S, Mortinger H (1989) Fatal dog bite injuries. Beitr Gerichtl Med 47:487–495 [in German]
Presutti RJ (2001) Prevention and treatment of dog bites. Am Fam Physician 63(8):1567–1573
Pretty IA (2008) Forensic dentistry: 2. Bitemarks and bite injuries. Dent Update 35(1):48–61
Pretty IA, Sweet D (2000) Anatomical location of bitemarks and associated findings in 101 cases from the United States. J Forensic Sci 45(4):812–814
Pretty IA, Sweet D (2010) A paradigm shift in the analysis of bitemarks. Forensic Sci Int 201(1–3):38–44
Pretty IA, Turnbull MD (2001) Lack of dental uniqueness between two bite mark suspects. J Forensic Sci 46(6):1487–1491
Pretty IA, Anderson GS, Sweet DJ (1999) Human bites and the risk of human immunodeficiency virus transmission. Am J Forensic Med Pathol 20(3):232–239
Rawson RD, Koot A, Martin C et al (1984) Incidence of bite marks in a selected juvenile population: a preliminary report. J Forensic Sci 29(1):254–259
Revis DR, Burke A, Cunha BA (2009) Human Bite Infections. eMedicine, http://emedicine.medscape.com/article/218901-overview. Accessed on 2010
Richardson AC (1993) Cutaneous manifestations of abuse. In: Reece RM (ed) Child abuse – medical diagnosis and management. Lea & Febiger, Philadelphia, pp 167–184
Rothwell BR (1995) Bite marks in forensic dentistry: a review of legal, scientific issues. J Am Dent Assoc 126(2):223–232
Schweich P, Fleisher G (1985) Human bites in children. Pediatr Emerg Care 1(2):51–53
Senn DR (2011) Chapter 1 History of bitemark evidence. In: Dorion R (ed) Bitemark evidence – a color atlas and text, 2nd edn. CRC Press, Boca Raton, pp 3–24
Sims BG, Grant JH, Cameron JM (1973) Bite-marks in the 'battered child syndrome'. Med Sci Law 13(3):207–210
Sognnaes RD (1977) Forensic stomatology. N Engl J Med 296(4):197–203
Stockheim J, Wilkinson N, Ramos-Bonoan C (2005) Human bites and blood exposures in New York City schools. Clin Pediatr (Phila) 44(8):699–703
Stornello C (1991) Transmission of hepatitis B via human bite. Lancet 338(8773):1024–1025
Stump J (2001) Bites, animal. eMedicine Journal 2(8)
Sweet D, Pretty IA (2001) A look at forensic dentistry – part 2: tooth as weapons of violence – identification of bitemark perpetrators. Br Dent J 190(8):415–418
Trube-Becker E (1973) Bissspuren bei Kindesmisshandlungen [Traces of human bites in child abuse]. Beitr Gerichtl Med 31:115–123
Trube-Becker E (1977) Bite-marks on battered children. Z Rechtsmed 79(1):73–78
Tsokos M, Byard RW, Püschel K (2007) Extensive and mutilating craniofacial trauma involving defleshing and decapitation: unusual features of fatal dog attacks in the young. Am J Forensic Med Pathol 28(2):131–136
Tsuji A, Ishiko A, Kimura H, Nurimoto M et al (2008) Unusual death of a baby: a dog attack and confirmation using human and canine STRs. Int J Legal Med 122(1):59–62
Turk J (2010) Behavioural phenotypes. Contact a family, http://www.cafamily.org.uk/medicalinformation/additionalmedicalinformation/behaviouralphenotypes.html. Accessed on 2011
Vale GL, Noguchi TT (1983) Anatomical distribution of human bite marks in a series of 67 cases. J Forensic Sci 28(1):61–69
Wagner GN (1986) Bitemark identification in child abuse cases. Pediatr Dent 8(1):96–100
Warnick AJ, Biedrzycki L, Russanow G (1987) Not all bite marks are associated with abuse, sexual activities, or homicides: a case study of a self-inflicted bite mark. J Forensic Sci 32(3):788–792
Whittaker DK (2004) Bite marks – the criminal's calling cards. Br Dent J 196(4):237
Wikipedia (2011a) Bite. http://en.wikipedia.org/wiki/Bite. Accessed on 2011
Wikipedia (2011b) Indentured servant. http://en.wikipedia.org/wiki/Indentured_servant. Accessed on 2011
Wright JC (1985) Severe attacks by dogs: characteristics of the dogs, the victims, and the attack settings. Public Health Rep 100(1):55–61
Yanai O, Goldin L, Hiss J (1999) Fatal rat bites. Harefuah 136(8):611–613, 659, 658 [Article in Hebrew]

9 Forensic Photography in Suspected Child Abuse

André van den Bosch, Frans Bel, and Hubert G. T. Nijs

9.1 Why?

> ... all notes (whether about the history or examination), diagrams and photographs (made as part of the examination) are part of the medical record and may be part of the criminal record. They must always therefore be as accurate as possible – a poorly written or inaccurate record has strong potential to unfairly prejudice a complainant and create a miscarriage of justice. (RCPCH 2008).

Photography of physical findings should be a routine procedure in child abuse cases. (Forensic) photography serves several purposes (Hobbs et al. 1999; RCPCH 2006). Primarily, it is meant to be a diagnostic tool, which is meant to document the findings during a physical examination:

- Photodocumentation of the presence of visible physical findings:
  - Injuries (bruises, abrasions, lacerations, burns)
  - Genital and anal signs (usually injuries or infection)
  - Normal variants, congenital abnormalities, and dermatological findings
  - Aspects of growth and development
  - Overall appearance, including demeanor, emotional signs, or signs of neglect
- Photodocumentation of the absence of physical findings, in other words documentation of unaffected parts of the body (parts without injuries or skin abnormalities)

In addition to these aspects, photodocumentation provides valuable information, which supports the protection of the child, if necessary. It enables objective discussion of cases, second opinion evaluations, and peer review (anonymized) by professionals (medical colleagues, law enforcement, court, and other professionals). When used as evidence in court procedures, photodocumentation can support written and oral evidence. Photodocumentation can also be used in discussions about concerns of child abuse with those who bear responsibility for the child, especially the parents or guardians of the child. Finally, photodocumentation provides material for teaching and research purposes.

9.2 Good Medicolegal Practice: Informed Consent and Patient Confidentiality

Specific and fully informed consent is required. The person who is responsible for the photodocumentation, for example, the referring clinician or police officer, should obtain a written consent from the child or the child's legal representative(s), for

A. van den Bosch (✉)
Department of Forensic Medicine, Netherlands Forensic Institute, The Hague, The Netherlands

F. Bel, RMF
Medical Photographer, Erasmus MC – Sophia Rotterdam, The Netherlands

H.G.T. Nijs
Section Forensic Pediatrics, Department of Forensic Medicine, Netherlands Forensic Institute, The Hague, The Netherlands

R.A.C. Bilo et al., *Cutaneous Manifestations of Child Abuse and Their Differential Diagnosis*, DOI 10.1007/978-3-642-29287-3_9, © Springer-Verlag Berlin Heidelberg 2013 example, parents, caregivers, or court appointed guardian, before a visual record is made. Preferably (depending on the judicial system and on the age of the child), informed consent of the child and of both parents should be obtained. The parents and the child (if appropriate) should be informed why the photographs are taken (documentation, consultation, protection, medical education and research, or combinations of purposes) and how the photographs will be stored. They should be reassured that photodocumentation is highly confidential, will be carefully looked after, and will not be copied without permission of the person, who is responsible for the photodocumentation (RCPCH 2006).

Informed consent and confidentiality are important features in clinical as well as in forensic photography, for example, in case of suspected child abuse. If consent is obtained before the examination, a photograph of the written consent form can be added to the series right after the ID or insurance pass (Sect. 9.4.3). In some situations, for example, a medical urgency or uncertainty about the legal status of the child, it is necessary to photograph the abnormalities or lack of abnormalities before consent can be obtained. In that case, one should always try to get consent afterward.

If a child or the parents refuse to give permission for photodocumentation, this should be respected and documented in detail. In that case, the presence and absence of physical findings should be documented accurately in words and careful line drawings (RCPCH 2008). In the United Kingdom, a physical examination of the anogenital area, including the photo- or video-documentation of the area, without consent of the child or the parents/legal representatives of the child may constitute an assault (Mitchels and Prince 1992).

9.3 When and by Whom?

Photographs should be taken, according to standardized procedures (Sect. 9.4), during the physical examination. In some cases, it is indicated to take photographs on consecutive hours/days, especially in cases of patterned injuries, such as bitemarks or hand imprints on cheeks. Such injuries can become more visible and recognizable over the course of several hours/days.

Preferably, photographs are taken by a (forensic) medical photographer (or a specialized forensic police photographer) (RCPCH 2006). With modern digital technology, however, a properly trained physician will be able to take photographs by himself or herself or organize photodocumentation by medical staff, according to accepted quality standards for (forensic) medical photography (Sect. 9.4).

If a (forensic) medical photographer is available, the examining doctor is responsible for clear and detailed instructions to the photographer of what should be documented and in which way the physical finding should be documented. The photographer is responsible for the photographic quality of the photographs. The instructions of the doctor determine the (forensic) medical value of the photographs.

If a (forensic) medical photographer or a well-trained physician is not (immediately) available, the presence and absence of medical findings should be recorded in writing, as long as accepted and correct medical terminology is used, with the use of age-specific body diagrams or (when not available) anatomically correct sketches.

Whenever photographs are used in child abuse cases, whether in civil or criminal court procedures, legal verification is required stating that the photographs are of the child in question, when and where they were taken and by whom. Guidelines of taking photographs should be available in writing at the institution, as they may be referred to in case the origin, content, or quality of the photographs are questioned during the course of law.

9.4 How?

> Many practices fail to achieve good quality photographs, so measures to improve quality are needed. (Bikowski 2011)

9.4.1 The Circumstances and Photographic Conditions

Photographs should be taken in a well lit and quiet room (no mess or busy background). A neutral (blue, green, or gray) wall or sterile blue or green wrap may be used as background. Before starting the examination, the doctor should explain to the child (and the accompanying parents or other legal representatives of the child) what is going to happen and why photographs are made (RCPCH 2006).

The use of an assistant, for example, a police officer (in case of a criminal investigation) or nurse can be very useful if available to allay anxiety in the child/victim and to assist in handling the child and achieving the required body positions during photography. An assistant may assist the photographer by handling the measuring scale or by improving the lighting conditions. In case of (suspicion of) sexual abuse, presence of a female assistant also acts as a chaperone and is essential for both support and reassurance and to prevent false allegations.

9.4.2 The Photographic Equipment

Professional modern digital [mirror single lens reflex (SLR)] cameras, with interchangeable lenses are preferred, as these cameras have better optical characteristics and use a larger chip than compact cameras. However, the quality of compact cameras nowadays, or Micro Four Third system cameras, means that they are quite usable and in most medical settings preferable to mirror single lens reflex cameras because of their ease of use and cost. All photographs should be digitally endorsed with the date and time of capture, regardless of the camera type (FFLM 2010).

For experienced photographers using professional digital SLR cameras, the following preset conditions should be applied (assuming sufficient light circumstances):

1. Macro lens, with a fast maximum aperture (light sensitive) usually 60 mm f/2.8 and 105 mm f/2.8
2. Light sensitivity of ISO 400–1000 and ISO 2000 in case of full-frame cameras (to allow for a narrow aperture yielding high depth of field at acceptable shutter speeds). With the newer technological improvements even higher ISO values may be used; if so, use two values below the maximum to avoid "color noise."
3. RAW file format (RAW/JPG-fine combination or RAW-compressed)
4. Camera on "M" (manual, for aperture and shutter speed)
5. Measure light on gray scale
6. Adjust white balance using a gray or white scale (using the camera's preset white balance)
7. Take a photograph of a color scale (e.g., X-rite Colorchecker®)

For less experienced photographers using compact cameras, and in medical settings such as an emergency department, the following conditions should be fulfilled:

1. Zoom function, with macro mode ("rose" or "tulip" permanently, allows focusing from 0 to 1.5 m)
2. Light sensitivity with a maximum of ISO 400–800
3. JPG-fine file format
4. Disable auto-flash function
5. Use "P" (program)
6. Use automatic white balance
7. Enable movement reduction (anti-shake, "hand")

It is highly advised to become familiarized with the equipment before undertaking any real (forensic) casework. Practicing needs time but costs no money.

With technological development, new modalities arise. In clinical settings, for example, a smartphone with a high-resolution camera, for example, the iPhone®, is used for several purposes, including making "clinical" photographs. Although the optics cannot, by definition, be as good as the optics of a digital SLR camera or even a compact camera, it is possible to take clinically usable photos with a smartphone, like the iPhone®. However, the use of nonofficial devices such as smartphones or personal digital cameras for forensic purposes should be avoided (FFLM 2010). At least, the use should be limited to situations in which there is no other equipment available. The collected data should immediately be stored safely and removed from the device.

9.4.3 Standardized Order of Photographing

As mentioned before, a standardized order should be applied for correctly identifying the identity of the child, (un)affected body parts, the injuries, and to prevent discussion during the course of law. An experience-based and literature-based order is given below (ABFO Guidelines 2008; Pretty 2008; Shrewsbury Group 2009; Ricci 2011):

1. Take a photo of an ID or insurance pass.
2. Take a portrait photo.

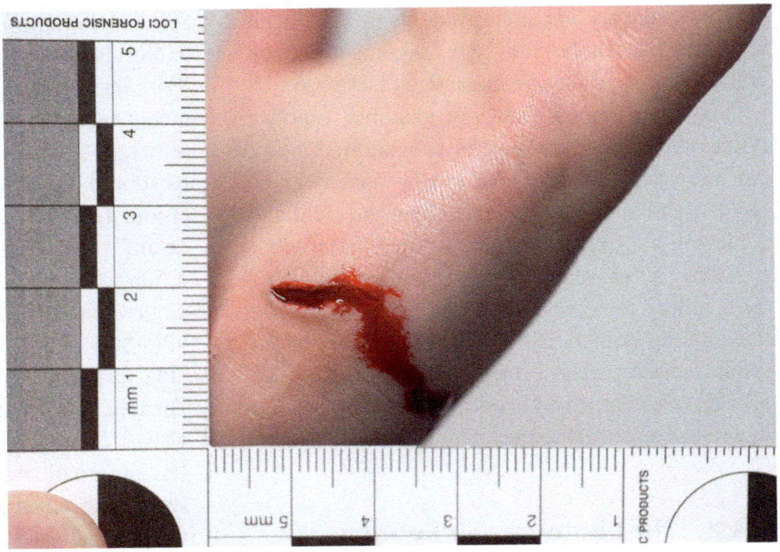

Fig. 9.1 L-shaped measuring scale

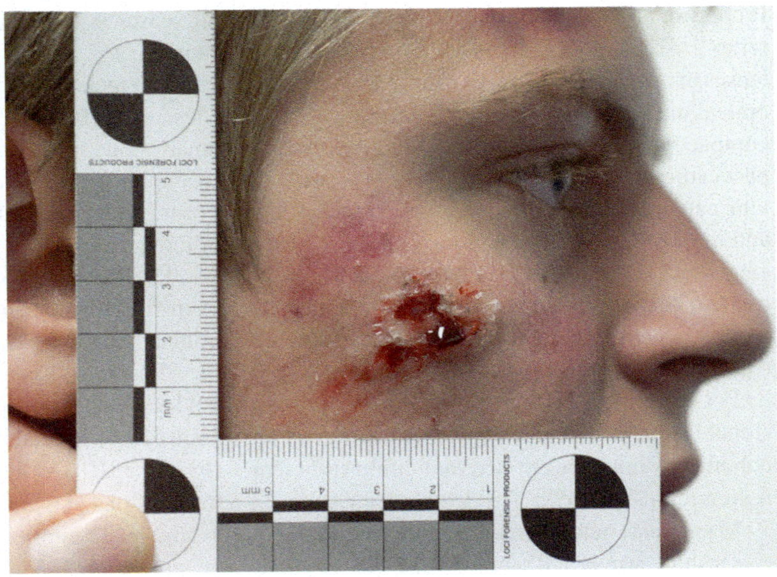

Fig. 9.2 L-shaped measuring scale

3. Take several overviews, from top to bottom (to enable recognition of the body part in question) (or take an overview from an entire body side in case of a small child).
4. Take an overview of a specific region of interest (try to incorporate several anatomical landmarks for reference purposes).
5. In case of patterned injuries, make some mid-range exposures (to capture the entire pattern, and relations to other body parts, clothing, or jewelry).
6. Take close-ups of the specific region of interest, at a 90° angle to the surface and by properly applying a measuring scale (Figs. 9.1 and 9.2).
7. Finally, take a photo of the same ID or insurance pass.

Try to take all photos with the same anatomic alignment (head up, no mixing of left and right). Steps 1 and 7 may look superfluous. However, in using this order, one can be confident, and state confidently in the course of law, that all photos between steps 1 and 7 are from the same child.

Steps 4 (overview) and 6 (close-up) should be taken from the same viewpoint to allow for identification of the body location in the close-up image. In addition to step 6 (90° to the surface), sometimes additional angled viewpoints are useful (e.g., 30° to the surface) in creating contour revealing shadows or swelling and by eliminating flashlight (if used) or glare.

When using SLR cameras, it is advised to focus manually rather than using autofocus (the autofocus uses areas with large contrast, which may be a different area to the body part of interest). It is advised not to use flash equipment. If the available light is insufficient, external lighting source, or day light (if possible), may be applied. If flash equipment is needed for overview pictures, mount an external flash and use bounced lighting by the ceiling or a wall (sideways or backward). Straightforward use of a flash light (at 90° to the surface) may ruin the visibility of the injury due to creating a "hot spot" or glare (photo). If flash equipment is needed for close-up pictures, for example, for bruises or burns, the use of a ringlight or ringflash should be considered.

Because digital photography is cheap, one should take more than one photo per step with slight variations in angle and distance. In case of forensic photography, the dogma is "more is better." However, the series of photos should always have a recognizable order, as explained above.

By using the above guidelines, the series of photos as a whole has the optimal constellation to be recognized as belonging to the same child, while the affected body parts and injuries (or absence of injuries) can be identified correctly in overviews and close-ups.

In using the measuring scale, several precautions should be taken into account. One should always position the scale in the same (virtual) plane as the injury (Figs. 9.3, 9.4, and 9.5). The edges of the injury should be visible entirely, and the scale should be positioned at least 5–10 mm from the edges. Any overlap of the scale with the injury is unacceptable (Fig. 9.6).

When there is some directionality in the injury, make sure one axis of the measuring scale runs parallel with that direction and that the measuring indications are close to (directed at) the injury. In this way, the dimensions of the injury can be read off at once.

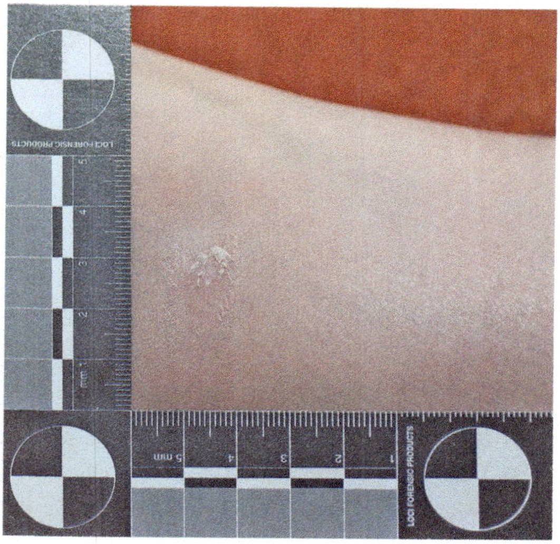

Fig. 9.3 Right: same virtual plane

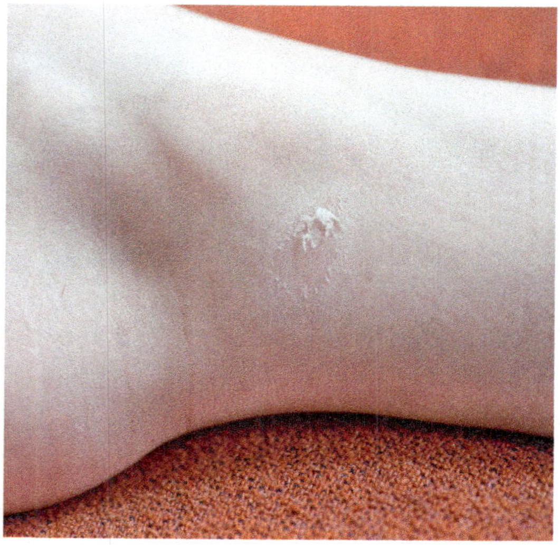

Fig. 9.4 Right: sharp. Wrong: no measuring scale

On curved body parts, like an arm, leg or buttock, a flexible measuring scale can be used (e.g., from paper at do-it-yourself companies). Photographs should then be taken in several directions following the curvature of the body part. Also, semi-adhesive, easy removable, flexible

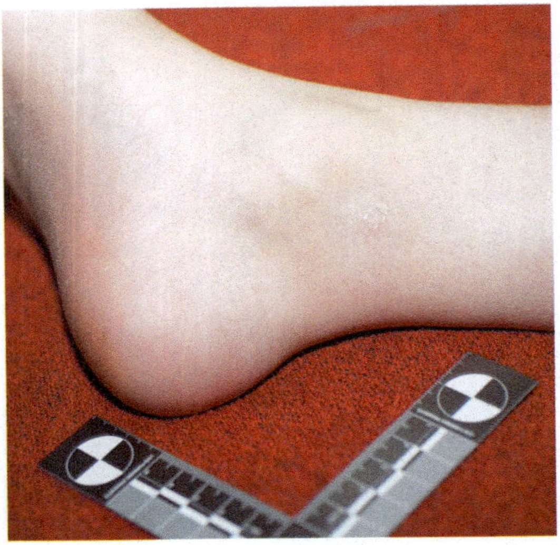

Fig. 9.5 Wrong: not the same virtual plane

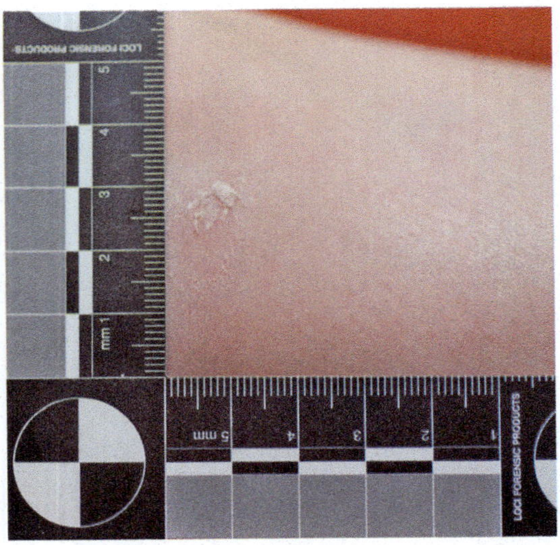

Fig. 9.6 Wrong: overlap

scales are available (Figs. 9.7 and 9.8), as shown below.

9.4.4 Storage

Photographs can be stored in printed form and as digital images (e.g., in JPEG or TIFF format, but preferably combined with the original RAW files) on a PC, DVD, or CD. The Faculty of Forensic and Legal Medicine (FFLM 2010) developed guidelines for the management of intimate images (photographic, digital, or video/DVD images of the genitalia or anus obtained using a colposcope or similar technology). These guidelines can also used in case of forensic imaging of injuries in children who are suspected victims of other types of child abuse.

Whatever working format is chosen, the images should be stored in a safe place as soon as possible and according to local policy (RCPCH 2008; FFLM 2010). Preferably, one should choose two separate safe places (e.g., in different buildings) for storage, but this may be an ideal not always achievable. Institution policy guidelines should be issued to ensure the privacy of the patient and the physical integrity of the digital data.

Access to the data should be limited to dedicated persons. This may be accomplished by storing data on a dedicated area, for example, once a day or once a week guarded with user rights on the intranet of the institution. After transferring the data to the PC, the data card of the camera should be reformatted in a way that it will not be possible to recover data erased from the data card. The camera (data card) should never leave the institution. The use of shared home or public computers for this purpose must be avoided (FFLM 2010).

Where the images are stored to external media such as DV tape, CD-rom, or DVD, then these media must be stored in a secure location that is accessible by properly authorized individuals only (FFLM 2010). The use of memory sticks or other flash media to store or share images should be avoided as they are easily lost or stolen (FFLM 2010).

Special attention should be paid to the proper identification of the photos. The hospital identification code (HIC) could be used in this regard, for example, a subdirectory called HIC, with renamed files like HIC_001.jpg. Guidelines should be issued which medical disciplines have access to the data.

It may be considered practical to print a few of the most relevant photos to be kept in the patient's paper file. In case of a completely digitized medical record, sometimes (depending on

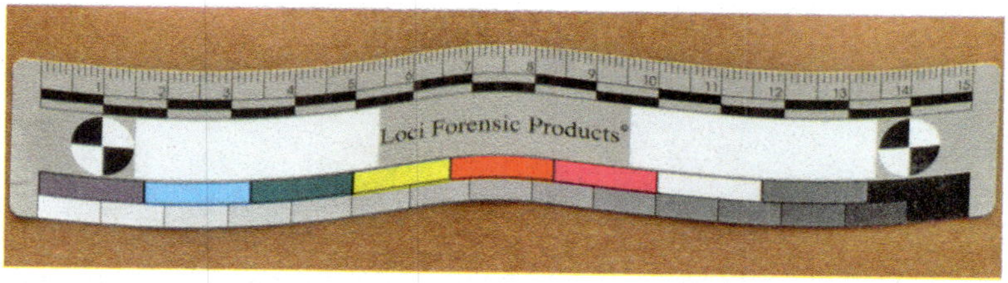

Fig. 9.7 Semi-adhesive flexible measuring scale, following body curves on lower back

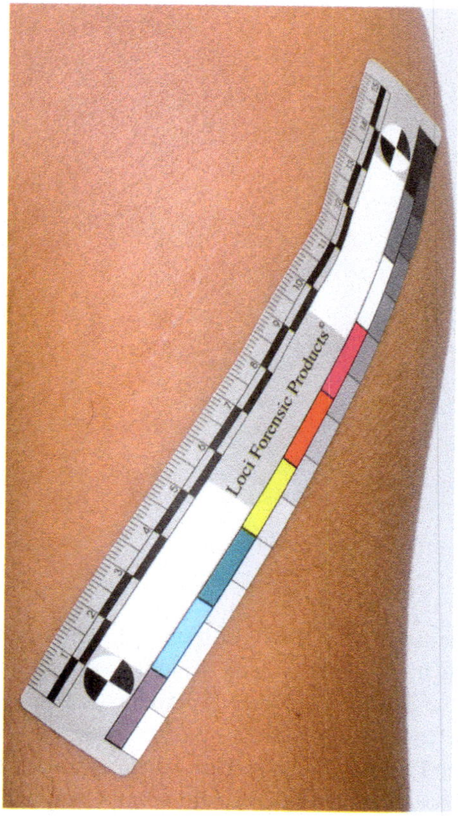

Fig. 9.8 Semi-adhesive flexible measuring scale, following body curves on right upper arm

the capacity of the system) photos may be coupled by HIC. Because of concerns about the "abuse" of intimate images (for other than forensic medical purposes) obtained during the physical examination of victims of sexual abuse, it is strongly advised to use line drawings in the patients paper file instead of intimate images (FFLM 2010). Images of faces must never be combined in the patient's paper file with intimate images (FFLM 2010).

9.5 Special Items

9.5.1 Tell-Tale Injuries

Special attention should be paid in documenting tell-tale injuries, such as bite marks or patterned injuries. Criteria such as adequate close-ups, at 90° to the surface and additionally taken from different angles, should be regarded with extra care (ABFO 2008). When at a later stage the question arises of comparing the marks or injuries with a questioned object (implement such as a belt or a dental print from a suspect), high-quality photos are required both of the injuries and, with the same quality criteria, of the object. In that case, the comparison of a patterned injury or mark with an object can be made using photographic techniques (by rescaling the images to the same level of magnification, e.g., similarly dimensioned X- and Y-axis, and by using two semitransparent layers with photo-enhancement software) (Figs. 9.9, 9.10, 9.11, 9.12, 9.13, and 9.14).

9.5.2 Anogenital Findings

> Highly sensitive medical images (e.g., of genitalia) should be treated with respect for the child's feelings. (RCPCH 2006)

9.5.2.1 The Setting

It should be noted that children, or their parents, may be embarrassed by the situation. Physical examination of the child can be difficult. Making pictures or a video can be even more embarrassing. However, with the right attitude, assistance, and reassurance, it should be possible to examine almost all

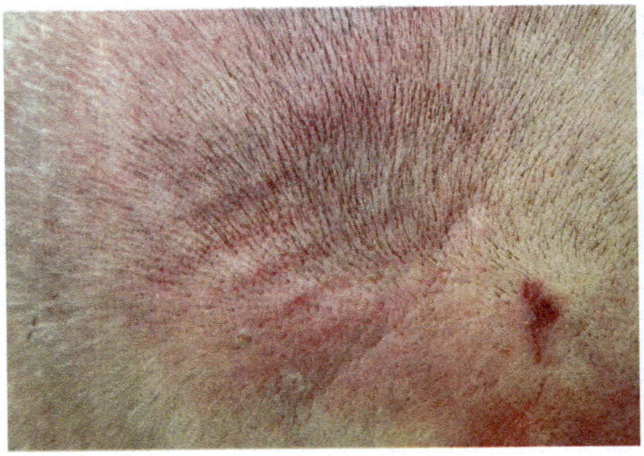

Fig. 9.9 Pattern injury

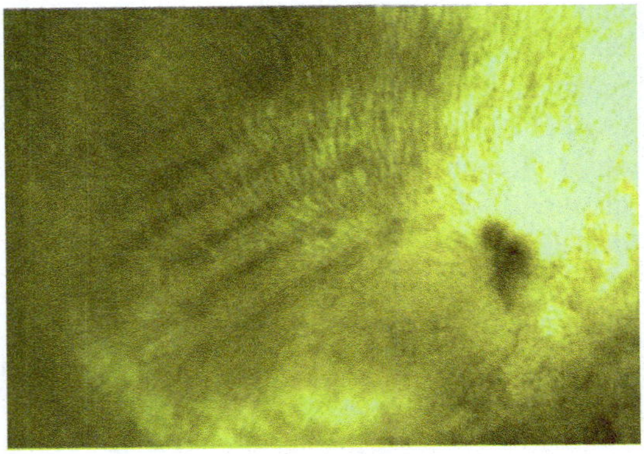

Fig. 9.10 Pattern injury, using forensic light

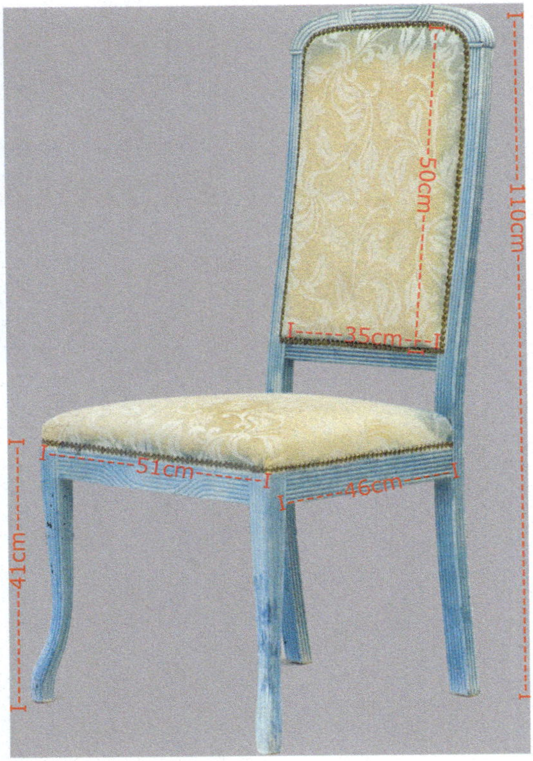

Fig. 9.11 Hit with a chair leg?

children. However, if a child is very resistant, the child should never be forced.

9.5.2.2 Colposcope

The use of a colposcope is now widely recommended for forensic examinations of the anogenital area in case of suspected child sexual abuse. A colposcope is a noninvasive instrument providing, with adjustable light illumination, a magnified image and with the possibility of readily obtainable digital photo- or videodocumentation (RCPCH 2008). Preferably, a colposcope with an integral eyepiece measuring device should be used, which enables to measure physical findings, if necessary.

The examining doctor should include comprehensive and contemporaneous notes and line drawings of the physical findings in the patient's paper file even if photo- or videodocumentation has been obtained (RCPCH 2008). According to Adams et al. (2001), colposcopic photographs may not reliably document subtle color changes. If the examining doctor is convinced, that this is the case, this should be noted in the patient's file. There is also a risk of overinterpretation of minor signs if the forensic colposcopic evaluation is done by an unexperienced professional (RCPCH 2008).

9.5.2.3 Videodocumentation

Because photographs often will not reflect the dynamic changes observed during the examination of the anogenital area of a child, (colposcopic) high-definition videodocumentation is becoming more common. Videodocumentation in itself is a dynamic process which is able to record movements, while photodocumentation is static and records in fact one single snapshot or a series of snapshots. High-quality digital photographs ("video stills") can be reproduced from the videoregistration, which enables the examining doctor to select exactly the findings seen

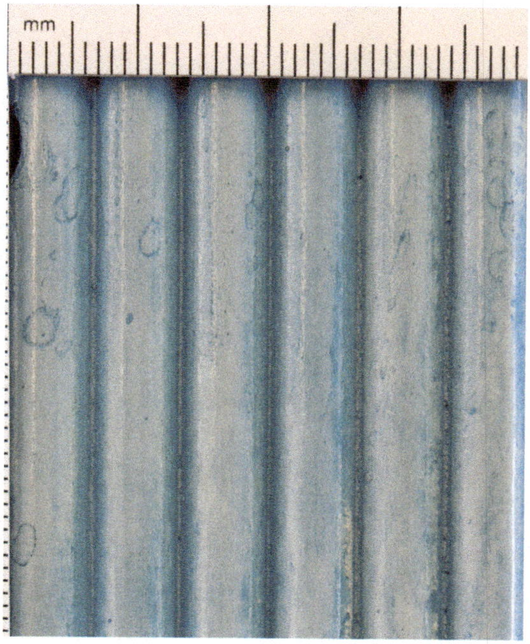

Fig. 9.12 Detail of one of the chair legs

during the physical examination. A tripod and good lighting conditions are needed to produce stable images. Also, sound recordings are possible, which may be useful for further investigation by CPS or police.

9.5.2.4 Photodocumentation Without the Use of a Colposcope

Photodocumentation of the anogenital area without using the colposcope poses several problems with regard to the lighting, available working space, and applying the measuring scale.

The lighting poses a potential problem because relevant anatomical structures like the hymen are not always located superficially and the risk of "shadowing," underexposure, or blurred images is high. If there is no colposcope available, a flexible external light source may be helpful (e.g., ringflash or ringlight with LEDs). Using flash in the anogenital area, however, may cause severe light reflections (hot spots or glare), which may ruin the entire image. Preferably, a LED ringlight with continuous light should be used.

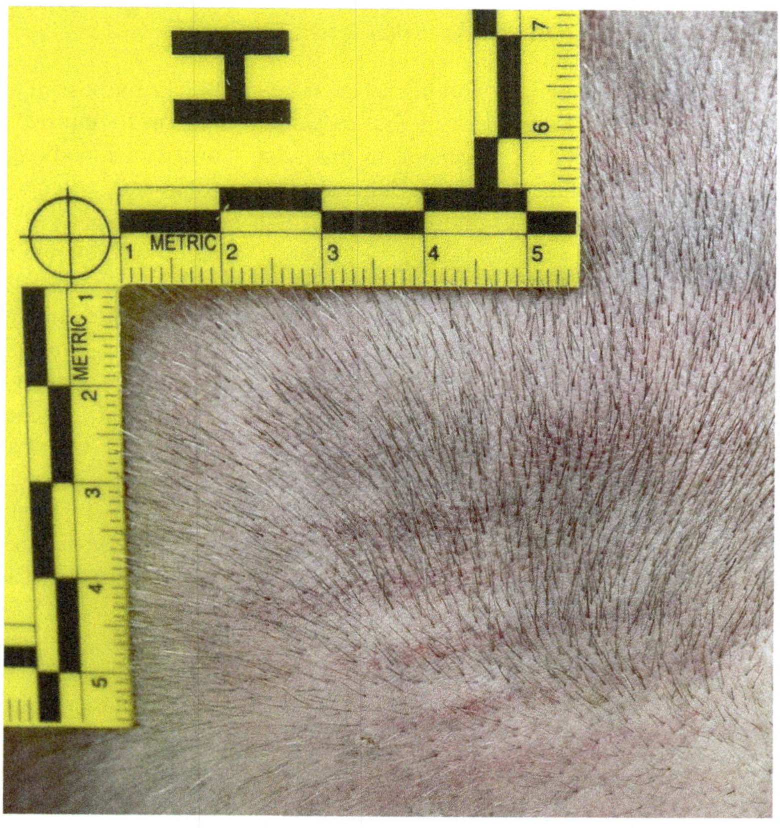

Fig. 9.13 The injury without overlay

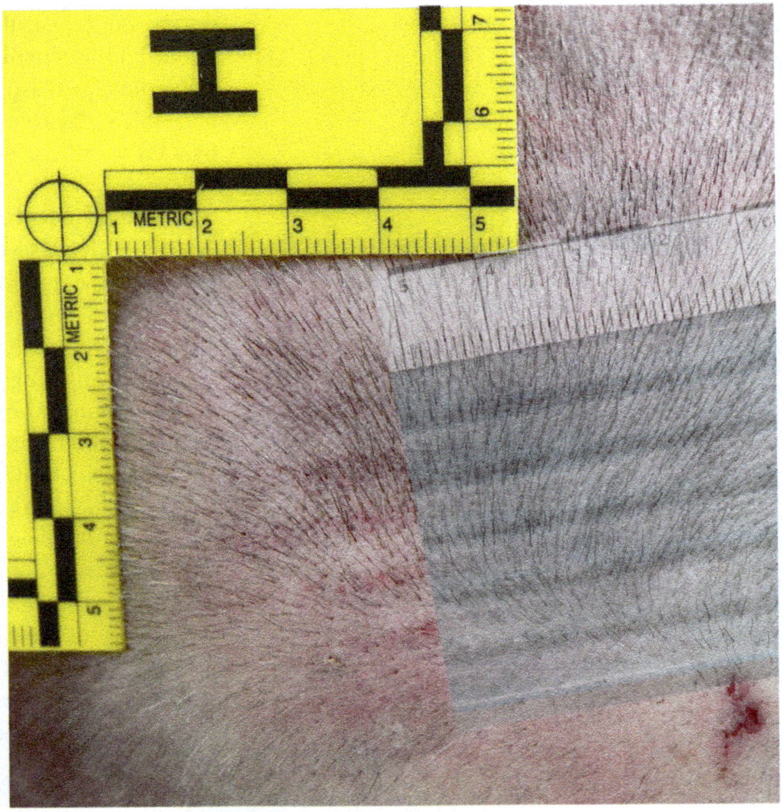

Fig. 9.14 Comparing injury (with overlay of the object): a match with the chair leg

Because of the limited working space, it may be difficult to make pictures of the anogenital region with a digital SLR camera. In that case, one may use a compact camera. Guidance (and prior practice) of the examining physician or nurse is required.

A measuring scale is often not used in photography of the anogenital region. Besides the limited amount of space, structures inside the body like the hymen do not allow the use of a measuring scale in the same plane as the structure. Sometimes, as a compromise, the measuring scale may be adhered to the groin to have some reference.

9.6 Photo-Enhancement or Adjustment

Software modification of any image should in general be avoided, but if necessary (e.g. if underexposed) recorded. (RCPCH 2006)

The purpose of photo-enhancement or adjustment is to improve the visibility of affected and unaffected body parts, by improving contrast (light/dark, colors) of the entire photograph. Any application of photo-enhancement or adjustment should be mentioned in the report or patient file. One should always describe the followed enhancement procedure in the report. To keep the report concise, only the adjusted photos may be used in the report with an additional remark that, if requested, "original" (unadjusted) RAW data (photos) can be supplied. Original RAW data should always be stored unmodified.

Sometimes, local adjustments are made to highlight the skin findings or to improve the visibility of the findings. If local adjustment is used, the followed procedure should be described in the report, and the original photographs should always be added to the report. Special features, which may be used to further enhance visibility (pattern recognition) (Figs. 9.15, 9.16, 9.17, and 9.18), are:

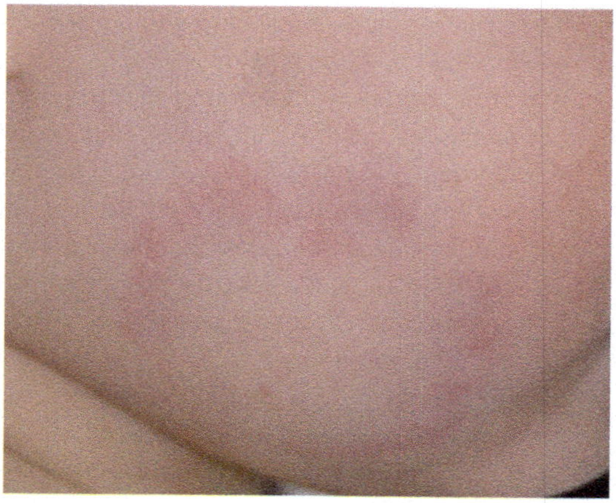

Fig. 9.15 Original picture: hardly recognizable pattern injury (= Fig. 8.4)

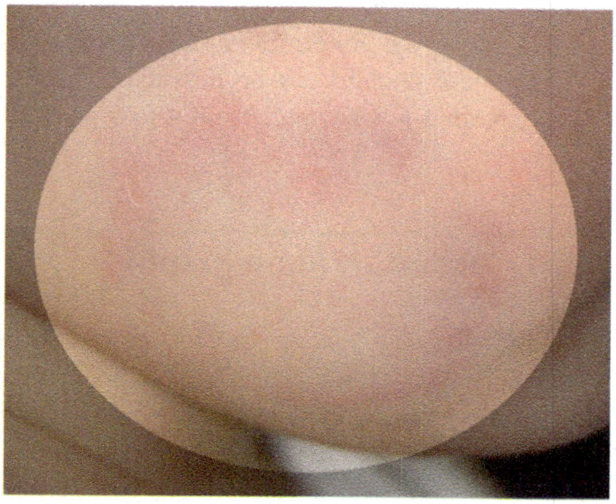

Fig. 9.16 Adapting of levels (= Fig. 8.5)

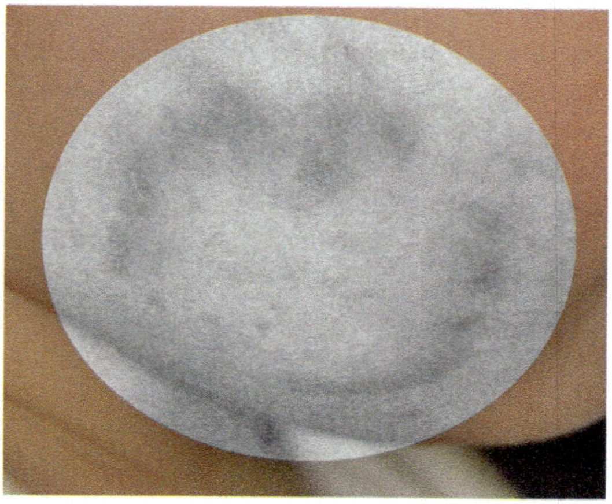

Fig. 9.17 Uncoloring: *black/white* conversion (= Fig. 8.6)

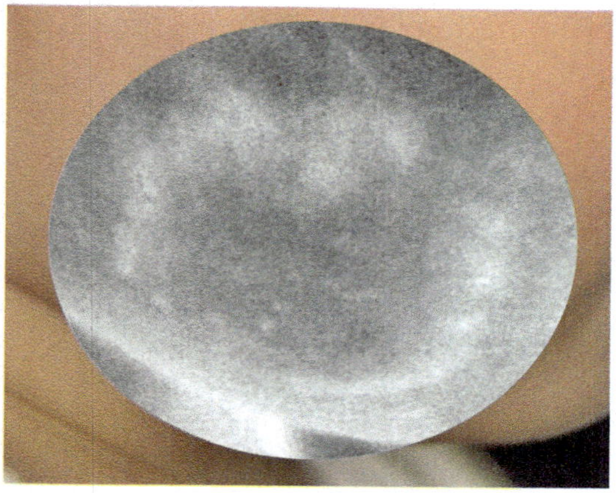

Fig. 9.18 Uncoloring: *black/white* negative (= Fig. 8.7)

- Adapting of levels, autolevel, and autocontrast
- Uncoloring: change full color images to black and white images and change levels
- Color or black and white negative conversion

Because of the absence of a measuring scale, the findings seen in Figs. 9.15, 9.16, 9.17, and 9.18 only have a limited forensic value. The pattern is suggestive for a bitemark (severity scale 2, see Chap. 8), but the finding cannot be used in identifying or excluding a suspect.

9.7 The Use of Wood's Lamp and Forensic Light Sources in Child Abuse

Wood's lamp illumination (ultraviolet light at a wavelength of approximately 365 nm) has been reported to be useful in identifying bruises that are faint or not visible to the naked eye (Vogeley et al. 2002).

A forensic light source is made up of a powerful lamp that contains ultraviolet, visible, and infrared light components (Crimescope 2003) (Fig. 9.19). These light sources are used in numerous forensic investigations. In child abuse, light sources can also be used during physical examination to investigate the presence of (body) fluids such as blood, saliva, semen, urine, vaginal secretions, and sweat. In the absence of other

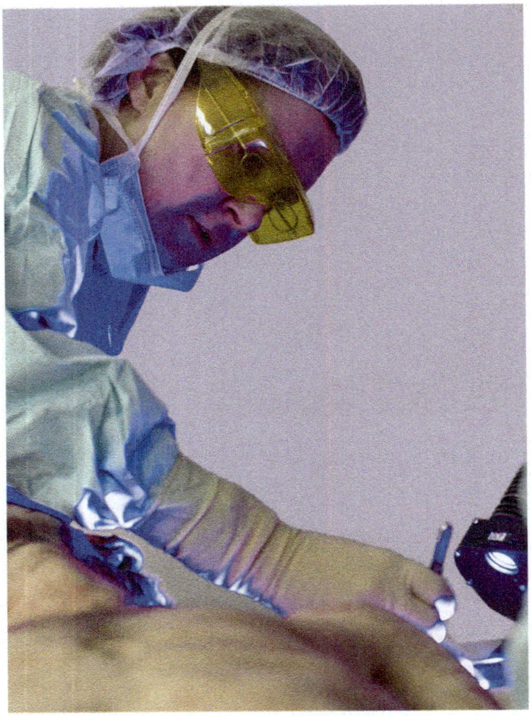

Fig. 9.19 Using forensic light during a forensic autopsy

aids, a forensic light source may reveal old and new bruises, bite marks, and patterned wound details that are invisible when illuminated by normal white light (Crimescope 2003) (Figs. 9.20, 9.21, 9.22, 9.23, and 9.24). Healed burns may still be visible after a number of years. This may take multiple color bands (wavelengths) because different colors will penetrate skin to different depths, and consequently, depending on the depth of the bruise or the wound, one would need to adjust the color band (wavelength) on the instrument. Deep wounds may require infrared illumination for adequate skin penetration (Crimescope 2003). Successful identifications of bite marks (faint, old, and difficult to recognize) have been made 6 months after injury (Smock 2000).

The use of these forensic light sources is promising but not without problems:

- Scientific evidence underlining the proposed advantage of identifying healed cutaneous injuries in children is still lacking. For this reason, the findings can only be used as an indication of earlier injuries but not as proof.
- To use forensic light sources properly, one needs professional, experienced, and well-equipped photographers.
- The use in living children may also lead to problems when used. The investigation needs to be conducted in an almost dark room to allow enough yield of light. This implies long shutter times and the use of a tripod. The child will have to stop moving for a longer period (including breathing or otherwise), especially if the observed abnormalities have to be photographed. A child can be instructed to keep his breath a few seconds from 4 to 5 years of age.

9.8 Digital 3D Photography

A promising new feature in clinical medicine (especially dermatology and plastic/reconstructive surgery) and in forensic medicine (including child abuse) is 3D (three-dimensional) photography. In 3D photography, a compact stereovision camera is used. This type of camera captures two images, differing by a few degrees, each time a picture is taken (Bikowski 2011). The two images are digitally combined to form a single composite image in 3D, which simulates three dimensions instead of two in conventional photography (Bikowski 2011). Experience in forensic medicine is limited, as of this writing (2012). The advantage may be a better visualization of curved body parts (e.g., the buttocks), special body areas (e.g., the neck), and body cavities (e.g., the mouth and the anogenital area).

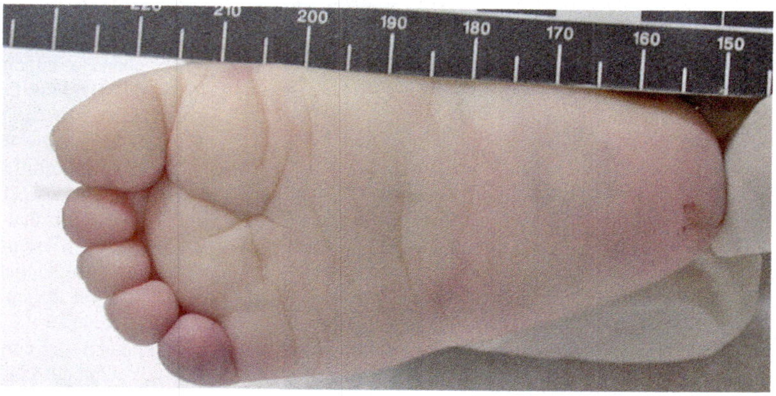

Fig. 9.20 Original picture: unexplained bruising (hardly visible)

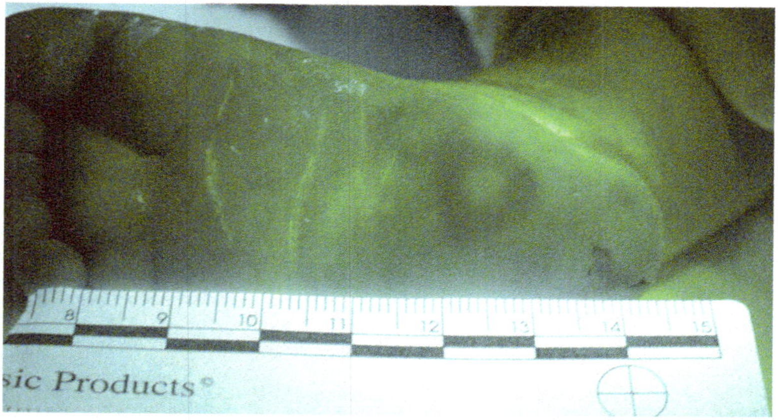

Fig. 9.21 Using forensic light: pattern injury

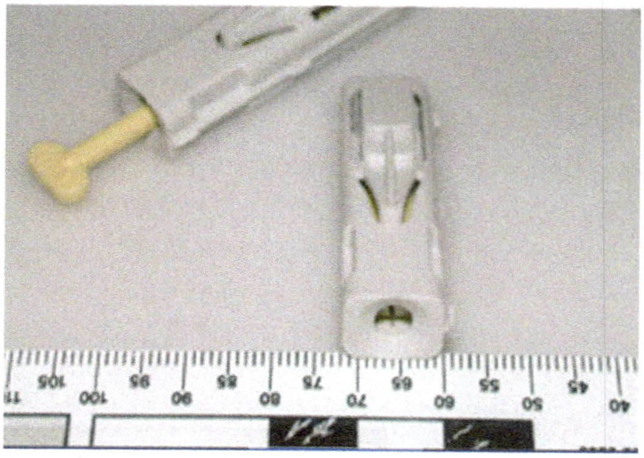

Fig. 9.22 Bruising caused by the use of a medical device

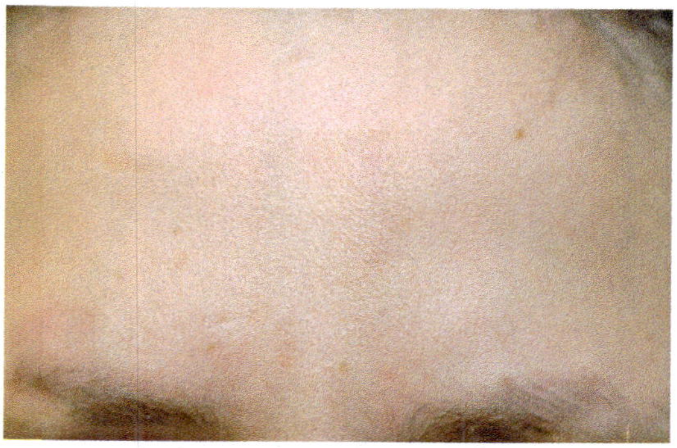

Fig. 9.23 Hardly visible bruising on the forehead (= Fig. 3.10)

Fig. 9.24 Using forensic light: rectangular pattern (= Fig. 3.11)

References

ABFO (American Board of Forensic Odontology) (2008) Bite mark guidelines. http://www.abfo.org. Accessed on 2010

Adams JA, Girardin B, Faugno D (2001) Adolescent sexual assault: documentation of acute injuries using photo-colposcopy. J Pediatr Adolesc Gynecol 14(4):175–180

Bikowski J (2011) Evolving technologies for clinical photography, a Q&A with Joseph Bikowski. Practical Dermatology. http://bmctoday.net/practicaldermatology/2011/09/article.asp?f=evolving-technologies-for-clinical-photography. Accessed on 2011

Crimescope (2003) Forensic Light Source Applications. http://www.crimescope.com/march%2015/Applications.htm. Accessed on 2009

FFLM (Faculty of Forensic and Legal Medicine) (2010) Guidance for best practice for the management of intimate images that may become evidence in court (Royal College of Paediatrics and Child Health/Association of Chief Police Officers/Faculty of Forensic and Legal Medicine), London. http://www.rcpch.ac.uk/sites/default/files/GuidanceonIntimateImages30JUNE2010.pdf

Hobbs CJ, Hanks HGI, Wynne JM (1999) Chapter 4. Physical abuse. In: Hobbs CJ, Hanks HGI, Wynne JM (eds) Child abuse and neglect, a clinician's handbook, 2nd edn. Churchill Livingstone, London, pp 63–104

Mitchels B, Prince A (1992) The children's act and medical practice. Jordan & Sons, Bristol

Pretty IA (2008) Forensic dentistry: 2. Bitemarks and bite injuries. Dent Update 35:48–61

RCPCH (Royal College of Paediatrics and Child Health) (2006) Chapter 11 Photography. In: Child protection companion, 1st edn. RCPCH, pp 81–84 http://haruv.org.il/_Uploads/dbsAttachedFiles/ChildProtComp.pdf

RCPCH (Royal College of Paediatrics and Child Health) (2008) The physical signs of child sexual abuse – an evidence-based review and guidance for best practice. RCPCH

Ricci LR (2011) Chapter 27. Photodocumentation in child abuse cases. In: Jenny C (ed) Child abuse and neglect. Diagnosis, treatment, and evidence, 1st edn. Elsevier Saunders, St. Louis, pp 215–221

Shrewsbury Group (2009) The West Midlands clinical photographic handbook – a complete photographic body atlas for clinical photographers. The Shrewsbury Group, Birmingham

Smock WS (2000) Recognition of pattern injuries in domestic violence victims. In: Siegel J, Knupfer G, Saukko P (eds) Encyclopedia of forensic sciences, 1st edn. Elsevier Academic Press, San Diego, pp 384–391

Vogeley E, Pierce MC, Bertocci G (2002) Experience with Wood lamp illumination and digital photography in the documentation of bruises on human skin. Arch Pediatr Adolesc Med 156:265–268

Index

R.A.C. Bilo et al., *Cutaneous Manifestations of Child Abuse and Their Differential Diagnosis*,
DOI 10.1007/978-3-642-29287-3, © Springer-Verlag Berlin Heidelberg 2013

The manufacturer's authorised representative in the EU is Springer Nature Customer Service Centre GmbH, Europaplatz 3, 69115 Heidelberg, Germany. If you have any concerns regarding our products, please contact ProductSafety@springernature.com

Printed and bound by CPI Group (UK) Ltd, Croydon, CR0 4YY
22/09/2026
02220957-0012